Self Assessment and Review of Forensic Medicine and Toxicology

[MCQs with Explanations and Discussions]

Anil Aggrawal

Director, Professor of Forensic Medicine
Maulana Azad Medical College
New Delhi

PEEPEE

PUBLISHERS AND DISTRIBUTORS (P) LTD.

Self Assessment and Review of Forensic Medicine and Toxicology

Published by
Pawaninder P. Vij and Anupam Vij
Peepee Publishers and Distributors (P) Ltd.
Head Office: 160, Shakti Vihar, Pitam Pura
Delhi-110034 (India)

Correspondence Address: 7/31, First Floor, Ansari Road
Daryaganj, New Delhi-110002 (India)
Ph: 41512412, 23246245, 9811156083
e-mail: peepee160@yahoo.co.in
e-mail: peepee160@gmail.com
www.peepeepub.com

join us on facebook.com/pp.publishers

First Edition: **2006**

Revised Reprint: 2020

ISBN: 978-81-88867-85-1

This book is dedicated to
Dr. Jason Payne-James
of Forensic Healthcare Services Ltd., UK,
whose association has always been an inspiration to me

Foreword

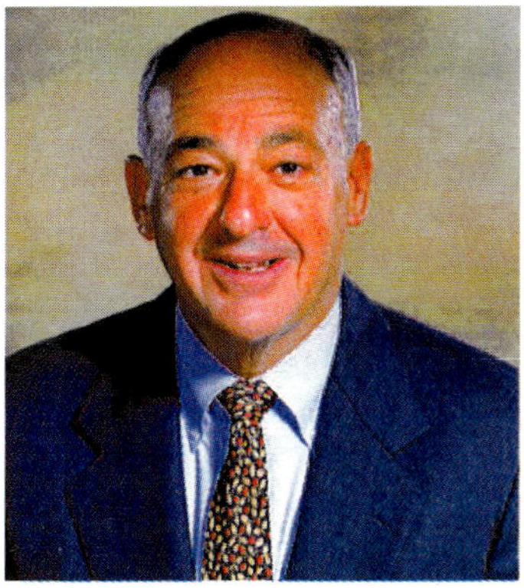

There are very few areas of professional endeavor that have grown and developed in recent decades to the extent that forensic medicine has. Although this psychologically fascinating and intellectually challenging subject has been appreciated and applied in some fashion by every significant civilization for more than three millennia, the technological advancements and societal recognition that we have witnessed regarding forensic medicine from the latter part of the twentieth century to the present time are truly phenomenal. Indeed, it can be reasonably argued that the degree of sophistication of medical-legal and forensic scientific principles and concepts, and the extent and manner in which they are utilized as an integral component of the civil and criminal justice systems, validly reflect and are correlative with the level of true democracy and adherence to basic universal rules of ethics and morality in that particular society. Law and medicine are arguably the world's two most ancient and noble professions. Thus, the interface and functional relationships of these two great bodies of knowledge and intellectual achievement are understandably essential components of any advanced civilization.

This excellent book by Professor Anil Aggrawal is a significant contribution to the forensic medical literature. The use of multiple choice questions as a teaching vehicle is an interesting and effective methodology. The discussions relating to the correct answers provide valuable information to medical and law students, as well as to practising physicians and attorneys who have a genuine interest in the subjects that relate to both fields of endeavor. The author, an eminent medical-legal expert, has structured a volume that contains a wealth of useful information. This book constitutes an effective academic springboard for graduate students and new practitioners in law and medicine who are desirous of learning what forensic medicine is all about. Succinct explanations and concise discussions relating to the correct answers of multiple choice questions that deal with a very vast array of medical-legal issues, from the most basic and traditional to the newest and most complex, make this book a very useful and worthwhile addition to the bookshelves of all physicians and attorneys.

Dr. Cyril H. Wecht, M.D., J.D.
Past President, American Academy of Forensic Sciences
Past President, American College of Legal Medicine

Foreword

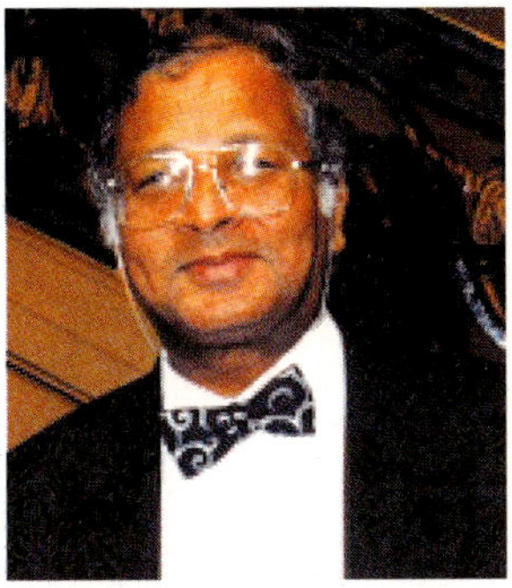

Every time I am asked to review a forensic textbook from India, I am amazed at the standard of undergraduate and postgraduate forensic teaching that exists in that country. It is good to know that the teaching of Forensic Medicine is alive, well and thriving in India. This is particularly so because the teaching of undergraduate Forensic Medicine is now virtually extinct here in Britain.

It is therefore with great pleasure that I write the foreword for this book of forensic Multiple Choice Questions (MCQs) compiled by Professor Anil Aggrawal. Having reviewed other books of this nature from India I can say that his book is rather innovative and breaks the traditional mould by its approach and presentation.

Anil has long experience of the subject both in and outside India. He is also well-known internationally in the world of Forensic Medicine. This is partly because of his pioneering Internet based forensic journal, which has a worldwide readership. I have no doubt that he is a well-known figure in the Indian world of Forensic Medicine as well.

Anil is also well travelled and I first met him many years ago when he worked with me in Edinburgh, Scotland. One thing that struck me about him then, was his questioning mind. The other thing that can be said about him is that he has an encyclopaedic knowledge of forensic matters, including trivia! (It must be said that his knowledge is not just confined to Forensic Medicine as one would gather from his Internet based book reviews!) His knowledge of the subject is clear from this book, which is well researched and complete with copious explanatory notes. This makes it a pleasure to read it in spite of the fact that it is a book of MCQs.

As I found out for myself as an examiner, MCQs are not easy to compile and require a lot of hard work and lateral thinking. Anil appears to have worked hard in producing this book.

Apart from the actual MCQs themselves the explanatory notes are quite enlightening. I am sure that this book will be well received by undergraduates as well as postgraduates.

Dr. Gyan C. A. Fernando
Home Office Forensic Pathologist
Devon and Cornwall
United Kingdom

Foreword

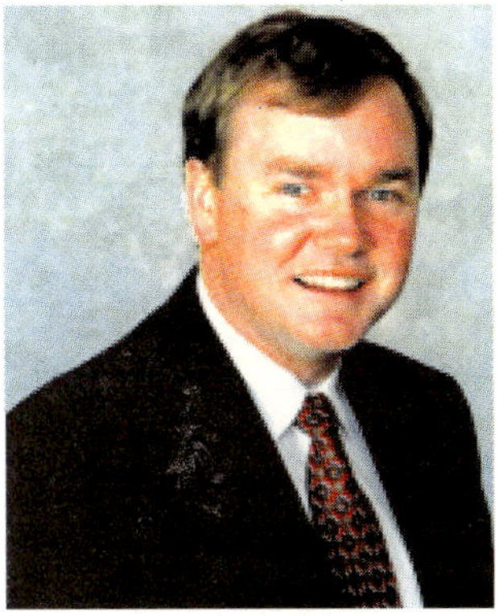

At some stage during their career, all medical practitioners and many other health professionals will be involved in the practice of forensic medicine. The involvement may be as simple as considering the appropriateness or otherwise of completing a death certificate. For others, the involvement may be considerably greater either by accident or by design. This application of medical knowledge for the purposes of the administration of the law is a long-established and very important but sometimes neglected discipline. Time is seeing this neglect change.

Generally, forensic medicine is synonymous with forensic pathology but it encompasses a number of speciality areas including forensic pathology, clinical forensic medicine, forensic psychiatry and psychology, forensic dentistry and toxicology and certain aspects of the law. The discipline has more recently attained significant prominence through the media with the coverage of high profile court cases, involvement in the aftermath of terrorist attacks, focal areas of genocide and the proliferation of forensic-based film and television productions.

A knowledge of this discipline is essential to the successful practice of all fields of medicine and its inclusion in the medical syllabus is universal. In keeping with other medical disciplines, MCQs are frequently and successfully used for forensic examinations. There are, however, very few books of specifically forensic MCQs for general use by students. Professor Aggrawal has an exceptional interest in forensic medicine and this is demonstrated in the preparation of this book, which has been undertaken with meticulous care. The chapters cover all the primary forensic areas including the relevant law.

The MCQs presented here offer the student a means of self-assessment and revision of the salient features of this field of medicine. It is an important and timely addition to the forensic literature.

Dr John AM Gall
BSc MBBS PhD FACLM DMJ (Clin & Path)
Forensic Physician
Australian Forensic and Medico-Legal Consultants
Melbourne, Australia

Preface

For postgraduate entrance examinations, the trend in this country – as well as in several others – is to set multiple choice questions. The aim of this book is to provide some core questions in forensic medicine and toxicology, which have appeared in last several years, as well as those, which could perhaps appear in future.

There are several MCQ books currently in the market, but I am aware of none, which explains why a given answer is correct. The result is that the student frequently finds himself cramming up the answer rather than understanding and assimilating the concept, which should be the aim of all good and rational teaching. This book not only attempts to give explanations to most questions but also gives additional information related to them.

During my 30 years in Forensic Medicine, I have acutely felt that Indian Forensic Medicine has been riddled with a number of inaccuracies, superstitions and myths. This is because we have – for reasons very inexplicable to me – shied away from challenging traditional beliefs, even if the contrary is obvious and staring right in one's face. For instance many of us still believe that rigor mortis does not appear in an infant less than seven months of age, while all of us have seen infants younger than this, and have surely noticed rigor mortis in them. This book attempts to discard all such old myths, superstitions, fancies and inaccuracies. This book follows the principle "Never use flawed science! Use your own observations and a little common sense!", one in which I have always believed.

The book is written with two particular segments in mind—firstly, the undergraduate student in his second professional who needs to quickly revise his text, and secondly, the undergraduate readying himself for the postgraduate entrance examination. I hope they would find it useful.

Although I have tried to check and crosscheck each fact with latest authentic references and by discussions with colleagues around the world, some inaccuracies or deficiencies may still be lurking around in the book. I would feel grateful if discerning students and readers point out these mistakes to me. I would also be looking for fresh questions, which have failed to find a place in this edition. This author can be reached via his website *www.anil.geradts.com*, *www.anilaggrawal.com* or directly via email at *dr_anil@hotmail.com.*

Finally a few acknowledgements. I would like to thank my dear friend Ravindra Saxena, who helped in innumerable ways to help shape this book. Mr. Jeevak Gupta, my dear student helped with diagrams. My thanks to him. I am deeply indebted to my wife Marygold and son Tarun who have been pillars of strength for me all through my life. They have rendered their wholehearted support while I was busy writing this book.

Anil Aggrawal
dr_anil@hotmail.com
www.anil.geradts.com

Contents

PART 1. FORENSIC MEDICINE

PART 1
FORENSIC MEDICINE

Plate 1

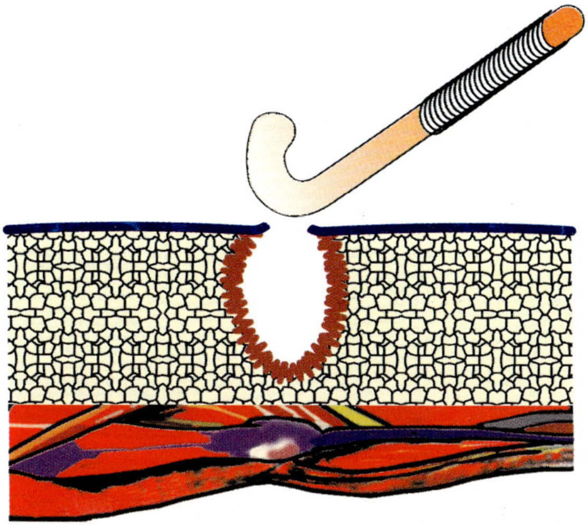

Fig. 11.5: Tear, the most general kind of laceration.

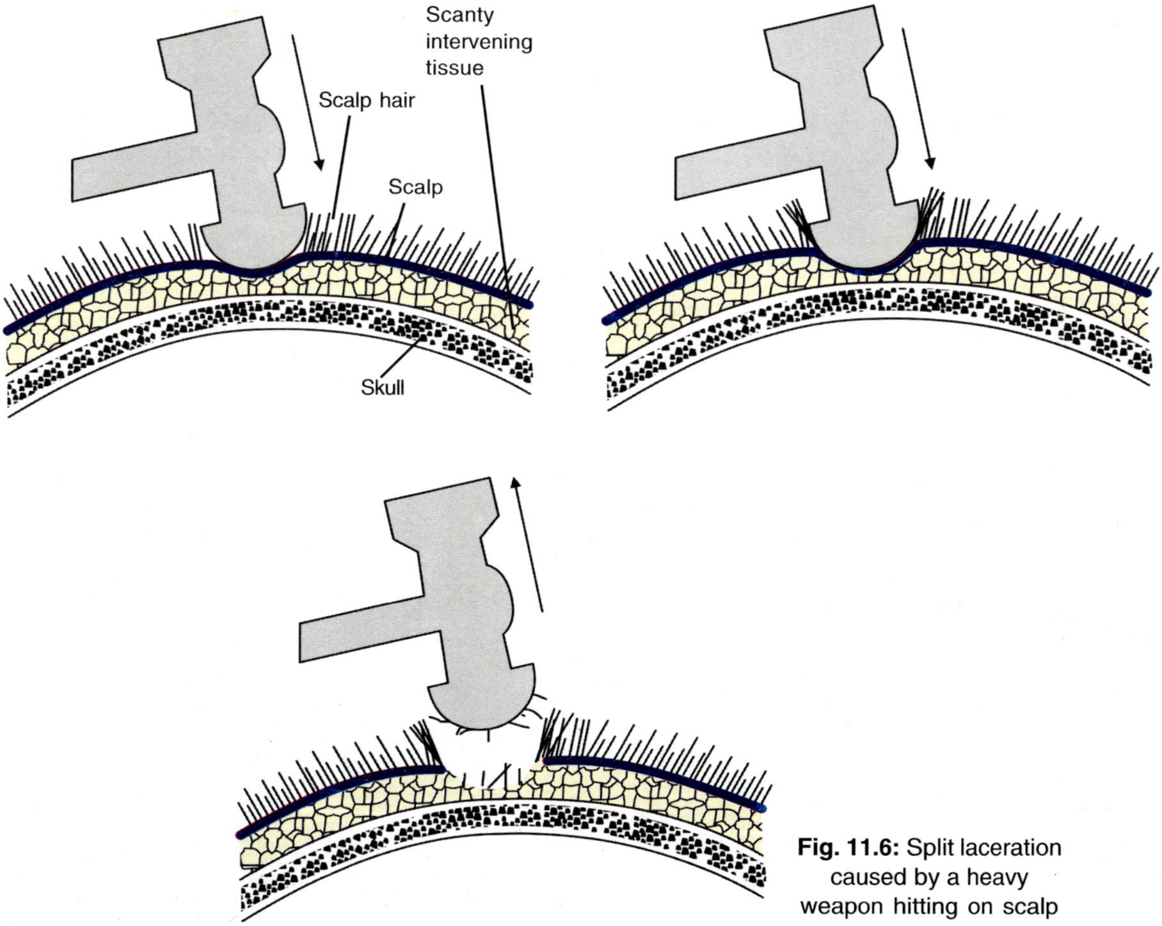

Fig. 11.6: Split laceration caused by a heavy weapon hitting on scalp

Plate 2

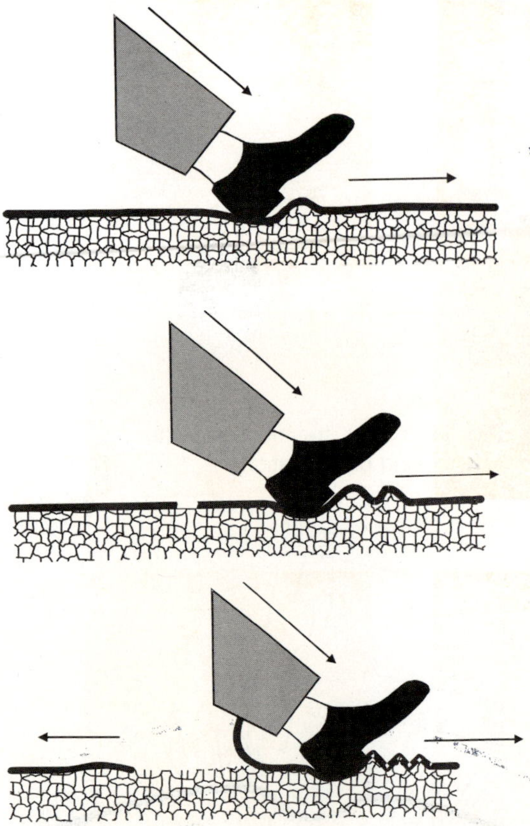

Fig. 11.7: Mechanism of a stretch laceration. Note that a large flap of skin is formed on one side

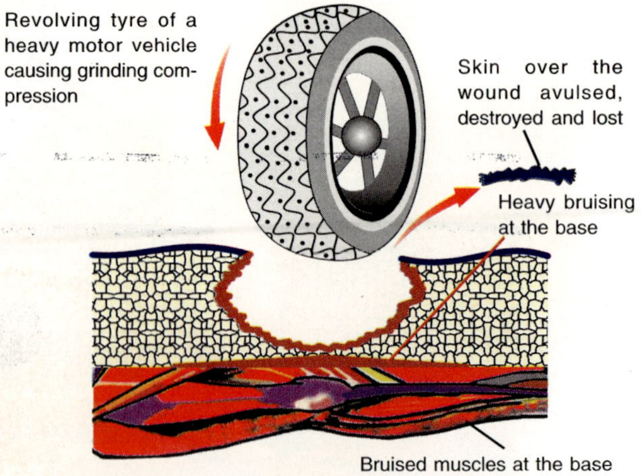

Fig. 11.9: Avulsion or flaying. Note that large areas of skin have been lost due to grinding compression.

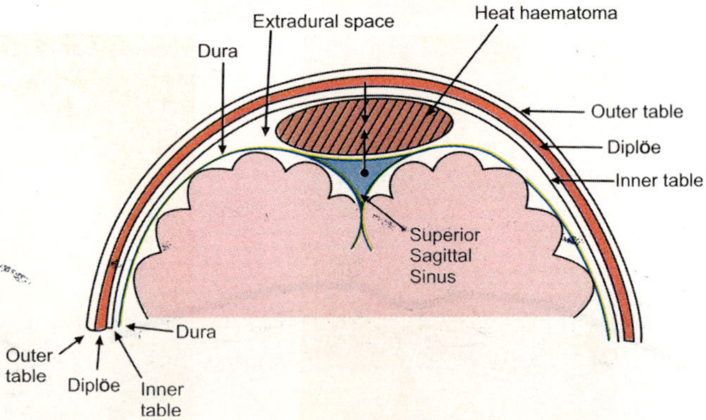

Fig. 13.2: A diagram of skull and brain, showing the position of heat hematoma. Note that the blood in heat hematoma comes from venous sinuses (superior sagittal sinus in the diagram) and from diplöe

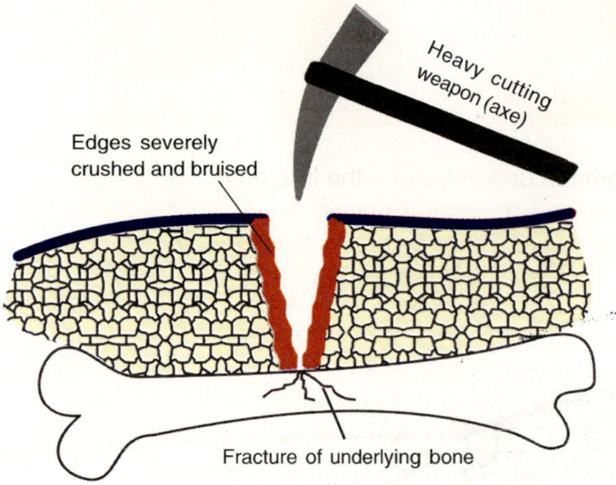

Fig. 11.8: Typical features seen in a cut laceration

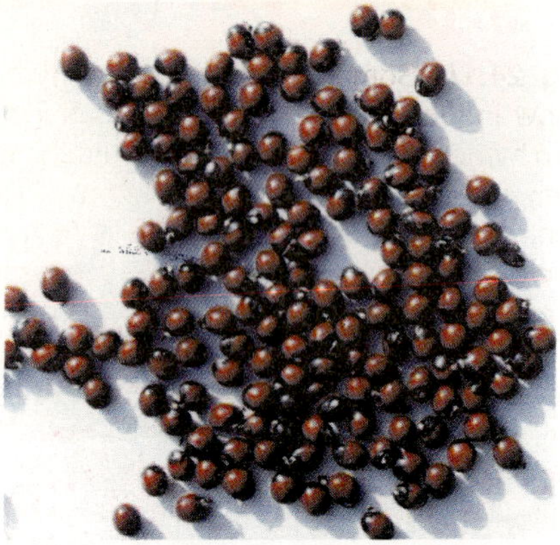

Fig. 37.1: *Ratti* seeds

Plate 3

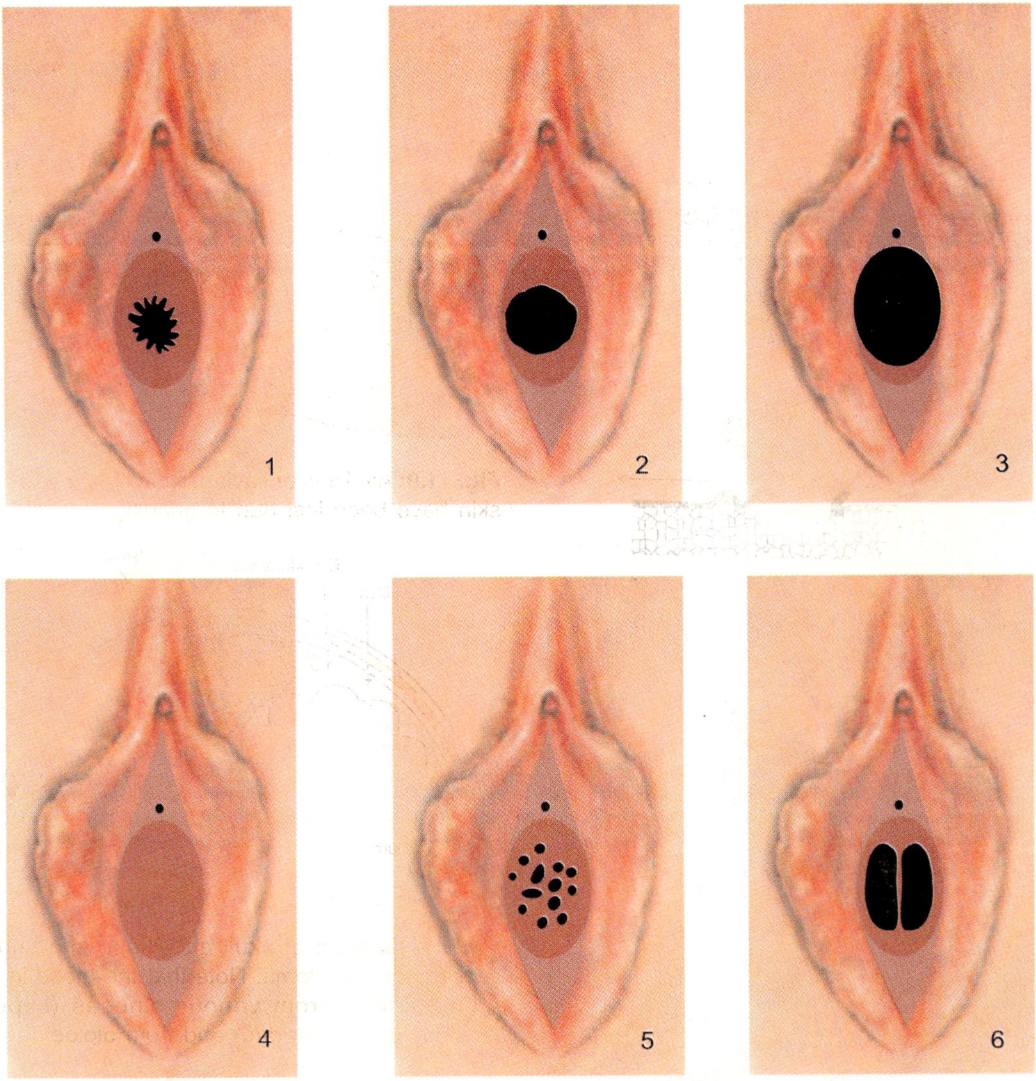

Fig. 24.1A: Some common types of hymen.(1) Fimbriated or denticular – the free edges of hymen show indentations, but the indentations do not reach the peripheral margin. Compare it with a torn hymen (11), where tears are reaching up to the periphery. This is the usual criteria to distinguish between these two types of hymen (2) Annular or Circular – the hymen has an almost circular central opening (3) Semilunar – The hymen looks like a crescent (4) Imperforate – The hymen has no opening at all. In such cases, at the onset of menstrual cycle, the doctor needs to make a surgical opening to let menstrual blood out. If this is not done, it may lead to collection of blood within the distensible vagina (hematocolpos) or uterus (hematometra) (5) Cribriform or Fenestrated - a hymen pierced by many small perforations. This type of hymen lets menstrual and other fluids out with no problem, but sexual activity and the insertion of tampons can be problematic (6) Septate - a hymen in which the opening is divided by a narrow septum. If the septum is somewhat broader, it has been called hymen bifenestratus or hymen biforis

Plate 4

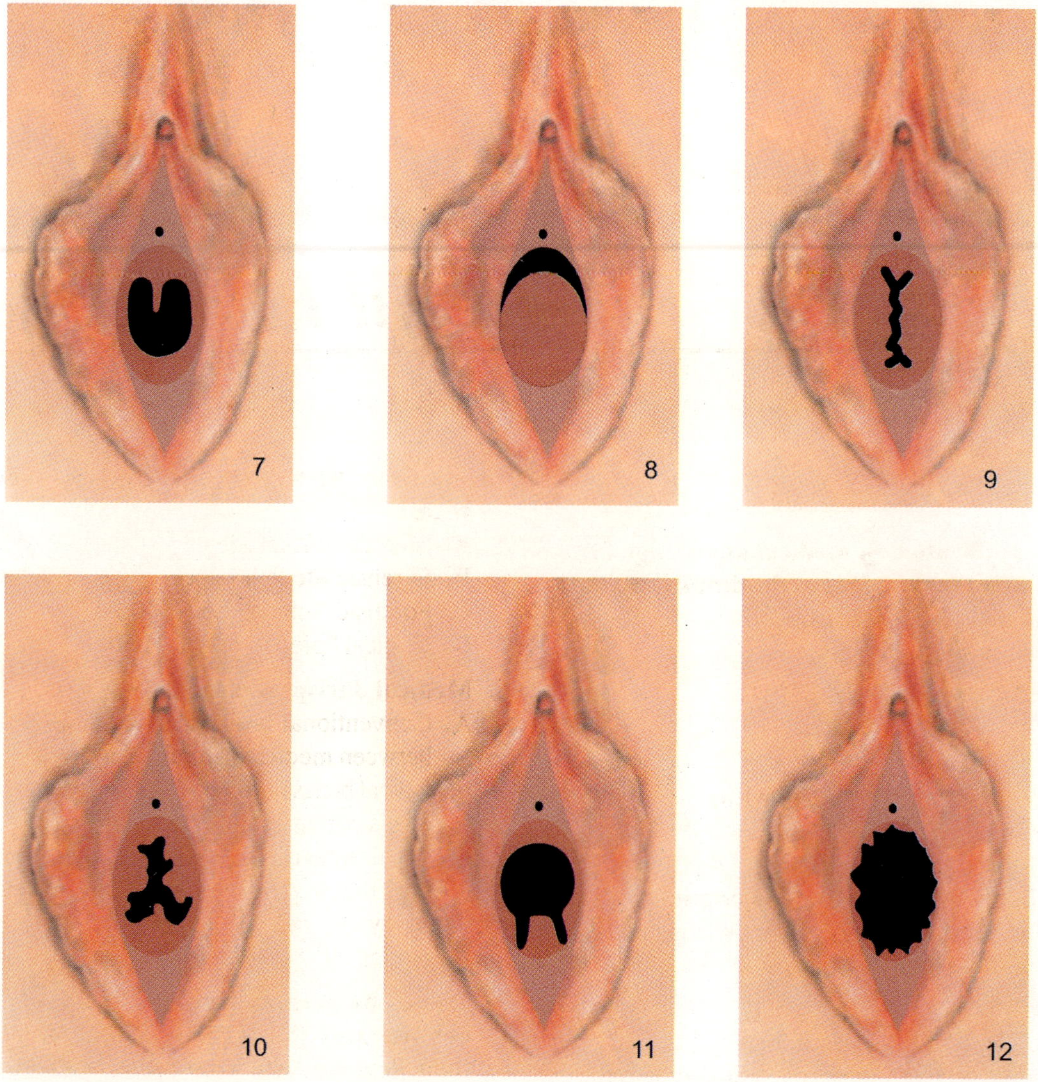

Fig. 24.1B: Some common types of hymen (7) Subseptate - a hymen in which the opening is partially filled by a septum growing out of one wall, but not reaching the other. It almost reminds one of throat with the uvula hanging down (8) Falciform - a sickle-shaped hymen (9) Vertical – the opening is almost vertical slit like (10) Irregular – No regular pattern can be made out (11) Normal injury at first coitus – hymen shows tears. Note that the tears reach the peripheral margin. This is an important feature to note. Please look at fimbriated hymen (1) and see that the indentations in that case do not reach up to the peripheral margin (12) Carunculae myrtiformes – In a woman having experienced multiple acts of intercourse, the hymen almost disappears giving rise to just small minuscule tags of tissue at the periphery

1 GENERAL ASPECTS

1 *Introduction and Legal Procedure*

GENERAL

1. The application of medical knowledge for the purposes of law and administration of justice is known as:
A. Forensic Medicine
B. Medical Jurisprudence
C. Medical Ethics
D. Medical Etiquette

2. Forensic Medicine deals with:
A. Crime and Punishment
B. Medicine and toxicology
C. Study of firearm and finger prints
D. Application of medical knowledge for the purposes of law and administration of justice

3. The word "Forensic" is derived from:
A. A Latin word meaning "belonging to the market place"
B. A Sanskrit word meaning "Crime detection"
C. A Greek Word meaning "application of medical knowledge in the detection of crime"
D. An Egyptian word meaning "clues"

4. Forensic Medicine is synonymous with:
A. Law
B. Medicine used in courts
C. Legal medicine
D. Autopsy

5. The term "State Medicine" is synonymous with:
A. Medical Jurisprudence
B. Forensic Medicine
C. Forensic Science
D. Clinical Forensic Medicine

6. Medical Jurisprudence deals with:
A. Conventional laws of courtesy observed between medical personnel
B. ethical behavior of the doctor with respect of his patients
C. Legal responsibilities of the physician with reference to physician-patient relationship
D. study of trauma illegally causes to a person

7. Moral principles which should guide members of the medical profession in their dealings with each other, with their patients, and with their State would together would be grouped as:
A. Medical Etiquette
B. Moral medicine
C. Principled Forensic Medicine
D. Medical ethics

8. Medical etiquette deals with:
A. Application of moral principles to the practice of medicine
B. Conventional laws of courtesy observed between members of the medical profession

C. Conventional laws of courtesy observed by a male doctor towards a female patient
D. Seeing an old and debilitated patient out of turn

9. Which of the following Bodies of law defines offences and prescribes punishment?
A. Indian Evidence Act
B. Indian Evidence Act
C. Code of Criminal Procedure
D. Indian Penal Code

INQUESTS

10. In which part of India, coroner's system of inquest is present?
A. in Madras
B. Nowhere in India
C. in Calcutta
D. in Mumbai

11. If death has occurred in police custody, it would be investigated by:
A. Deputy Inspector General of Police
B. Home Minister and officials under him
C. An executive magistrate
D. A judicial magistrate

12. The most common type of inquest held in India is:
A. Police inquest
B. Magistrate's inquest
C. Medical Examiner system
D. Coroner's inquest

13. Section 174 Cr.P.C. deals with:
A. Magistrate's inquest
B. Coroner's inquest
C. Police inquest
D. None of the above

14. Section 176 Cr. P.C. deals with:
A. Magistrate's inquest
B. Coroner's inquest
C. Exhumation
D. Sending the viscera for chemical analysis

15. Dowry death is investigated by:
A. Police Officer
B. Chief Judicial Magistrate
C. Judicial 1st Class Magistrate
D. District Magistrate

16. The term "*Panchanama*" refers to:
A. Order by a police officer compelling the witness to appear in police station
B. A local body of five people deciding criminal cases
C. Inquest report
D. Order by the court compelling the witness to appear before it

17. Medical Examiner System is vogue in:
A. Calcutta
B. Russia
C. USA
D. The European Union

18. Which of the following is the superior most form of inquest?
A. Police inquest
B. Magistrate's inquest
C. Medical Examiner system
D. Coroner's inquest

19. Which of the following types of inquest is not followed in India?
A. Medical Examiner system
B. Police inquest
C. Coroner's inquest
D. Both (A) and (C)

COURTS AND THEIR POWERS

20. Which is the highest Judicial Tribunal in India?
A. Rajya Sabha
B. Lok Sabha
C. Supreme Court
D. The President

21. The different criminal courts of India and their powers have been defined in:
A. Constitution of India

B. Indian Evidence Act
C. Criminal Procedure Code
D. India Penal Code

22. Which section of the Indian Penal Code (I.P.C.) prescribes the various punishments which can be awarded by the courts?
A. Section 44
B. Section 53
C. Section 54
D. Section 320

23. How many High Courts are there in India?
A. Only one
B. Ten
C. Twenty one
D. One in each State

24. Which of the following statements is correct regarding trial by jury in India?
A. It is only done in the Supreme Court
B. It is done only in High Court and Supreme Courts
C. It is done only in Mumbai
D. It has been abolished in India

25. In places where trial by jury is in vogue, the number of jurors is:
A. 5
B. 7
C. 9
D. Any of the above

26. The phrase "*voir dire*" refers to:
A. The process of declaring a witness hostile
B. The process of selecting a jury that is competent and not biased
C. The process of taking an oath
D. The stage of cross-examination

27. Which was the last case in India in which jury system was used?
A. The Indira Gandhi assassination trial
B. The Mahatma Gandhi assassination trial
C. Kawas Nanawati case
D. Mathura rape case

28. Which is the maximum sentence which a High Court Judge can pass?
A. He can pass any sentence authorized by law
B. Except death sentence, he can pass all sentences
C. He can pass imprisonment for life and a fine of upto Rs. 50,000
D. It varies depending upon his seniority

29. Death sentence can be awarded by:
A. First class magistrate
B. Second class magistrate
C. District and sessions judge
D. Chief Judicial magistrate

30. Which is the maximum sentence which a District and Sessions Judge (DSJ) may pass?
A. Death sentence
B. Life imprisonment
C. Imprisonment upto 7 years
D. Death sentence, but it must be confirmed by the High Court

31. Which of the following judicial officers can pass a maximum sentence of imprisonment of upto 10 years?
A. An Assistant Sessions Judge
B. Chief Judicial Magistrate
C. Judicial Magistrate of the first class
D. Judicial Magistrate of the Second Class

32. Which is the maximum sentence which a Chief Judicial Magistrate can pass?
A. Upto 10 years
B. Upto 7 years
C. Fine upto Rs. 25,000
D. Both (B) and (D)

33. Which is the maximum sentence which Judicial Magistrate of the First class may pass?
A. 5 years and a fine of Rs 3000
B. 3 years and a fine of Rs 5000
C. 1 year and a fine of Rs 1,000
D. 3 years and a fine of Rs 10,000

34. The maximum sentence which can be passed by a Judicial Magistrate of the Second class is:
A. Imprisonment of 1 year and Rs 1000
B. Imprisonment of 3 years and a fine of Rs 3000
C. Imprisonment of 1 year and/or fine of Rs 5000
D. Imprisonment of 1 year and/or fine of Rs 3000

35. Which is the maximum sentence which a Chief Metropolitan Magistrate can pass?
A. Upto 10 years
B. Upto 7 years
C. Fine upto Rs 25,000
D. Both (B) and (D)

36. Which is the maximum sentence which a Metropolitan Magistrate can pass?
A. Imprisonment for 5 years and fine of Rs 10,000
B. Imprisonment for 3 years and fine of Rs 3,000
C. Imprisonment for 1 year and fine of Rs 10,000
D. Imprisonment for 3 years and fine of Rs 5,000

37. Chief Metropolitan Magistrate has the same powers as that of:
A. An Assistant Sessions Judge
B. Chief Judicial Magistrate
C. Judicial Magistrate of the first class
D. Judicial Magistrate of the second class

38. Metropolitan Magistrate has the same powers as that of:
A. An Assistant Sessions Judge
B. Chief Judicial Magistrate
C. Judicial Magistrate of the first class
D. Judicial Magistrate of the first class

39. "Juvenile Justice Board" is presided over by:
A. Metropolitan magistrate
B. Judicial magistrate of the first class
C. Judicial magistrate of the first class who must be a woman
D. Either (A) or (B)

40. Immediate jurisdiction of land assessment comes under:
A. Supreme Court
B. Sessions Court
C. District Court
D. None of the above

41. Under which of the following sections does the court derive power to recall and reexamine any person already examined as a witness?
A. Section 45 Indian Evidence Act
B. The court does not hold this power under any law
C. Section 114 A Indian Evidence Act
D. Section 311 Cr.P.C.

MEDICAL EVIDENCE

42. The person who initiates a lawsuit is known as:
A. Plaintiff
B. Defendant
C. Public prosecutor
D. Complainant

43. Subpoena is a kind of:
A. Decomposed body tissue
B. Designation
C. Document
D. Court

44. A doctor may be called to testify as:
A. Ordinary witness
B. Expert witness
C. Physician who treated a patient
D. Any of the above

45. An expert witness is defined under which of the following sections?
A. Section 45 of Indian Evidence Act
B. Section 141 of Indian Evidence Act
C. Section 114A of Indian Evidence Act
D. Section 54 of Cr. P.C.

46. The word *subpoena* means:
A. penal erasure of name
B. Under penalty
C. Cross examination
D. Taking oath

47. Which of the following facts is true about *Subpoena duces tecum* ?
A. It compels a witness to give evidence and also bring with him certain documents in his possession
B. It means the medical witness can send reply by post
C. It means the medical witness can be examined via telephone, this being used only for very busy medical practitioners
D. The court officially personally accompanies medical witness to the court

48. Which of the following is an expert witness?
A. Fingerprint expert
B. Handwriting expert
C. Doctor who is authorized to conduct an autopsy
D. All of the above

49. The word *subpoena* is synonymous with:
A. Res ipsa loquitur
B. Res judicata
C. Summons
D. Solemn affirmation

50. Conduct money in civil cases is given by:
A. The lawyer who calls the witness
B. The party which calls the witness
C. The government
D. The opposite party to that which calls the witness

51. Conduct money in criminal cases is given by:
A. The lawyer who calls the witness
B. The opposite party to that which calls the witness
C. The accused
D. The court

52. If a doctor receives subpoena from more than one court simultaneously, which of the following rules should he normally observe?
A. Criminal courts have priority over civil courts
B. Higher courts have priority over lower courts
C. Civil courts have priority over criminal courts
D. Both (A) and (B) above

53. Medical evidence is recorded in a certain sequence. Which of the following sequence is the correct sequence?
A. Examination-in-Chief, Cross-examination, Oath, Questions asked by the Judge, Reexamination
B. Oath, Questions asked by the Judge, Examination-in-Chief, Cross-examination, Reexamination
C. Oath, Examination-in-Chief, Cross-examination, Reexamination, Questions asked by the Judge
D. Oath, Cross-examination, Examination-in-Chief, Reexamination, Questions asked by the Judge

54. In oath taking the witness has to keep his/her hand on a holy book. This does not apply to:
A. A medical man
B. A lawyer
C. A minor
D. An atheist

55. If a medical witness refuses to take oath before giving evidence:
A. He may be imprisoned for upto 6 months and/or fined upto Rs. 1000
B. He would only be asked to solemnly affirm
C. His evidence would be taken without oath
D. His evidence would not be taken, and he would be asked to leave the court

56. Which of the following is the *main* purpose of cross-examination?
- **A.** To help the accused win the case
- **B.** To help the judge understand the case
- **C.** To confuse the witness
- **D.** To test the accuracy of statement of witness

57. Perjury means:
- **A.** Contempt of court
- **B.** Cases tried with the help of jury
- **C.** To act according to law
- **D.** False evidence given by a witness after taking oath

58. Under which of the following sections is perjury defined?
- **A.** Section 191 I.P.C.
- **B.** Section 191 Indian Evidence Act
- **C.** Section 191 Cr. P.C.
- **D.** Section 193 I.P.C.

59. If a doctor issues a false medical certificate, under which of the following sections will he be prosecuted?
- **A.** Section 197 of I.P.C.
- **B.** Section 197 of Cr.P.C.
- **C.** Section 198 of I.P.C.
- **D.** Section 201 of I.P.C.

60. Which of the following witnesses can not testify in a court of law?
- **A.** A child below 12 years
- **B.** A prosecuted criminal
- **C.** A lunatic who can not understand questions because of his lunacy
- **D.** All of the above

61. Which of the following is the best definition of a leading question?
- **A.** A question suggesting the answer which the person putting it wishes to receive
- **B.** A question which leads a medical witness to confusion
- **C.** A question which is which is asked out of context
- **D.** A question which belongs outside the expertise of the medical witness

62. Section 141 of the Indian Evidence Act, 1872:
- **A.** Defines rules for taking oath
- **B.** Defines a leading question
- **C.** Bars an insane person to give evidence in a court of law
- **D.** Gives the correct sequence in which medical evidence should be recorded

63. Leading questions are generally permitted in:
- **A.** Examination-in-Chief
- **B.** Cross-examination
- **C.** Reexamination
- **D.** All of the above

64. During which part of the recording of medical evidence are leading questions *normally* not allowed?
- **A.** Examination-in-Chief
- **B.** Cross-examination
- **C.** Reexamination
- **D.** Both (A) and (C)

65. The defence witness in a murder trial is cross-examined by:
- **A.** Public Prosecutor
- **B.** Defence Counsel
- **C.** Police Officer
- **D.** Judge

66. Cross-examination of the prosecution witness is done by:
- **A.** Public prosecutor
- **B.** Defence counsel
- **C.** Judge
- **D.** Any of the above

67. Dying deposition is superior to Dying declaration because:
- **A.** Deposition is always done in writing while declaration is always orally
- **B.** Deposition is always done in the presence of some responsible person like a medical officer
- **C.** Dying persons always speak the truth
- **D.** It is made on oath in presence of accused and the defence counsel can cross-examine the dying man

68. Which one of the following is not followed in India?
A. Recording a dying declaration
B. Recording a dying deposition
C. Conducting a police inquest
D. Conducting a magistrate's inquest

69. Dying declaration can be recorded by:
A. Medical officer
B. A person trained in law
C. A police officer
D. Any of the above

70. Evidence that would, if uncontested, reasonably establish a fact or raise a presumption of a fact is called:
A. Hearsay evidence
B. Direct evidence
C. Prima facie evidence
D. Indirect evidence

71. Evidence that is NOT drawn from direct observation, but is *derived* from other facts is known as:
A. Circumstantial evidence
B. Direct evidence
C. Indirect evidence
D. Hearsay evidence

72. Second hand evidence, i.e. evidence that is not what the witness knows personally, but what someone else told him or her is best described as:
A. Faulty evidence
B. Tertiary evidence
C. Hearsay evidence
D. Third-party evidence

73. Which of the following is an example of *Res gestae*?
A. Involuntary exclamations or acts made at the time the offense was committed
B. Making false statement under oath
C. Asking leading questions during examination-in-chief
D. Questions asked by the judge

OFFENCES AND PROCEDURES OF CRIMINAL TRIALS

74. Which of the following is defined in section 2(c) of the Criminal Procedure Code?
A. Bailable offence
B. Cognizable offence
C. Non-cognizable offence
D. Judicial proceeding

75. All are cognizable offence *except*:
A. Murder
B. Rape
C. Attempted suicide
D. None of the above

76. Which of the following is a cognizable offence?
A. An offence for which the maximum punishment is life imprisonment
B. An offence for which one could be imprisoned up to 3 years
C. An offence for which only fine is imposed
D. An offence for which a police officer can arrest a person without a warrant from magistrate

77. Which of the following is not a cognizable offence?
A. Rape
B. Voluntarily causing grievous hurt
C. Attempted suicide
D. Voluntarily causing hurt

78. Which of the following would be called a Summons-case?
A. A case relating to an offence for which summons can be issued to a medical witness
B. A case relating to an offence for which summons can be issued to the guilty person within 5 days
C. A case relating to an offence for which the maximum punishment is imprisonment for a term of two years

D. A case in which doctor has to attend the court immediately on an emergent basis

79. Which of the following would be called a Warrant-case?

A. A case relating to an offence for which warrant can be issued to a medical witness

B. A case relating to an offence punishable with death, imprisonment for life or imprisonment for a term exceeding two years

C. A case relating to an offence in which search warrants are issued by the court

D. A case relating to such a serious and grave offence that the doctor has to attend the court immediately on an emergent basis

80. If a man eater lion enters a village and kills a villager, and the villagers subsequently stone the lion to death, the case will be dealt with in the:

A. High Court

B. Sessions court

C. Veterinary court

D. None of the above

SENTENCES

81. Which of the following facts is correct in case a woman sentenced to death is found to be pregnant?

A. Her sentence must be commuted to life imprisonment by the High Court

B. Only the Supreme court can commute the sentence to life imprisonment, and it is binding on the Supreme Court

C. The sentence is postponed till the delivery of the child by the District and Sessions Judge

D. The High Court may postpone the sentence for any period, and may if it thinks fit, commute the sentence to imprisonment for life

MULTIPLE ANSWER TYPE (PGI, CHANDIGARH PATTERN)

82. If a patient survives after having given dying declaration, what is the status of the dying declaration?

A. The statement is valid for 48 hours

B. It cannot be admitted under section 32 of Indian Evidence Act

C. It can be used for corroboration of testimony in court under section 157 of the Indian Evidence Act

D. It is valid if it was given to magistrate, otherwise it is invalid

E. It is valid if it was reduced to writing and signed by the declarant, otherwise it is invalid

83. By which of the following methods is judicial sentence of death carried out in India?

A. Hanging

B. Guillotine

C. Garroting

D. Burking

E. Lethal injection

84. A dumb witness:

A. Is not allowed to testify in a court of law

B. Can testify by signs in an open court

C. By producing a previously written statement

D. By writing in an open court

E. Is sent to a speech therapist and is allowed to testify only when he is able to speak

85. Essential elements for recording the dying declaration are:

A. It should be written in patient's own language

B. Signatures of the dying person on the statement is very essential

C. It should be sent to *illaqa* magistrate in a sealed envelope

D. The medical practitioner should certify that he or she is insane

E. Leading questions are not permitted

ANSWERS

GENERAL

1. A.
2. D.
3. A. The word is derived from the Latin word *"Forensis"*, meaning "belonging to the market place" or "forum". In ancient Rome, cases were tried and pleaded at the "forum" or public meeting place.
4. C.
5. B. ***Related fact:*** State medicine refers to medical knowledge used for the purposes of the State. It is the duty of the State to investigate various criminal matters. Since Forensic medicine caters to that, it is sometimes referred to as "State Medicine". This term however is not much in vogue today.
6. C.
7. D. Ethical behavior is not legally enforceable. It is a self-imposed duty on the doctor himself. Some examples of good ethical behavior are (a) not criticizing the professional ability of another doctor (b) dealing with the female patients with utmost respect (c) not administering narcotic drugs to the patients for the sake of satisfying their addictive behavior.
8. B.
9. D.

INQUESTS

10. B. Coroner's inquest is nowhere held in India now. The last city to abolish it was Mumbai, where it was abolished on 29th July 1999.
11. C. ***Additional facts:*** Executive magistrate would also conduct an inquest when death has occurred in jail, during police interrogation, police lock-up or during police firing.

    Variant of this question: In case of lock up, the inquest is held by (a) A police officer (b) Magistrate (c) Panchayat officer (d) District attorney.

    The answer is (b) Magistrate.
12. A.
13. C.
14. A.
15. D. Section 174(4) specifically specifies which magistrates are empowered to hold inquests. They are (i) District Magistrate (ii) Sub-divisional Magistrate and (iii) Any other Executive Magistrate specifically empowered in this behalf by the State Government or the District Magistrate. Note that Judicial Magistrates are not included.
16. C. ***Related fact:*** Traditionally a police officer investigating a murder case, used to record information from five (Hindi: *Panch*) witnesses. These witnesses were preferably some respectable people from the locality who were supposed to speak the truth. The report thus prepared was called panchanama. Now usually statements from two witnesses are recorded.
17. C.
18. C.
19. D.

COURTS AND THEIR POWERS

20. C. ***Related fact:*** The President is not the Judicial Tribunal, although he can hear the mercy petition in case of condemned criminals.

21. C.

22. B. These punishments are (i) Death (ii) Imprisonment for life (iii) Imprisonment for a lesser period, which could be of two descriptions – namely simple and rigorous (iv) Forfeiture of property and (v) Fine.

23. C. Much against popular belief, High courts do not exist in every state. Many states together have a single High Court. For instance the Guwahati High Court caters to all the seven States of North East (Arunachal Pradesh, Assam, Manipur, Meghalaya, Mizoram, Nagaland and Tripura). Mumbai High Court caters to the State of Maharashtra and Goa (as well as Union Territory of Dadra and Nagar Haveli and Daman and Diu).

High Courts are not necessarily located in the State Capitals. For instance the High Court of Uttar Pradesh is located at Allahabad (not at Lucknow, which is its capital). Other High Courts not located at State capitals are Chhattisgarh High Court at Bilaspur, Kerala High Court at Ernakulam, Madhya Pradesh High Court at Jabalpur, Orissa High Court at Cuttack, Rajasthan High Court at Jodhpur and Uttranchal High Court at Nainital.

Between 28 States and 7 Union Territories of India there are a total of 21 High Courts at present.

24. D.

25. D. The list of jurors is prepared by the court. It has to be an uneven number.

26. B. ***Related facts:*** The phrase "*voir dire*" [pronounced as *vwahr* (with a near-silent "r") *deer*] is derived from French, meaning "to see to speak". In English it has come to mean "to speak the truth".

The process refers to the interrogation of prospective jurors by the attorneys and judge in court. *Voir dire* determines whether any of the jurors are biased and/or cannot deal with the case's issues fairly, or if there is just cause to not allow a juror to serve (such as knowledge of facts; acquaintanceship with parties, witness or attorneys; occupation which might lead to bias; prejudice against the death penalty; or similar experiences). The purpose of *voir dire* is to provide the attorneys with a feeling for the jury panel's personalities and likely views. Sometimes, the judge will ask the majority of the questions, while in some courts, lawyers have substantial latitude and time to make inquiries. The judge can dismiss jurors if not found suitable. Attorneys may discard others in "peremptory" challenges without indicating a reason (Peremptory Challenge refers to a limited number of challenges each side in a trial can use to eliminate potential jurors without stating a reason. May not be used to keep members of a particular race or sex off the jury).

In England, the process of *voir dire* consists of the single question: "Can you give a fair hearing to both the crown and the defense?" Any prospective juror who affirmatively answers the question is impaneled on the jury.

27. C. ***Related facts:*** Until 1959 India had a jury based system. The landmark Kawas Nanavati case changed it all. Kawas Nanavati, a Commander in the Indian Navy, was accused of murdering his wife's (a British lady Sylvia Nanavati) lover Prem Ahuja. The evidence was against Nanavati. However, he was a young and handsome man who the public (and parts of the press) looked upon as some sort of "hero". The jury declared him not guilty by 8:1.

The verdict was considered perverse by the Sessions judge RB Mehta who referred the case to the Bombay High Court. The High Court found him guilty too and sentenced Nanavati to life imprisonment. Nanavati appealed to the Supreme Court, but lost.

Because the jury in the sessions court was thought to be unduly influenced by the press (notably Rusi Karanjia's paper *Blitz*) to give a verdict in favour of Nanavati, jury trials in India were abolished.

28. A. This is given in ***Section 28(1) of Cr.P.C.***

29. C. District and Sessions Judge (DSJ) can pass a death sentence. But remember it must be confirmed by the High Court. A few facts about DSJ may be mentioned here. He is the highest judicial authority below a High Court judge. He is known as a District Judge when he presides over a civil case, and a Sessions Judge when he presides over a criminal case.

30. D. This is given in ***Section 28(2) of Cr.P.C. Section 366 of Cr.P.C.*** further says that when the Court of Sessions passes a sentence of death, the proceedings shall be submitted to the High Court and the sentence shall not be executed unless it is confirmed by the High Court.

31. A. This is given in ***Section 28(3) of Cr.P.C.***

32. B. This is given in ***Section 29(1) of Cr.P.C.***

33. D. This is given in ***Section 29(2) of Cr.P.C.*** Previously First class magistrate could pass a sentence of 3 years and a fine of Rs. 5000, but by a new amendment in 2005, he can now impose a fine upto Rs. 10,000.

34. C. This is given in ***Section 29(3) of Cr.P.C.*** Previously First class magistrate could pass a sentence of 1 year and a fine of Rs. 1000, but by a new amendment in 2005, he can now impose a fine upto Rs. 5,000.

35. B. Chief Metropolitan Magistrate sits in Metropolitan cities (like Delhi) and has the same powers as the powers of a Chief Judicial Magistrate (Please refer also to question 32).

36. D. A Metropolitan Magistrate sits in Metropolitan cities and has the same powers as the powers of a Judicial Magistrate of the 1st Class.

37. B. This is given in ***Section 29(4)*** of the Cr.P.C.

38. C. This is given in ***Section 29(4)*** of the Cr.P.C.

39. D. ***Related facts:*** Section 4 of the *"The Juvenile Justice (Care of Protection of Children) Act, 2000"* discusses about the constitution of the Juvenile Justice Board. It consists of three persons

i. Metropolitan Magistrate or a Judicial Magistrate of the first class. He is designated as the Principal Magistrate.

ii. Two social workers, of whom at least one shall be a woman.

This Board has all the powers of a Judicial Magistrate of the first class, i.e. it can pass a sentence of 3 years and a fine of Rs. 5000 only.

The term "Juvenile Justice Board" is often substituted by "Juvenile Court" in many MCQ books. This is incorrect. The Juvenile Justice Act does not talk about the term "Juvenile Court" at all, although in common parlance it is usual to refer to the Juvenile Justice Board as Juvenile Court.

The Act prescribes qualifications for both the magistrate and the social workers. No magistrate can be appointed as a member of the Board unless he has special knowledge or training in child psychology or child welfare. No social worker can be appointed as a member of the Board unless he has been actively involved in health, education, or welfare activities pertaining to children for at least seven years.

40. C.

41. D. ***Related fact:*** Under section 311 Cr.P.C. not only can any court recall and reexamine any person already examined, it can indeed summon any person as a witness, even if not directly connected with that case, if the court thinks that it is essential to the just decision of the case. The court can do this at any stage of trial.

MEDICAL EVIDENCE

42. **A.** ***Related fact:*** The person who initiates a lawsuit by filing a complaint is called the plaintiff. When the document that initiates a lawsuit is a *petition rather than a complaint,* the initiating person is usually referred to as the petitioner rather than the plaintiff. A petition is a request, directed to a court or administrative tribunal, seeking some sort of relief such as a court order.

43. **C.**

44. **D.**

45. **A.**

46. **B.**

47. **A.** Subpoena is of two types: (i) *Subpoena ad testificandum:* It compels a witness to attend and give evidence and (ii) *Subpoena duces tecum:* It compels a witness to give evidence and also bring with him certain documents in his possession (usually the post-mortem or the medicolegal report) specified in the subpoena.

48. **D.**

49. **C.**

50. **B.**

51. **D.**

52. **D.**

53. **C.**

54. **D.** Normally a person affirms in the name of God, by putting his hand on a holy book. But if he is a non-believer in God as an atheist, he would be required only to solemnly affirm.

55. **A.** This is in accordance with Section 178 of I.P.C.

56. **D.** Although the witness is quite commonly seen to be confused during the cross-examination, this can not be considered the purpose of cross examination. The main purpose of cross examination remains to test the accuracy of statement of witness.

57. **D.**

58. **A.** ***Related fact:*** Punishment for perjury is defined under section 193 of I.P.C. It is imprisonment of either description (i.e. either simple or rigorous) for a period of upto 7 years and fine.

59. **A.** ***Related fact:*** The punishment to the doctor under this section would be 7 years and fine. If a patient used such a certificate, he would be punished under section 198 of I.P.C. and the punishment would be the same.

60. **C.** Section 118 of the Indian Evidence Act, 1872, clearly states that everyone can testify in a court of law, unless the court considers that one can not understand questions put to them, or give rational answers to those questions because of very young age (note that no age is specified), extreme old age or some disease of body or mind. Even a lunatic can give evidence if he is not prevented by his lunacy to understand questions, or give rational answers to them.

61. **A.**

62. **B.** It defines a leading question like this: Any questions suggesting the answer which the person putting it wishes to receive or expects to receive is called a leading question.

63. **B.** This is in accordance with section 143 of IEA.

64. **D.** This is in accordance with section 142 of IEA.

65. **A.**

66. **B.**

67. **D.**

68. **B.**

69. **D.** ***Related facts:*** Dying declarations are made under section 32(1) of *Indian Evidence Act.* No guidelines are laid down under this section as to who can record the statement. This means that virtually anyone can record

the statement. The statement can even be oral, tape-recorded, or may even be made on phone to someone!

Other general guidelines regarding dying declarations—based on various court judgments—are as follows:

- It is an example of hearsay evidence. It is admitted on the principle of necessity.
- Doctor should certify that the declarant is fit to make a statement. A certificate to this effect may not be necessary. Even if the Magistrate verifies from the doctor that the injured is in senses and fit to make a statement, it is alright.
- Deceased unable to speak→questions put and signs/gestures made in reply are admissible as dying declaration.
- Dying declaration narrated in one language (Punjabi), but recorded in another (Urdu)→Admissible.
- It should preferably be in the form of questions and answers.
- No leading questions may be asked.
- Dying declaration made by a minor can be believed.
- FIR/report by deceased to police (deceased dying subsequently) is a dying declaration.
- Complaint made in writing to police expressing apprehension of death at the hands of certain persons. Complainant dies subsequently. It is a dying declaration.
- Dying declaration→Only cause of death is admissible. If the statement is not relating to the cause of death or circumstances of his death, statement is inadmissible.
- Dying declaration should contain information for HIS OWN cause of death. If A made certain statements with respect to the death of B and A dies subsequently→Statement of A is inadmissible.
- Dying declaration is inadmissible if the declarant survives. He will have to come to the court and face proceedings normally. However according to **section 157 of Indian Evidence Act,** dying declaration may be taken as a corroborative evidence to the testimony given in court.
- Dying declaration may be made not only in homicide, but also in cases of suicide.
- Dying declaration need not be made in expectation of death. Even if the person did not apprehend that he would die, a statement made by him about the circumstances of his death would be admissible. Letters of bride burnt to death revealing instances of torture and intention of her husband and mother-in-law to murder are admissible as dying declaration. However it has been opined by courts that an apprehension of approaching death gives a sanction of oath to the statement.
- Conviction has been done solely on dying declaration in a number of cases.
- Incomplete dying declaration (declarant dying during the course of making statement)→may be admissible if it sufficiently identifies the accused. If there were two accused A and B. Dying declaration does not sufficiently identify A, but it completely identifies B, it would be admissible in connection with B.
- Dying declaration must be taken as a whole.
- Dying declaration of a dacoit can be used against other dacoits (or accomplices).
- Dying declaration recorded by the police in the presence of medical officer. Medical officer need not attest the statement.

70. C. ***Related facts:*** *Prima facie* is Latin for "at first view." For instance, a plaintiff can establish a *prima facie* case of race discrimination by establishing that (1) he or she belongs to a racial minority; (2) he or she applied and was qualified for a job for which the employer was seeking applicants; (3) he or she was rejected for the position despite his or her qualifications; and (4) the position remained open after his or her rejection and the employer continued to seek applications from other people with similar qualifications to the plaintiff. *[McDonnell Douglas v. Green, 411 U.S. 792, 802 (1973)].*

71. A. If a person slept at night, seeing that the environment around his house was completely dry, and on waking up he finds that all around his house and locality, everything is ankle deep in water, it would be very reasonable for him to conclude that it rained heavily in the night. Since he did not actually see rain and is just deriving this fact from other observations, it is a circumstantial evidence that it rained in night (had he got up in the night and seen it actually raining, it would have been direct evidence).

The same situation can now easily be understood in a legal setting. Consider the following facts:

- A couple is known to be hostile to each other.
- The wife is seen to buy arsenic allegedly for killing rats on a particular day.
- The husband dies of arsenic poisoning the next day.
- Police raids the house and finds that there is arsenic in the food, which the wife prepared.
- Arsenic is also found in one of the cupboards of the wife, but is somewhat lesser in amount than what she actually bought.

It would be very reasonable to suspect that she gave arsenic to the husband. Since no one actually saw her giving arsenic, it is only circumstantial evidence. If someone had actually seen her mixing arsenic in her husband's food, and then giving the food to him, it would have been direct evidence.

Circumstantial evidence is generally admissible in court unless the connection between the fact and the inference is too weak to be of help in deciding the case. Many convictions for various crimes have rested largely on circumstantial evidence.

72. C. ***Related facts:*** In general, hearsay may not be admitted in evidence, but there are two notable exceptions (i) Dying declarations and (ii) Res gestae. Res gestae are involuntary exclamations or acts made at the time the offense was committed and are so closely connected to the main fact in issue as to be a part of it. These utterances or acts are not planned, but are forced from the individual by the excitement of the moment. The ground of reliability upon which such declarations are received is their spontaneity; they are the facts talking through the party. For example let us imagine that A is passing through a dark and narrow lane and he hears B running around violently and exclaiming C has stabbed him. B dies subsequently without making any further statement. As far as A is concerned, the fact that C stabbed B is "hearsay evidence", but since it was made by B in the "heat of the moment", it is an example of res gestae and admissible as valid evidence.

73. A. For further explanations, please see question 72.

OFFENCES AND PROCEDURES OF CRIMINAL TRIALS

74. B. ***Related fact:*** In the First Schedule of the Cr.P.C. a detailed list of all cognizable and non-cognizable offences are given.

75. D. ***Related fact:*** Cognizable offence is defined in section 2 (c) of Criminal Procedure Code as an offence in which a police officer may arrest a person without warrant. This provision is reserved for more serious offences, where the police must arrest the offender immediately, lest there is a risk of offender escaping. Section 2 (l) of Criminal Procedure Code defines the "non-cognizable offence", and this is defined as an offence in which a police officer has no authority to arrest without warrant. This applies to less serious offences.

The Criminal Procedure Code gives two schedules at the end (which are much like appendices at the end of a book). Of these the first schedule gives a classification of all offences. All offences are classified under three headings (i) whether they are cognizable or not (ii) whether bailable or not and (iii) which court can try them (e.g. sessions court, first class magistrate or any magistrate etc.).

Major examples of **non-cognizable offences** are (i) Bribery (S. 171 E, I.P.C.) (ii) Causing miscarriage with woman's consent (S. 312 I.P.C.) [causing miscarriage without woman's consent comes under S. 313 I.P.C.; this is cognizable] (iii) Voluntarily causing hurt (S. 323 I.P.C.) and (iv) Intercourse by a man with his wife not being under twelve years of age.

Murder, theft, robbery and dacoity are some examples which fall under cognizable offence, i.e. the police office can arrest a person accused of these offences without warrant from a magistrate. One of the biggest misunderstandings among students is that attempt to commit suicide is a non-cognizable offence. It is not. Attempt to commit suicide is a cognizable offence.

However it (attempt to commit suicide) is a bailable offence, while both murder and rape are non-bailable offences.

76. D.

77. D.

78. C. Summons-case has been defined in Section 2 (w) of *Criminal Procedure Code.* The procedure for trial in a Summons case is slightly different, being guided by sections 251-258 of Cr.P.C.

79. B. Warrant-case has been defined in Section 2 (x) of *Criminal Procedure Code.* The procedure for trial in a Warrant case is slightly different, being guided by sections 238-250 of Cr.P.C.

80. D. ***Related facts:*** It is not an offence to kill an animal who has fatally attacked a human being.

SENTENCES

81. D. This is prescribed in section 416 Cr. P.C.

MULTIPLE ANSWER TYPE (PGI, CHANDIGARH PATTERN)

82. B, C. Section 32 of the *Indian Evidence Act* refers to cases in which statements have been made by persons who are dead or cannot be found. Since the person has survived, his dying declaration under section 32 cannot be admitted. However under section 157 of the *Indian Evidence Act*, dying declaration may be used for corroboration of victim's testimony in court.

83. A. ***Related facts:*** This is known as judicial hanging and is different from ordinary hanging used by potential suicides. In judicial hanging, the victim is made to fall from some distance after a noose has been fixed around his neck. This causes his cervical vertebrae to break and injure spinal cord, causing immediate death.

84. B,D. According to section 119 of the *Indian Evidence Act*, a witness who is unable to speak may give his evidence in any other manner in which he can make it intelligible, as by writing or by signs; but such writing must be written and the signs made in *open* court. Evidence so given shall be deemed to be oral evidence.

85. E. Regarding choice (D)→Medical officer need only certify that the patient was fit to make a statement. No need to prove or certify that a person is sane or insane, since everybody is considered sane unless proved otherwise. Note that the choice (D) mentions about doctor certifying that the patient is insane. This is obviously absurd.

2 Law in Relation to Medical Men; Medical Ethics

GENERAL

1. **Law which is laid down by state legislatures or Parliament is known as?**
   A. Law of torts
   B. Statute law
   C. Law of courts
   D. Common law
2. **Law which is laid down by the Judges by their judgements is:**
   A. Law of torts
   B. Statute law
   C. Law of courts
   D. Common law
3. **The law of torts is created by:**
   A. Parliament
   B. State legislatures
   C. President
   D. Courts of law
4. **The main law which deals with procedures to be followed in a criminal case is:**
   A. Cr.P.C.
   B. Indian contract Act
   C. Indian evidence Act
   D. I.P.C.

ACTS RELATING TO MEDICAL PROFESSION

Consumer Protection Act 1986

5. **A district consumer redressal forum can entertain claims for compensation up to a maximum of:**
   A. Rs. 50,000
   B. Rs. 1 lakh
   C. Rs. 5 lakh
   D. Rs. 20 lakh
6. **State consumer redressal commissions can entertain claims for compensation:**
   A. Up to Rs. 1 lakh only
   B. Up to Rs. 25 lakh only
   C. Between Rs. 5 lakh and 20 lakh
   D. Between Rs. 20 lakh and one crore
7. **The National Consumer Redressal Commission can entertain claims for compensation only when they are of more than:**
   A. Rs. 15 lakh
   B. Rs. 20 lakh
   C. Rs. 1 crore
   D. Rs. 5 crore

INDIAN MEDICAL COUNCIL AND STATE MEDICAL COUNCILS

8. Which of the following statements regarding the composition of Indian Medical Council is not correct?

A. One member from each state other than a Union territory is nominated by the Central Government

B. One member from each state where a State Medical Register is maintained is selected by persons among themselves, enrolled in the said Register

C. Five members are elected from amongst persons enrolled in any of the State Medical Register

D. Eight members are nominated by the Central Government

9. Which of the following facts about Medical Council of India is correct?

A. The President and Vice President of the Council are elected from amongst the members of the Council

B. The President is elected but the Vice President is nominated by the Central Government

C. The President is nominated by the Central Government but the Vice President is elected

D. Both the President and Vice President are nominated by the Central Government

10. Which of the following regarding the Executive Committee of the Medical Council of India is correct?

A. It holds office for a period of six years

B. It comprises of the President, Vice President, Secretary and Joint Secretary

C. It comprises of the President, Vice President and 25 other members

D. It comprises of the President, Vice President and 7-10 other members

11. Disciplinary control of the medical profession is maintained by:

A. The hospital in which doctor is working

B. Indian Medical Association

C. The Supreme Court

D. State Medical Council

12. The responsibility of maintaining standards of medical education in India is that of:

A. State Medical Association

B. Medical Council of India

C. National Board of Examinations

D. Indian Medical Association

13. Which one of the following is not a function of State Medical Councils?

A. Issue of warning notices

B. Maintenance of Medical Register

C. Disciplinary Control of Medical Profession

D. Maintenance of Standards of Medical education

PRIVILEGES/DUTIES OF MEDICAL PRACTITIONERS

14. Which one of the following is NOT a privilege (right) of a Registered Medical Practitioner?

A. Running a drug store or medical shop

B. Right to add title, description etc. to his name

C. Possessing and supplying dangerous drugs to his patients

D. Recovery of fees from his patient

15. All of the following are examples of *privileged communication except*:

A. A child suffering from congenital AIDS —doctor informs the school authorities

B. A syphilitic is taking bath in a public pool —doctor informs the owner of the pool

C. Engine driver is color blind—doctor informs the state transport authority

D. A airplane pilot is having hypermetropic —doctor informs the administration of the airplane company

16. Which of the following is an example of *privileged communication*?
A. Doctor is appointed on the panel of the Life Insurance Corporation. He reveals the information that the person taking the policy is suffering from some life threatening disorder
B. Patient sues the doctor for not treating him properly. During the trial, the doctor reveals to the court that the patient is suffering from an incurable disorder
C. A teenager suffering from suicidal tendencies. The doctor reveals this condition to his parents
D. All of the above

17. A doctor should not take fees for issuing the following certificate:
A. Certificate to a government employee
B. Death certificate
C. Certificate given to a poor patient
D. Certificate given to a psychiatric patient

PROFESSIONAL NEGLIGENCE

18. All of the following are related to medical negligence *except*:
A. Section 304A I.P.C.
B. Section 37 I.P.C.
C. Section 351 I.P.C.
D. Section 312 I.P.C.

19. Professional death sentence is:
A. Death sentence given to a professional such as a doctor
B. Permanent erasure of a doctor's name from the medical register
C. Expulsion of a doctor from the professional body to which he belongs
D. Expulsion of an intern from a hospital for gross negligence, so he can not get his medical degree

20. Professional death sentence can be passed by:
A. Supreme Court
B. Consumer Court
C. Medical Superintendent of a Hospital
D. State Medical Council

21. For civil negligence in treating a patient, a doctor may be:
A. Fined
B. Imprisoned
C. Both imprisoned and fined
D. Required to pay compensation

22. A civil wrong is known as:
A. *Mutatis mutandis*
B. *Pari passu*
C. *Tort*
D. *Ultra vires*

23. Example of *res ipsa loquitur* is:
A. A drug for external use prescribed for taking by mouth
B. Death due to anesthesia
C. Operating a patient without a post-graduate degree in surgery
D. Tetanus infection to an indoor patient

24. An intern is conducting a laparotomy under supervision of his Head of Department of Surgery. An artery forceps is left in the abdominal cavity because of which the patient suffers ill health and agony. The patient files a criminal case against the hospital, the intern and the Head of Department. Which of the defences can the intern effectively take?
A. *Res ipsa loquitur*
B. *Respondent superior*
C. *Novus actus interveniens*
D. *Res judicata*

25. If the damage to the patient has been caused, where the doctor was NOT negligent, but the patient was negligent, this situation may best be described as:
A. Civil Negligence
B. Negligence of the patient

C. Criminal negligence
D. Contributory negligence

26. If the damage to the patient has been caused where both doctor and the patient have been negligent at the same time, the situation may best be described as:
A. Criminal negligence
B. Ethical Malpraxis
C. Vicarious liability
D. Contributory negligence

27. Law does not consider one of the following doctrines in a charge of criminal negligence. Identify it:
A. Contributory negligence
B. Vicarious liability
C. Novus actus interveniens
D. *Res ipsa loquitur*

28. Contributory negligence is a valid defence to the doctor in:
A. Civil negligence
B. Criminal negligence
C. Both civil and criminal negligence
D. Ethical misconduct

29. A conduct on the part of a medical practitioner during the practice of his profession, which would be reasonably regarded as disgraceful or dishonourable by his professional colleagues of good repute and competency is known as:
A. Civil negligence
B. Criminal negligence
C. Professional misconduct
D. *Res ipsa loquitur*

30. In a case the doctor as well as the patient have been negligent. The patient suffers damage as a result. However the doctor had a clear and unambiguous opportunity to avert the damage caused by the patient's own negligence. The doctor takes the defence of contributory negligence by the patient. Which of the following rules/doctrines act against the doctor in this case?
A. The avoidable consequences rule
B. The last clear chance doctrine
C. Therapeutic misadventure
D. Corporate negligence

31. The doctor is found negligent in a particular case. The patient suffers damage as a result. Later he (the patient) himself becomes negligent too and aggravates his injury. The patient claims compensation for the aggravated injury caused as a result. The doctor can take advantage of which of the following rules/doctrines?
A. The last clear chance doctrine
B. The avoidable consequences rule
C. *Res Judicata*
D. *Novus Actus Interveniens*

32. Dichotomy means
A. Fee splitting
B. Summons
C. Civil wrong
D. Employment of touts

33. Unexpected complications of medical procedures is termed as:
A. Therapeutic misadventure
B. Vicarious liability
C. Therapeutic privilege
D. Diminished liability

34. Repeated advertisements in newspapers by a medical practitioner is an example of:
A. Infamous conduct
B. Civil malpraxis
C. Criminal negligence
D. Privileged communication

EUTHANASIA

35. The original meaning of the term "Euthanasia" in Greek is:
A. Nice death
B. Homicide
C. Suicide
D. Cruel death

36. If the life support systems of a severely defective infant is turned off to put an end to his life, this would be called:
A. Infant euthanasia
B. Involuntary euthanasia
C. Non-voluntary euthanasia
D. Both (B) and (C)

37. In Indian law, which of the following forms of euthanasia is allowed?
A. Voluntary
B. Involuntary
C. Non-voluntary
D. None

38. In Indian law, euthanasia is same as:
A. Murder
B. Abetment of suicide
C. Attempt to commit murder
D. Excusable homicide

CONSENT

39. Consent is legally defined in which of the following legal statutes:
A. Indian Consent Act
B. Indian Evidence Act
C. Code of Criminal Procedure
D. Indian Contract Act

40. A 20-year-old young female comes to a male gynaecologist for pelvic examination. The consent for examination is:
A. Implied consent
B. Written consent
C. Verbal consent
D. Informed consent

41. If an unconscious patient needs to be operated upon immediately to save his life, and relatives are not traceable for taking consent, which of the following procedures must a doctor follow?
A. He should operate without consent
B. At least two doctors must consent
C. Consent taken from police officer
D. Consent taken from Medical Superintendent of the Hospital

42. The minimum age required to give consent for surgery is:
A. 7 years
B. 12 years
C. 16 years
D. 18 years

43. If a doctor performs an emergency surgery in an unconscious patient, without consent from the relatives because they were not available, which of the following statutes of law provide him protection?
A. Section 53 Cr.P.C.
B. Section 88 I.P.C.
C. Section 92 I.P.C.
D. He gets no protection because although he may be morally right, he has committed a legal wrong

44. What is the doctrine of *"in loco parentis"*?
A. Consent for life-threatening operations in case of minors can only be taken from a parent and not from a legal guardian
B. If the question is of a life-threatening operation on a minor, both parents must consent
C. Consent of any one of the two parents is sufficient for ordinary operations
D. In Emergency surgery, the person immediately in-charge of the minor such as a teacher or warden can give consent

45. Under section 53 Cr.P.C., which of the following persons, can be examined by a medical practitioner without consent?
A. An insane person
B. A woman who has been raped
C. A minor
D. An arrested person

46. If a doctor is examining a female under section 53 Cr.P.C., which of the following conditions must be satisfied?
A. The police officer accompanying her should be female
B. The doctor should either be a female, or if male, he should be under the supervision of a female doctor

C. The examination must be made in a police station and not in any other place

D. All of the above

INTERNATIONAL DECLARATIONS AND CONVENTIONS

47. The Hippocratic oath was first formulated by Hippocrates, who was a.........?

A. Roman physician

B. Indian physician

C. Greek physician

D. Egyptian physician

48. Which of the following conventions or declarations formulated a modernized version of Hippocratic oath?

A. Geneva Conventions 1949

B. Declaration of Helsinki, 1964

C. Declaration of Tokyo, 1975

D. Declaration of Geneva, 1948

49. For which of the following persons is it legal to use Red cross emblem for trade or business?

A. A registered nurse

B. A registered allopathic doctor

C. Medical men of the armed forces

D. All of the above

50. The declaration of Tokyo, 1975 by World Medical Association adopted guidelines for medical doctors regarding which of the following issues?

A. Torture and other cruel treatment in relation to detention and imprisonment

B. Always taking informed consent from the patient

C. Keeping the ethical values of doctors at the highest level

D. It was basically a resolve among doctors to keep themselves abreast of latest developments

51. Which of the following professionals can legally use the Red Cross emblem to further their profession?

A. Allopathic doctors

B. Homeopathic doctors

C. Members of the medical service of an army

D. All of the Above

HUMAN EXPERIMENTATION

52. Which of the following conventions or declarations drew up a code of ethics on human experimentation?

A. Geneva Conventions 1949

B. Declaration of Helsinki, 1964

C. Declaration of Tokyo, 1975

D. Declaration of Geneva, 1948

MULTIPLE ANSWER TYPE (PGI, CHANDIGARH PATTERN)

53. Which of the following sections are related to medical negligence?

A. S 327(2) Cr.P.C.

B. S 336 I.P.C.

C. S 337 I.P.C.

D. S 338 I.P.C.

E. S 114 A IEA

ANSWERS

GENERAL

1. **B.** Also known as Codified Law.
2. **D.**
3. **D.**
4. **A.** ***Related facts*:** All law can broadly be divided in two—substantive law and procedural law. While substantive law deals with rights and duties, procedural law relates to procedures. *Indian Penal Code* and *Indian Contract Act* are mainly substantive laws, while *Criminal Procedure Code* (Cr.P.C.) and *Indian Evidence Act* are mainly procedural laws.

   Remember the following basic facts about three most important bodies of law relevant to medical students:

   Indian Penal Code (I.P.C.): Framed by British, and came into force on 6 October 1860. Has 23 chapters and 511 sections. Chapter 16 (sections 299-377) deals with offences affecting human body and is most relevant to medical practitioners. Important sections such as 299, 300, 304A, 309, 312, 319, 320, 336, 337, 337, 351, 363, 375, 376 and 377 fall under this chapter.

   Criminal Procedure Code (Cr.P.C.): Came into force on 25 January 1974. Has 37 chapters and 484 sections and two schedules. Very few sections of this law are relevant for medical students, most notable being 53, 54, 174 and 176.

   Indian Evidence Act (IEA): Came into force on 15 March 1872. Has 11 chapters and 167 sections. Prescribes rules as to procedures for tendering evidence in a court of law.

ACTS RELATING TO MEDICAL PROFESSION

Consumer Protection Act 1986

5. **D.** Previously, the district forum could entertain claims for only upto 5 lakh, but by an amendment of 2002, which came into force with effect from 15 March 2003, the jurisdiction is now 20 lakh [Section 11(1) of *Consumer Protection Act 1986]*.
6. **D.** Previously, the State Commissions could entertain claims between Rs. 5 lakh and Rs. 20 lakh, but by an amendment of 2002, which came into force with effect from 15 March 2003, the jurisdiction is now between 20 lakh and 1 crore [Section 17(1)(a)(i) of *Consumer Protection Act 1986]*.
7. **C.** Previously, the National Commission could entertain claims of more than Rs. 20 lakh, but by an amendment of 2002, which came into force with effect from 15 March 2003, the jurisdiction is now more than 1 crore [Section 21(a)(i) of *Consumer Protection Act 1986]*.

INDIAN MEDICAL COUNCIL AND STATE MEDICAL COUNCILS

8. **C.** ***Related fact*:** The composition of the Medical Council of India is an important fact to remember. It is constituted by members chosen in five different ways. Of these nomination is made in two methods and election in rest of the three. Nomination is only made by Central Government. The composition is like this:

i. One member from each state other than a Union territory is **nominated** by the Central Government in consultation with the respective State Government.

ii. One member from each University is **elected** from amongst the members of Medical Faculty of the university by members of its Senate.

iii. One member from each state where a State Medical Register is maintained is **selected** by persons among themselves, enrolled in the said Register.

iv. Seven members are **elected** from amongst persons enrolled in any of the State Medical Register.

v. Eight further members are **nominated** by the Central Government. Note that here, no consultation is made by the Central Government with anyone else.

9. A.

10. D. ***Related fact***: The Executive Committee does not hold office for a period more than five years. The Council appoints a Registrar and a Secretary for its day-to-day functioning.

11. D.

12. B.

13. D.

PRIVILEGES/DUTIES OF MEDICAL PRACTITIONERS

14. A. ***Related fact***: Other privileges of a doctor are: Right to dispense medicines. Regarding right to choose a patient, the doctor does not have an unconditional right. According to latest Supreme Court verdicts, a doctor **must** treat a patient in emergency. He does not have a right to choose a patient in such cases. He has to administer treatment.

15. A. Normally a doctor should not divulge information about his patient to others. This is known as the doctrine of Professional Secrecy. However in certain special circumstances he can divulge the information to others, especially when the community at large is in danger. In choices (B), (C) and (D) above the community at large is in danger, but not in choice (A) above.

16. D. Disclosures made in doctor's self interest (choice B above) and patient's self interest (choice C above) are also included in privileged communication.

17. B. ***Related facts***: According to Section 10 (3) of the *Registration of Births and Deaths Act, 1969*, if the medical practitioner has attended a patient during his last illness, and if that patient has expired, the medical practitioner shall issue the certificate without charging any fee. Under section 23 (3) of the same Act, any medical practitioner who neglects or refuses to issue a certificate under the above section shall be punishable with fine which may extend to fifty rupees.

PROFESSIONAL NEGLIGENCE

18. B. ***Related fact***: This question is very frequently asked by students. Section 304A I.P.C. is causing death by rash and negligent act. Section 351 is assault, which is just making any threatening gesture (Actual touching of the body is dealt with by Section 350, which is Criminal Force). If a doctor examines a patient without his or her consent, he may be charged under section 351. Section 312 is causing miscarriage intentionally.

19. B.

20. D.

21. D.

22. C. ***Related facts and definitions:*** All these four terms are legal terms, of which most relevant to forensic medicine is "tort". Tort means civil wrong, such as applying the plaster so tightly that gangrene sets up in foot.

It might be helpful to know the meaning of other distracters.

The meaning of *mutatis mutandis* is "with the necessary changes having been carried out". It is generally used in the context of making allowances for differences in small, inessential details when comparing cases that are substantially the same. For example: "What is said of the army here is to be taken also to apply *mutatis mutandis*, to the air force and the navy."

Pari passu is Latin for "with equal step" *(par, equal; passus,* step). It means "at an equal rate of progress". In legal context it means "equitably" or "without unfair preference". Examples: "Expand the state and [its] destructive capacity necessarily expands too, *pari passu*", or "proceed with warlike measures and conciliatory measures *pari passu*".

Ultra vires means "beyond the legal power or authority of a person or official or body etc" or "beyond the scope or in excess of legal power or authority" such as "an *ultra vires* contract". This phrase is used frequently in relation to acts or enactments by corporations in excess of their chartered or statutory rights.

The opposite is *intra vires.*

23. A. ***Related fact*****:** Other valid choices could be (i) a swab or instrument found on X-ray to be in the abdominal cavity (ii) amputation of the wrong limb.

24. B. ***Additional comments*****:** Respondent superior literally means "Let the superior reply". An intern is only liable to conduct surgeries and prescribe drugs under the supervision of a full fledged doctor, and he can take this defence. Another example: If a dog bites a man and the man files a case against the owner of the dog, the owner of the dog can not say, "go and hang my dog". The sufferer has a right to say, "let the superior (in this case–owner) reply."

25. B.

26. D.

27. A.

28. A. It is very important to remember that the doctor can take the plea of contributory negligence *only* in cases of civil negligence, i.e. where the patient has demanded monetary compensation from him. If there is a criminal case against the doctor such as under Sec 304A of I.P.C., the doctor *can not* take the defence of contributory negligence.

29. C.

30. B. The "last clear chance doctrine" is an important limitation to the doctrine of contributory negligence. Here if it is shown that the defendant (doctor in this case) had a "Last Clear Chance" to avert the damage caused to the patient, and he did not avail of this chance, the doctor loses his defence of contributory negligence.

A good example of "last clear chance doctrine" is the Mississippi case of *Fuller v. Illinois Central R.R.*, (1911). Although this is a non-medical case, it serves to explain the concept very well. In this case the plaintiff (Fuller) used a dirt track which crossed a railway line to get to his home. At the time of the accident the train was half an hour late, and so was running much faster than usual. The train gave its usual signal nine hundred feet from the crossing that alerted the train station further down the track of its imminent arrival. Almost immediately afterwards, the plaintiff, over seventy years old, began to cross the tracks in his horse and cart. He had looked neither left nor right and was killed instantly.

Here undoubtedly the old man was negligent in causing his own death. Thus the railway company could take the defence of contributory negligence. However the driver of the train still had the "last clear chance" to stop the train and save the old man. If he had exercised reasonable care and prudence, he could have avoided the accident. The defendant had the "last clear chance" to avoid the accident but did not act upon it. So railroad company was found guilty.

31. B. The "doctrine of avoidable consequences" or the "avoidable consequences rule" states as follows:

'Where one party to a contract (doctor in the above case) commits a breach of contract, the other party (the patient) is required by the "avoidable consequences" rule of damages to make all reasonable efforts to minimize the loss he sustains as a result of the breach, and he (patient) can charge the party in default (doctor) with such damages only as, with reasonable endeavors and expense and without risk of additional substantial loss or injury, he could not prevent.'

Here the patient could have avoided the consequences by not being negligent. But he did not do so. The doctor gets the benefit here.

32. A.

33. A.

34. A. This is a violation of the Code of Medical Ethics. Such a violation is called serious professional misconduct or infamous conduct. Some authors call it ethical malpraxis or ethical negligence, but it is not a widely accepted term and should best be avoided.

EUTHANASIA

35. A. The Greek prefix *"eu"* means good, well, true or nice [it is seen in such words as eugenics (good breeding) and euphoria (good feeling)]. *Thanatos* is the Greek word for death. Thus the actual meaning of euthanasia is "good death" or "nice death". By extension, it has come to mean mercy killing.

36. C. *Voluntary euthanasia* is when a person is suffering greatly and has given his consent for death. *Non-voluntary euthanasia* is *different* from involuntary euthanasia. Non-voluntary euthanasia refers to a situation where the person is incapable of making his wish known (as in comatosed persons, mentally retarded individuals and severely defective infants). *Involuntary euthanasia* on the other hand means killing against the wishes of the person, i.e. compulsory. Many opponents of euthanasia believe that most cases of so-called voluntary euthanasia are actually cases of involuntary euthanasia, i.e. they are forced to give consent for dying.

37. D.

38. A. ***Related facts*:** Euthanasia is specifically barred by at least 3 sections of Indian Penal Code—Sections 88, 89 and 92 I.P.C. All acts of euthanasia in India would be viewed as murder.

CONSENT

39. D. ***Related fact:*** Consent is defined in section 13 of this Act (this fact can indeed form another MCQ question). The definition is: *Two or more person are said to consent when they agree upon the same thing in the same sense.*

40. A.

41. A.

42. D. This is rather a tricky question. The usual convention is that a person can give consent for general physical examination after 12 years and for surgery after 18 years. The difference in these ages needs an explanation. Section 88 of the *Indian Penal Code*, which is specifically meant for doctors—when read with section 90 of I.P.C.—suggests that the valid age of consent is 12 years, if the act is done in good faith for the benefit of the person (e.g. surgery). Thus it would appear that a person can give valid consent for surgery at 12 years. However in such cases, although a criminal charge can not be brought against the doctor, a civil suit can still be brought against him, because a child below 18 years can not enter into a valid contract. Thus the correct answer to the above question is (D).

43. C.

44. D. ***Related fact***: *"In loco parentis"* is a Latin phrase, which when translated in English means "In place of a parent". Thus teacher or warden can act in place of a parent, if they are not immediately available for giving consent.

45. D. ***Related fact***: Following provisions must be remembered in connection with Section 53 Cr.P.C. (i) The person must be arrested on a charge of committing an offence (ii) requesting police officer should not be below the rank of sub-inspector or any person acting in good faith in his aid and under his direction (iii) examination must be such as is reasonably necessary in order to ascertain the facts which may afford useful evidence (iv) reasonable force to do such examination may be applied.

46. B. ***Related fact***: This is provided in Section 53(2) Cr. P.C.

INTERNATIONAL DECLARATIONS AND CONVENTIONS

47. C.

48. D. ***Related fact***: This was Adopted by the 2nd General Assembly of the World Medical Association, Geneva, Switzerland, in September 1948. Amended by the 22nd World Medical Assembly, Sydney, Australia, August 1968, and by the 35th Assembly in Venice, 1983.

49. C.

50. A. ***Related fact***: It was the 29th assembly of the World Medical Association (WMA), which was held in 1975 at Tokyo, Japan, which adopted this declaration. The declaration adopted at this assembly basically asserted that no doctor would participate in the practice of torture or other forms of cruel, inhuman or degrading procedures. It was modified in 2005. Mnemonic: T for Tokyo and T for Torture.

A note on Assemblies of the World Medical Association:

World Medical Association held its 1st assembly in 1947 at Paris, France. Since then it has been holding annual assemblies at different cities. Only one assembly, the 16th (1962) has been held in India, and that was in New Delhi. For a brief period, the assemblies were held biannually (1981 and 1983).

In several of these assemblies, important ethical declarations have been adopted by the World Medical Association, which are important from our view point. Most of these have been modified by further assemblies, but they are always known by the very first place (and year) where they were first adopted. Most important of these declarations are:

1. **Declaration of Geneva (1948)→** Adopted by the 2nd assembly at Geneva, Switzerland. Amended in 1968, 1983, 1994 and 2005. It is a modernized version of Hippocratic oath. Also known as *Physician's Oath.* It basically prescribes an oath to bc taken by medical doctors at the time of being admitted as a member of the medical profession. Mnemonic: (G)eneva→(H)ippocratic oath. 'G' is followed by 'H' in English alphabet.
2. **International Code of Medical Ethics (1949)→**Adopted by the 3rd General Assembly of the World Medical Association at London, England in October 1949. It was amended by the 22nd World Medical Assembly Sydney, Australia (August 1968) and the 35th World Medical Assembly Venice, Italy (October 1983). It prescribes duties of physicians in general, duties of physicians to the sick and duties of physicians to each other.
3. **Declaration of Helsinki (1964)→** Adopted by the 18th WMA General Assembly held at Helsinki, Finland in June 1964, and subsequently amended five times (1975, 1983, 1989, 1996 and 2000). These prescribe ethical Principles for Medical Research Involving Human Subjects (Human Experimentation). Mnemonic: (H)elsinki→(H)uman experimentation.
4. **Declaration of Sydney (1968)→** Adopted by the 22nd World Medical Assembly at Sydney, Australia in August 1968. It is a statement on when to pronounce death. The assembly recognized that two recent developments namely (a) the ability to maintain by artificial means the circulation of oxygenated blood through tissues of the body which may have been irreversibly injured and (b) the use of cadaver organs such as heart or kidneys for transplantation, necessitated a proper definition of death. It was decided that ECG was the most helpful diagnostic aid in the diagnosis of death, and If transplantation of an organ is involved, the decision that death exists should be made by two or more physicians and the physicians determining the moment of death should in no way be immediately concerned with performance of transplantation. Mnemonic: Si(d)ney →(D)eath.
5. **Declaration of Oslo (1970)→**Adopted by the 24th World Medical Assembly held at Oslo, Norway in 1970. It is a statement on therapeutic abortion. One of the principles adopted was that "abortion should be performed only as a therapeutic measure". However Indian parliament passed MTP Act only next year (1971), where MTP was allowed on virtually every case (The Act came into force on April 1, 1972). The famous American case of abortion [Roe v. Wade 410 US 113 (1973)] was decided on 22 January 1973. So at least in the area of medical termination of pregnancy, India was definitely the leader. Mnemonic: (O)slo→ Ab(o)rtion.
6. **Declaration of Tokyo (1975)→**Adopted by the 29th World Medical Assembly at Tokyo, Japan in October 1975 and amended in 2005. These prescribe Guidelines for Medical Doctors Concerning Torture and Other Cruel, Inhuman or Degrading Treatment or Punishment in Relation to Detention and Imprisonment. Mnemonic: (T)okyo→(T)orture.

Other important declarations worth mentioning are as follows (with first year as the year of adoption and subsequent years indicating years of amendments):

1. Declaration of Lisbon on the Rights of the Patient (1981, 1995, 2005).
2. Declaration of Venice on Terminal Illness (1983).
3. Declaration of Madrid on Professional Autonomy and Self-Regulation (1987).
4. Declaration of Hong Kong on the Abuse of the Elderly (1989, 1990).
5. Declaration of Malta on Hunger Strikers (1991, 1992).
6. Declaration of Hamburg Concerning Support for Medical Doctors Refusing to Participate in, or to Condone, the Use of Torture or Other Forms of Cruel, Inhuman or Degrading Treatment (1997).
7. Declaration of Ottawa on the Right of the Child to Health Care (1998).
8. Declaration on Ethical Considerations Regarding Health Databases (2000).
9. Declaration of Washington on Biological Weapons (2002).

51. C. ***Related fact*:** Red Cross Act, 1938 Section 4: On and after the date of the establishment of the Society it shall not be lawful for any person to use for the purpose of trade or business or any other purpose whatsoever, without the consent of the Minister for Defence, the heraldic emblem of the red cross on a white ground formed by reversing the Federal colours of Switzerland or any emblem closely resembling such heraldic emblem, or the words "Cros Dearg", "Cros na Geinéibhe", "Red Cross" or "Geneva Cross" or any words closely resembling the words "Cros Dearg", "Cros na Geinéibhe", "Red Cross" or "Geneva Cross".

HUMAN EXPERIMENTATION

52. B.

MULTIPLE ANSWER TYPE (PGI, CHANDIGARH PATTERN)

53. B,C,D. *Related facts*: If death has occurred due to medical negligence of a doctor, he may be charged under section 304 A I.P.C. But if death has not occurred (e.g. if a doctor has amputated a wrong leg due to negligence) he may be charged under sections 336, 337 and 338 of I.P.C.

S 336. Act endangering life or personal safety of others: Whoever does any act so rashly or negligently as to endanger human life or the personal safety of others, shall be punished with imprisonment of either description for a term which may extend to three months, or with fine which may extend to two hundred and fifty rupees, or with both.

Example: Doctor conducts a delivery under influence of alcohol→Delivery occurs safely. The doctor is yet liable to be charged under this section, because he was rash and negligent in attending a patient under influence of alcohol.

S 337. Causing hurt by act endangering life or personal safety of others: Whoever causes hurt to any person by doing any act so rashly or negligently as to endanger human life, or the personal safety of others, shall be punished with imprisonment of either description for a term which may extend to six months, or with fine which may extend to five hundred rupees, or with both.

Example: Doctor does not test for penicillin sensitivity→Gives injection→patient suffers from anaphylaxis→saved by doctor→patient does not die→the doctor is still liable to be charged under this section, because the patient suffered from hurt.

S 338. Causing grievous hurt by act endangering life or personal safety of

others: Whoever causes grievous hurt to any person to doing any act so rashly or negligently as to endanger human life, or the personal safety of others, shall be punished with imprisonment of either description for a term which may extend to two years, or with fine which may extend to one thousand rupees, or with both.

Example: Doctor amputates a wrong leg, or removes the wrong kidney→He is liable to be charged under this section, because patient has suffered grievous hurt.

S 327(2) Cr.P.C. and S 114 A IEA do not fall under medical negligence. For details about them, see chapter 25 (Sexual offences, and sex perversions).

3 Personal Identity

GENERAL

1. The first modern system of criminal identification was:
A. Superimposition of the skull
B. Finger prints
C. Bertillonage
D. Lip prints

2. The term "*Corpus delicti*" includes the following *except*:
A. Body of the victim
B. Photographs of the deceased showing fatal wounds
C. Clothing showing marks of weapons
D. Inquest report

3. Davidson body is an indicator of:
A. Age
B. Sex
C. Race
D. Height

4. In which of the following cells is Davidson body observed?
A. Neutrophils
B. Basophils
C. Monocytes
D. All body cells except RBCs

5. Which of the following statements about the chilotic line are correct?
A. It is present on the femur and is useful in the determination of race
B. It is present on the femur and is useful in the determination of sex
C. It is present on the hipbone and is useful in the determination of race
D. It is present on the hipbone and is useful in the determination of sex

6. What is the meaning of the word *Corpus delicti*?
A. Dead body
B. Body of crime
C. Enquiry made by the police
D. Dereliction of duty

7. Surest or the most reliable method of identification is:
A. DNA Profiling
B. Dactylography
C. Gustafson's method
D. Anthropometry

RACE

8. If maximum breath of the skull is taken as "B", its maximum Length as "L", and its maximum height as "H", the Cephalic index would be denoted by which of the following formulae?
A. (B/L) × 100

B. (H/L) × 100
C. (L/B) × 100
D. (L+B/L) × 100

9. A skull will be called dolichocephalic if its cephalic index is:
A. Less than 60
B. Between 70-74.9
C. Between 75-79.9
D. 80 and above

10. Cephalic index gives clue to determine:
A. Age of the person
B. Sex of the person
C. Race of the person
D. Height of the person

11. From various measurements of the skull, race can be measured in:
A. 50-60% of cases
B. 65-70% of cases
C. 85-90% of cases
D. 100% cases

12. The Brachycephalic (short) type of skull is seen in
A. Mongolians
B. Europeans
C. South Indians
D. Negroes

13. The Cephalic index of Indians is between:
A. 70-75
B. 75-80
C. 80-85
D. 85-90

14. Brachycephaly may result as a result of premature fusion of:
A. Sagittal suture
B. Coronal suture
C. Parietal suture
D. Lambdoid suture

15. Crual index is calculated as:
A. $\frac{\text{Length of radius}}{\text{Length of humerus}} \times 100$
B. $\frac{\text{Length of tibia}}{\text{Length of femur}} \times 100$
C. $\frac{\text{Length of tibia}}{\text{Length of fibula}} \times 100$
D. $\frac{\text{Length of (humerus + radius}}{\text{Length of (femur + tibia)}} \times 100$

SEX

16. X-chromosome can usually be demonstrated by:
A. Quinacrine staining
B. Feulgen reaction
C. Gustafson's method
D. Gettler's test

17. Y-chromosome can be demonstrated by:
A. Quinacrine staining
B. Gustafson's method
C. Gettler's test
D. Sudan red

18. "Barr bodies" were first demonstrated by:
A. Robert Koch
B. Priestley
C. Huxley and Smith
D. Mary Barr and Ewart Bertram

19. If a person has been accused of gagging someone, and the gagging material has been recovered from the accused's house, detection of buccal epithelium on the gagging material may help:
A. To establish the sex of the victim
B. To establish the sex of the accused
C. To ascertain the age of the victim
D. To ascertain the age of the accused

INTERSEX

20. In gonadal agenesis, the nuclear sexing is:
A. Female

B. Male
C. Female in some cells, while male in others
D. Negative

21. Chromosomal pattern in Turner's syndrome is:
A. 46/XO
B. 45/XO
C. 47/XXY
D. 45/YO

22. Chromosomal abnormalities are seen in all of the following *except*:
A. Intersex
B. Concealed sex
C. Klinefelter's syndrome
D. Down's syndrome

23. Colonel Victor Barker's case was a case of:
A. Intersex
B. Concealed sex
C. True Hermaphrodite
D. Female pseudohermaphrodite

SEX FROM BONES

General

24. Which of the following bones give maximum accuracy in sexing?
A. Pelvis
B. Skull
C. All the long bones together
D. Sternum

25. If the entire skeleton is available, the accuracy in estimating the sex is:
A. 80%
B. 90%
C. 98%
D. 100%

Skull

26. Which of the following aspects of a skull help to differentiate sex?
A. Digastric groove
B. Frontal eminence
C. Foramen magnum
D. All of the above

27. Skull of a male differs from that of a female by all of the following *except*:
A. Capacity is greater than 1500 cc in males
B. Muscular markings over occiput are less marked in males
C. Orbits are square in males
D. Frontal eminence is smaller in males

28. Which of the following fact regarding human skull is wrong?
A. Until the age of puberty there is little difference between the skull of the two sexes
B. Sexual dimorphism is less marked in mankind than in gorilla, orang utan and many species of baboon
C. The capacity of the male skull is about 10% more than that of the female
D. Teeth are larger in females

29. Which of the following is true of a male skull?
A. Orbits have rounded margins
B. Mastoid process is round
C. Foramen magnum is smaller
D. Both (A) and (B)

Pelvis

30. Which of the following facts regarding pelvis is INCORRECT?
A. Preauricular sulcus is more prominent in males
B. Acetabulum is larger in males
C. Obturator Foramen is triangular in females
D. Greater Sciatic foramen is larger, wider and shallower in women

31. Preauricular sulcus is used for the determination of:
A. Race

B. Sex
C. Age
D. Both race and sex

AGE

Teeth

32. Which of the following statements regarding the 3rd Molar is correct?
A. It first erupts in right lower quadrant
B. It first erupts in left lower quadrant
C. It first erupts in right upper quadrant
D. There is no significant difference in the age of eruption in the four quadrants

33. Which of the following teeth is not present in human primary dentition?
A. Molars
B. Premolars
C. Canines
D. Incisors

34. The dental formula of children is:
A. 2123/2123
B. 2102/2123
C. 2102/2102
D. 2123/2102

35. The dental formula of adult human beings is:
A. 2123/2123
B. 2102/2123
C. 2102/2102
D. 2123/2102

36. First deciduous tooth appears at the age of:
A. 6-8 months
B. 12-14 months
C. 17-18 months
D. 6-7 years

37. Permanent lateral incisor appears approximately at the age of:
A. 4-5 years
B. 6 years
C. 8 years
D. 11 years

38. A child has a total of 24 teeth. His probable age is:
A. Less than 6
B. Between 6 to 9 years
C. Between 6 to 11 years
D. Between 12 and 18 years

39. If a child has 20 permanent teeth and 4 temporary teeth, his age is likely to be:
A. 6 years
B. 8 years
C. 10 years
D. 14 years

40. Which of the following is the age of mixed dentition?
A. 4 to 6 years
B. 7 to 10 years
C. 6 to 11 years
D. 6 to 18 years

41. Which of the following permanent teeth are most erratic in eruption and of little value in determining age?
A. Third molar
B. Premolars
C. Second molars
D. Incisors

42. Which of the following are also known as "wisdom teeth" ?
A. Incisors
B. Second molars
C. Third molars
D. Both second and third molars

43. Age from teeth is estimated by:
A. Galton system
B. Rule of Hasse
C. Trotter and Glesser's formula
D. Gustafson's method

44. Which of the following is NOT a criteria used in Gustafson's method?
A. Root resorption
B. Periodontosis

C. Width of enamel prisms
D. Secondary dentin formation

45. Gustafson's method for age determination from teeth is most useful in which one of the following age groups?
A. <5 years
B. 6-10 years
C. 11-15 years
D. Above 25 years

46. Which is the MOST useful single criterion in Gustafson's method?
A. Transparency of the root
B. Root resorption
C. Cementum apposition
D. Attrition

47. Shovel shaped teeth are most commonly seen in:
A. Caucasoid race
B. Mongoloid race
C. Negroid race
D. Australian Indians

BONES

General

48. Total weight of adult male skeleton is:
A. 3 kg
B. 4.5 kg
C. 7.5 kg
D. 9.5 kg

49. Total weight of adult female skeleton is:
A. 3 kg
B. 4.5 kg
C. 7.5 kg
D. 9.5 kg

50. If angle of mandible is obtuse, it means that the bone belongs to:
A. Adult male
B. Adult female
C. Young female child
D. Elderly person

51. The two halves of mandible join together by:
A. 5-6 month of intrauterine life
B. 5-6 month of extra uterine life
C. 2nd year of life
D. 5-6 years of life

52. The mental foramen is close to alveolar margin in:
A. Infancy
B. Adult
C. Old age
D. Both infancy and old age

Ages of Ossification

53. Ossification center for lunate appears at:
A. Birth
B. 2 years
C. 4 years
D. 8 years

54. Ossification center for lunate appears at nearly the same time as:
A. Capitate
B. Hamate
C. Pisiform
D. Trapezium

55. Head of humerus unites with the shaft at the age of:
A. 12 years
B. 14 years
C. 16 years
D. 18 years

Other Unions

56. Anterior fontanelle closes:
A. Just after birth
B. At 2 months
C. By 8 months
D. By 2 years

57. Posterior fontanelle closes:
A. Just at birth
B. By 2 months

C. By the end of first year
D. By the end of second year

58. The greater cornu of the hyoid bone unites with the body:
A. Between 10 and 20 years
B. Between 20 and 30 years
C. Between 30 and 40 years
D. Between 40 and 60 years

59. Coronal suture is completely obliterated by:
A. 25 years
B. 40 years
C. 55 years
D. 75 years

SECONDARY SEXUAL CHARACTERS

60. In an adolescent male, hair appear in the following order—from earliest to last:
A. Axilla–face–pubis
B. Pubis–face–axilla
C. Pubis–axilla–face
D. Face–pubis-axilla

MEDICOLEGAL IMPORTANCE

61. A person is called a Juvenile or child when he is below the age of:
A. 12 years
B. 14 years
C. 16 years
D. 18 years

62. A person becomes a major under Indian Majority Act 1875, when he completes the age of:
A. 16 years
B. 18 years
C. 21 years
D. 25 years

63. Under the Indian Railways Act, 1989 the minimum age for criminal responsibility is:
A. 3 years
B. 5 years
C. 7 years
D. No such age has been prescribed under this Act

64. According to Indian Penal Code, the minimum age for criminal responsibility is:
A. 7 months
B. 5 years
C. 7 years
D. 12 years

65. According to section 83 of the Indian Penal Code, a child between ....years and ....years who has not attained sufficient maturity of understanding to judge of the nature and consequence of his conduct on that occasion, would NOT be held responsible for any crime.
A. 5, 7
B. 7, 12
C. 12, 16
D. 14, 18

MISCELLANEOUS

66. Rule of Haase is used to determine:
A. The Age of fetus
B. Height of an adult
C. Race of a person
D. Identification

67. Which of the following facts is CORRECT?
A. C-R length of a fetus of 4 calendar months is 16 inches
B. C-H length of a fetus of 7 lunar months is 49 cms
C. C-R length of a fetus of 5 lunar months is 25 inches
D. C-H length of a fetus of 3 lunar months is 9 cms.

68. Boyde's method is used to determine:
A. Age

B. Sex
C. Race
D. Height

STATURE

69. Which of the following facts regarding the stature of the body is correct?
A. Immediately after death, the body may shorten by about 2-3 cm.
B. Immediately after death, the body may lengthen by about 2-3 cm.
C. Change is stature after death occurs only when the deceased was engaged in struggle at the time of death
D. There is absolutely no change in stature after death

70. Which of the following formulae has been tried to determine the stature from fragmentary long bones?
A. Dupertuis and Hadden's formula
B. Steele's formula
C. Karl Pearson's formula
D. Trotter and Glesser's formula

71. The multiplication factor for estimation of height from femur is:
A. 3.6
B. 4.4
C. 5.3
D. 6.0

ANTHROPOMETRY

72. Anthropometry was started by:
A. Sir Francis Galton
B. Alphonse Bertillon
C. William Herschel
D. John Galton

73. Which of the following criteria were included in the Bertillon system?
A. Descriptive data
B. Body marks
C. Body measurements
D. All of the above

74. How many measurements of the body were taken in Bertillon system?
A. 5
B. 7
C. 11
D. 14

75. The system of identification known as *Portrait parlé* was devised by:
A. Sir William Herschel
B. Sir Francis Galton
C. Scotland Yard
D. Alphonse Bertillon

DACTYLOGRAPHY

76. The most common type of fingerprints are:
A. Loops
B. Arches
C. Whorls
D. Composite

77. Least common type of fingerprints are:
A. Loops
B. Whorls
C. Arches
D. Tombs

78. How many points of similarity between two fingerprints have to be established before the two can be said to be identical?
A. 6
B. 16
C. 25
D. The figure varies from country to country

79. Identification by poroscopy was started by:
A. William Herschel
B. Sir Francis Galton
C. Edmond Locard
D. Alphonse Bertillon

80. Each millimeter of friction ridge contains how many pores?
A. 1-2 pores
B. 9-18 pores
C. 100-200 pores
D. About one million pores

81. Edgeoscopy refers to the use of following for identification:
A. Fingerprint patterns on the edges of fingers
B. Ridge edges in conjunction with other friction ridge detail
C. Ridge patterns on the forehead
D. Ridge patterns on the soles

82. Of the following, which ones are plastic prints?
A. Invisible fingerprints
B. Barely visible fingerprints
C. Blood stained fingerprints
D. Fingerprints made on soap

83. Dactylography was invented by:
A. Sir Francis Galton
B. Sir William Herschel
C. Juan Vucetich
D. Hem Chandra Bose

84. World's first fingerprint bureau was established in:
A. London
B. Paris
C. Calcutta
D. Madras

OTHER CRITERIA

85. Cheiloscopy is the study of:
A. Palato prints
B. Nail prints
C. Foot prints
D. Lip prints

86. Which of the following facts regarding a scar is NOT correct?
A. An abrasion does not result in a scar
B. A scar remains vascular up to 6 months
C. A scar is devoid of elastic tissue
D. A scar is devoid of sweat glands

87. A scar remains tender upto:
A. One week
B. Three weeks
C. Six weeks
D. Six months

88. Tattoos can be removed by:
A. Surgery
B. Carbon dioxide snow
C. Laser beam
D. All of the above

89. Sydney Shark case is famous for:
A. Anthropometry
B. Tattoo marks
C. Superimposition
D. Lip prints

90. Trichology is the study of:
A. Hair
B. Tattoos
C. Scars
D. Complexion and features

91. Tattoos are useful in identifying:
A. Dead bodies
B. Living persons
C. Decomposed bodies
D. All of the above

92. Hair grows at the rate of:
A. 0.004 mm/day
B. 0.04 mm/day
C. 0.4 mm/day
D. 4.0 mm/day

93. An obliterated tattoo can best be detected by:
A. Treating the suspected area with a 0.1% nitric acid
B. Histological study of the regional lymph nodes
C. Treating the suspected area with 2% hydrogen peroxide
D. All of the above

94. Nails grow at the rate of:
A. 0.001 mm/day
B. 0.01 mm/day
C. 0.1 mm/day
D. 0.8 mm/day

95. The layers of the human hair are:
A. Scales, cortex and medulla
B. Scales and cortex only
C. Scales and medulla only
D. Only dead scales

96. Which is the outermost layer in human hair?
A. Cuticle
B. Medulla
C. Cortex
D. Pigment layer

97. In which of the following layers are pigment granules found?
A. Cuticle
B. Medulla
C. Cortex
D. Outer scales

98. If the cross-section of a human hair is kidney shaped, the race is most likely to be:
A. Caucasoid
B. Negroid
C. Mongoloid
D. Either Caucasoid or Negroid

99. In an animal hair, pigmentation is:
A. Evenly distributed throughout cortex
B. More concentrated towards the inner medullary layer
C. More concentrated towards the outer cuticular layer
D. More concentrated towards both outside and inside, and completely absent in the middle

100. If the pigmentation in human hair tends to be localized around the outside, then the hair is most likely to be:
A. Caucasoid
B. Mongoloid
C. Negroid
D. Either Caucasoid or Negroid

101. If the medulla is fragmented, what information can be derived about the race of the person?
A. He is likely to be Caucasoid
B. He is likely to be Negroid
C. He is likely to be Mongoloid
D. No useful information about race could be derived from this fact

102. Callosities present on the center of the forehead of a person indicate his:
A. Sex
B. Race
C. Religion
D. Age

103. A convict whose family or relations were not known and no biological sample was available with jail authorities, escaped from jail. A dead body resembling the convict was found in nearby forest, but due to mutilation of face, identity could not be established. How can the positive identity that he is the same convict who escaped from jail be established?
A. Blood grouping
B. DNA profile
C. Anthropometry
D. There is no way his identity could be established

MULTIPLE ANSWER TYPE (PGI, CHANDIGARH PATTERN)

104. The skull in the male shows following features:
A. Glabella is more prominent
B. Orbits have rounded margins
C. Zygomatic arches are less prominent
D. Digastric groove is deeper
E. Frontal eminences are large

105. About frontal sinuses, which of the following facts are true?
A. They can be used for identification, especially in cases of air disasters
B. Frontal sinuses are absent in 5% cases
C. Frontal sinuses can be used for identification in males but not in females
D. Frontal sinuses are unilateral in about 1% cases
E. No two persons, not even identical twins have the same frontal sinus pattern

106. Dyes commonly used for tattooing are:
A. India Ink
B. Vermillion
C. Prussian blue
D. Ultramarine
E. Indigo

107. Which of the following facts about HUMAN HAIR are correct?
A. Cortex is thick–about 4-10 times as broad as medulla
B. Medulla is continuous and very prominent
C. Medullar index is less than 0.3
D. Cuticular scales are very large and have step like or wavy pattern
E. Precipitin test is specific for human

108. Which of the following statements about Barr bodies are true?
A. They were first described by Barr and Bertram in 1949
B. They are seen outside the nucleus
C. They are seen in vaginal cells of females and prostate cells of male
D. They are indicators of age, as they are mostly found in old people
E. The are found more commonly in Negroes than in Asiatic Indians and Caucasians

109. Which of the following statements about Gustafson's method are correct?
A. It is used to estimate the race of an individual
B. It uses teeth as a criteria
C. It can only be used in the living
D. It uses six criteria
E. It is applicable only in children

110. Which of the following are successional teeth?
A. Incisors
B. First molar
C. Canines
D. Premolars
E. Second molar

111. Which of the following facts about identical twins are incorrect?
A. The have the same DNA profile
B. They have the same fingerprint pattern
C. They have the same blood group
D. They have the same HLA system
E. They have different fathers

ANSWERS

GENERAL

1. C.

2. D.

3. **B.** These bodies are named after William M. Davidson of King's college hospital medical school, London, who first described these bodies in 1954.

4. **A.** ***Related fact***: This body which appears like a drumstick is present only in neutrophils. Other relevant facts, which can form good MCQ questions are:

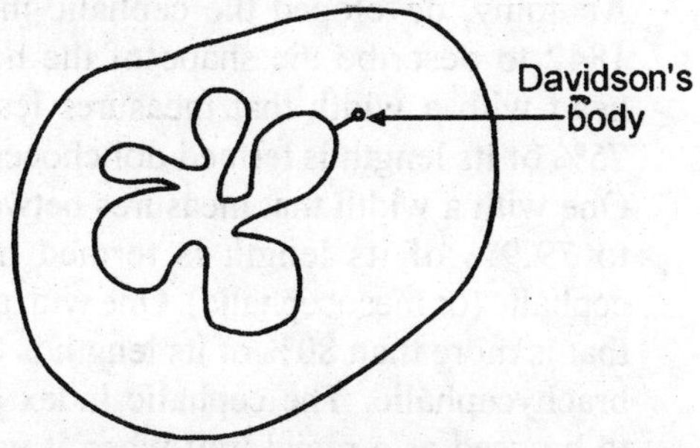

Fig. 3.1: Davidson's body seen as a drumstick in neutrophils

- Davidson's body is found only in neutrophil's of females and not those of males.
- It is NOT found in all neutrophils. The percentage of neutrophils in which it is found has been quoted variously by various authors. In his original paper published by William M. Davidson, he found on an average 6 Davidson bodies in 227 female neutrophils (about 3% of all female neutrophils), and none in 500 male neutrophils (0% in male neutrophils). So the correct figure is 3% of female cells [although some books have wrongly described this figure as 6%].
- The size of the round head at the end of the drumstick is 1.5 microns (diameter).
- The staining method that has to be used is Jenner-Giemsa method. Davidson certainly used this method. He stained a few slides with Feulgen method also.

5. **D.** ***Related fact***: Chilotic line is the line extended backwards from the iliopectineal eminence to the nearest point on the anterior margin of the auricular surface and then to the iliac crest. The auricular point divides this *chilotic line* into anterior (pelvic) and posterior (sacral) segments, each of which is expressed as a percentage of other. These *chilotic indices* display reciprocal values in the sexes, the pelvic part of the chilotic line being relatively prominent in the female, the sacral part in the male.

   (From Gr. *Cheilos*, a margin, lip, brim. Called so because it is at the brim of pelvis. Related word is *Cheiloscopy*, which is study of lip prints).

6. **B.** The meaning of *corpus delicti* is "body of crime" or "essence of crime". It is used mostly in relation to murder, and is used to denote that evidence, which confirms that the person is indeed dead.

   If for example, a person is found missing from a village, it would be difficult to conclude that he has been murdered, until and unless some evidence is brought forthwith which conclusively proves that the person is indeed dead. This could include his dead body, a photograph of his dead body, his blood stained clothes, his severed head etc. All these from corpus delicti.

7. B. ***Related facts***: This is a tricky question, many students choosing "DNA profiling" as the right answer. Since DNA is similar in identical twins, DNA profiling can not distinguish between them, while dactylography or fingerprints can distinguish between them too (since they are different even in identical twins). Sometimes choice (b) is replaced with "Galton method", which is also a correct choice (Dactylography is sometimes referred to as Galton system or Galton method).

Interesting fact: Besides fingerprints, another major identification criteria, that is different even in identical twins is the frontal sinus pattern.

RACE

8. A. ***Related facts:***

- Because differences in skin color were apparent when different human groups came into contact, skin color became one of the most common traits of racial classification.
- Johann Friedrich Blumenbach (1752-1840), German physiologist and comparative anatomist, frequently called the father of physical anthropology, proposed one of the earliest classifications of the races of mankind. He classified humans into four races. He used skin color [white (Caucasians), yellow (Mongolians), brown (Malayan), and black (Ethiopian)] as well as other traits, but emphasized that humans do not fall neatly into these categories. Some workers added a fifth category—red (American Indians). Later Anders Retzius (1796-1860), a Swedish Professor of Anatomy introduced the concept of cephalic index in 1842, but it too fell into disrepute.

9. B. ***Related facts:*** The skulls are traditionally classified as:

Table 3.1: Classification of skulls according to their cephalic indices

Skull type	*Cephalic index*
Dolichocephalic	70-74.9
Mesaticephalic	75-79.9
Brachycephalic	80 and above

10. C. It was once thought that race could be determined by cephalic index. Not many physical anthropologists today believe this.

11. C.

12. A. ***Related fact***: Believing that head shape was a stable "racial trait", **Anders Retzius** (1796-1860), a Swedish Professor of Anatomy, developed the cephalic index in 1842 to describe the shape of the head. A head with a width that measures less than 75% of its length is termed dolichocephalic. One with a width that measures between 75 to 79.9% of its length is termed mesaticephalic (or mesocephalic). One with a width that is more than 80% of its length is termed brachycephalic. The cephalic index ceased to be used as a racial trait when it was discovered that allegedly superior dolichocephalic northern Europeans shared a similar head shape with some so-called "inferior" African populations.

13. B. This is basically an absurd question, and should never have found a place in any MCQ book. The only justification of its inclusion here is that it has been asked so many times in examinations. The question is given here with what is generally expected to be the correct answer. However many authors think that "the population of the Indian subcontinent are allied with the European population in terms of anthropological kinship". If that is taken to be true, the correct answer should be (A).

Quite understandably, this is a controversial question. There are two basic problems in this question.

1. First and foremost is—whom does one consider a typical Indian? Is a Kashmiri with more Caucasoid features an Indian, or a Dravidian (Tamil) with more Negroid features an Indian, or a Manipuri with Mongoloid features an Indian? It is common knowledge that all three are Indians. If that be the case, then what is the point in asking the cephalic index of an Indian?
2. Secondly and still a very important point is that race is a very ill-defined concept. Not many physical anthropologists believe in this concept any more. Some feel that it is more a culturally defined concept than a biologically defined one. Or perhaps even a geographically defined concept.

   We might perhaps have to go into historical Background of race too for a better understanding.

   Because differences in SKIN color were apparent when different human groups came into contact, SKIN color became one of the most common traits of racial classification. Johann Friedrich Blumenbach (1752-1840), a German physiologist, anthropologist and comparative anatomist classified humans into four races. He used SKIN color (white, yellow, brown, and black) as well as other traits, but emphasized that humans do not fall neatly into these categories.

   Europeans believed that Caucasoids were the superior race, and from the very beginning they were out to find a biological trait to prove this. They found this in cephalic index, and immediately announced that cephalic index can indeed differentiate the so called "superior" race like Caucasoids from an "inferior" race such as Negroids. Believing that head shape was a stable "racial trait", a Swedish scientist Anders Retzius developed the cephalic index in 1842 to describe the shape of the head.

   According to him, a head with a width that measures less than 75% of its length is termed dolichocephalic; one with a width that measures between 75 to 79.9% of its length is termed mesocephalic; and one with a width that is more than 80% of its length is termed brachycephalic.

   Quite interestingly, Europeans dropped the concept of cephalic index like a hot potato, when they discovered that allegedly superior dolichocephalic northern Europeans shared a similar head shape with some so-called "inferior" African populations.

   Currently race is not an easily defined term – to the extent that many scientists do not believe in this term at all. Certainly it is not a biological construct. One great reason to think so is that the genetic variations within groups (say within several members of Caucasoids themselves) is vastly greater than the genetic variation between groups (i.e. between Negroids and Caucasoids).

   It is now amply clear that traditional racial traits have a continuous range of phenotypic variation and it is impossible to construct discrete phenotypic or genotypic boundaries around populations (such as cephalic index).

14. B. ***Related facts***: Normal skull growth occurs perpendicular to each suture. The primary factor that keeps sutures open is ongoing brain growth. If one or more cranial sutures fuse prematurely (craniosynostosis) it may result in an abnormal head shape.

Brachycephaly: Early bilateral coronal suture fusion.

Scaphocephaly: Early fusion of the sagittal suture.

Anterior plagiocephaly: Early fusion of 1 coronal suture.

Posterior plagiocephaly: Early closure of 1 lambdoid suture.

Trigonocephaly: Early fusion of the metopic suture.

15. B. The word "crural" comes from Latin *crus* meaning leg (this serves as a good mnemonic too). In this index the two major leg bones—one representing the lower part and the other representing the upper part are compared with each other. All indices (cephalic index, medullary index, sternal index, ischiopubic index etc.) are basically comparisons between two measurements (of bone, hair etc.), the shorter of which generally goes in the numerator. Thus in cephalic index, breadth—the shorter of the two measurements—goes in the numerator. Similarly in crural index length of the shorter bone —the tibia—goes in the numerator. By multiplying the ratio with 100, we basically try to represent this ratio as a percentage. Thus, crural index is a way of representing the length of tibia as a percentage of the length of the longer bone—the femur.

Crural index is important for determining the race, as it is different in different races. Crural index is also known as tibio-femoral index.

Other important indices which may be asked in MCQs are:

i. **Brachial index or radio-humeral index.** It is calculated as:

$$\frac{\text{Length of radius}}{\text{Length of humerus}} \times 100$$

Remember it—and all other indices-logically. Let us work this one out. Since the name is brachial, it must have something to do with upper arm (from Latin *Brachium*, arm; remember structures like brachial artery, brachio-radialis). Since it is an index, it has got to be a ratio between two unequal sized structures, and it must be multiplied by 100. The unequal sized structures in arm are humerus and radius (we leave out the ulna as radius is the major bone in the lower arm); of these radius is smaller. In all indices, smaller measurement goes up. Hence we get the formula mentioned above.

ii. **Intermembral index:**

$$\frac{\text{Length of (humerus + radius}}{\text{Length of (femur + tibia)}} \times 100$$

Intermembral index is a "comparison" of the two "members" of the body–the upper limb and the lower limb. Upper limb is smaller than the lower limb, so it would be expressed as a fraction of the lower limb. The length of the upper limb (in terms of the bones it comprises) is "humerus + radius". Similarly the length of the lower limb is "femur + tibia".

Generally upper limbs bear a ratio of 0.7 (or 70%) with the lower limbs. Persons having smaller arms in comparison with their own legs would have a lower intermembral index. This is a way to differentiate races. For instance, in Asiatic Indians, the intermembral index has been calculated as 67.27 (meaning their arms are 67.27% of their own legs). In Europeans this index turns out to be 70.4. A physical anthropologist could differentiate between the races by calculating these indices. Furthermore, just by looking at these indices, we can comment that Europeans have longer arms compared to Asiatic Indians.

iii. **Humerofemoral index:**

$$\frac{\text{Length of humerus}}{\text{Length of femur}} \times 100$$

Here "upper bones" of both limbs are compared. This index too is used to differentiate between races.

To recapitulate: four major indices which are used in determination of race are (i) crural index (i) brachial index (iii) intermembral index (iv) humerofemoral index.

Interesting fact: Although initially developed for determination of race, sports trainers now use these indices to sort out athletes who are at a natural advantage at certain sports. For instance, it is believed that an athelete, who has a large crural index would be a better runner. Similarly a person having a large brachial index could be a good "thrower" (shot put, javelin etc.), since he could extract greater mechanical advantage by generating the same amount of force.

Other indices of lesser importance are:

i. **Skelic Index**: (lower limb height × 100/ sitting height). The word comes from "skeleton". It is essentially a comparison of the lower half of the body (lower limbs) with the upper half (sitting height).

SEX

16. B. ***Additional info***: In Feulgen reaction, Acriflavin Schiff reagent is used for staining. X-chromosome is seen as a bright yellow spot.

17. A. ***Additional info:*** Y-chromosome, when stained with Quinacrine dihydrochloride demonstrates fluorescence.

18. D. For more on "Barr Bodies" please see question 108).

19. A. This is an old question, and the intended answer is (A). This can be done by looking at Barr bodies (see the previous question). However now a complete DNA profile of the victim can be made from a few buccal epithelial cells and a positive identity can be established.

INTERSEX

20. D.

21. B.

22. B. Concealed sex does not involve any chromosomal abnormalities. It is a case where a person of one sex (mostly a male) conceals his sex for some illegal purpose, say, to avoid the law. He would wear the clothes of opposite sex (say male wearing the clothes of a female) to look like a person of the opposite sex. This condition is different from transvestism, in which cross-dressing is not done with any evil design in mind; it is simply a psychiatric disorder.

23. B. ***Related facts:*** Colonel Sir Victor Barker's case is one of the most amazing cases of concealed sex. Barker (1895 – 1960) was born a female (Valerie Lilias Barker), who acted like a man between 1923 and 1929. In 1918, she married an Australian Officer Harold Arkell-Smith. She now became known as Valerie Lilias Arkell-Smith. The marriage however was a failure almost immediately. Later she married Ernest Pearce-Crouch - another Australian – with whom she had 2 children, a boy and a girl. In 1923, she left her second husband too (and her children) and on 14 November 1923, posing as a man (Sir Victor Barker), married a woman Elfrida Haward. Always living above his means, Sir

Victor was indicted for bankruptcy in 1929. It soon emerged that the 'Colonel' was a woman who had been passing herself off as an Army officer for years. She was charged with perjury and with making a false statement in a marriage register and in court. Elfrida abandoned her, claiming she had no idea her husband was a woman. Arkell-Smith was found guilty and sentenced to nine months imprisonment. She was thus able to conceal her sex for full six years (from 1923 till 1929) and it is possible that if she were not caught by law, she might have kept up the deception until her death. During the period she posed as man, she played for a cricket club, moved about in the streets in Khaki shorts with a shirt open at the neck, dropped in at pubs for drinks, and most of all, lived with another woman as her "husband"! For more on concealed sex, see question 22).

SEX FROM BONES

General

24. A.
25. D. ***Related fact***: According to Krogman, the accuracy in sexing the adult human skeleton is as follows: Entire skeleton, 100%; Pelvis alone, 95%; Skull alone 90%, Pelvis plus skull 98%, Long bones alone 80%.

Skull

26. D. ***Related fact***: Digastric groove is deeper in males. Frontal eminence is **small in males.** Foramen magnum is relatively large and **long** in males, and relatively small and round in females.
27. B. ***Related fact***: Both frontal and parietal eminences are less pronounced in the males. Orbits are also supposed to be relatively smaller in males, and relatively larger in females. Otherwise almost every other feature is more pronounced in males. This catch has to be borne in mind. Features in the skull which are more prominent in the males are (i) Digastric groove (ii) Frontal sinuses (iii) Zygomatic arch (iv) Glabella (v) Bony ridge along the upper border of external auditory meatus (vi) Mastoid process (vii) Occipital condyles (viii) Foramina (ix)Teeth (x) Foramen Magnum (xi) Palate is U-shaped (in female it parabola).
28. D.
29. D. ***Related fact***: Generally structures are rounded in females and pointed in males. The two notable exceptions are given in this question. Note that the **margins** are rounded in males. The orbits themselves are rounded in females and square in males!

Pelvis

30. A. ***Related fact:*** Preauricular sulcus is the site of attachment of **anterior sacroiliac ligament**, and is MORE PROMINENT in females.
31. B.

AGE

Teeth

32. D.
33. B.
34. C.
35. A.
36. A. ***Related facts and mnemonics***: Remember the following mnemonic for deciduous teeth:

South Indian Idlis, mothers can make.

South→Indicates lower teeth appear first (especially incisors)

Indian→Incisors, central (lower)→6 months
Incisors, central (upper)→8 months

Idlis→Incisors, lateral (upper)→10 months (Lateral incisors are an exception, in as much as the upper appear first)
Incisors, lateral (lower)→12 months

Mothers→Molars (first)→14 months

Can→Canine→18 months

Make→Molars (second)→24-30 months

Remember, the ages start at 6 months. After this one goes on adding 2 months to go to next step. Nothing appears at 16, 20 and 22 months.

37. C. *Related facts*: The order of appearance of permanent teeth, with a few months' variation on either side is like this:

Table 3.2: The order of appearance of permanent teeth

Tooth	Age of eruption
Molar, 1st	6 years
Incisors, Central	7 years
Incisors, Lateral	8 years
Premolar, 1st	9 years
Premolar, 2nd	10 years
Canine	11 years
Molar, 2nd	12 years
Molar, 3rd	18-24 years

These eruption ages are true for maxillary teeth. Generally speaking, the mandibular teeth would appear a few months earlier. The major exception is in the case of canines, which appear lot earlier – almost 2 years earlier. Thus the lower canine would appear at 9 years.

Premolars are an exception in the sense that they appear earlier in the upper jaw first. Thus lower first premolar would appear at 10 years, and lower second premolar would appear at 11 years.

The whole subject of dental eruption, especially that of permanent dentition may sound complex, but can thankfully be remembered by an interesting mnemonic.

Mama Is In Pain; Papa Can Make Medicine

The first letter of each word indicates the first letter of the maxillary tooth. The mnemonic can be decoded thus

Table 3.3: An easy mnemonic to remember ages of eruption of permanent teeth

Mama	Molar, 1st
Is	Incisor, 1st
In	Incisor, 2nd
Pain	Premolar, 1st
Papa	Premolar, 2nd
Can	Canine
Make	Molar, 2nd
Medicine	Molar, 3rd

Interestingly there is yet another good mnemonic for remembering the same sequence.

Mother is in bed; baby comes Monday morning

Here the letter 'b' in 'bed' and 'baby' should remind us of the word Bicuspid, which is sometimes used for Premolars. Rest of the letters are as in the previous mnemonic.

38. C. *Related fact:* This is a question which stumps many students. During examinations students are seen counting teeth in their minds, wasting much of their time. In reality this is a very simple question if the concept of superadded and successional teeth is kept in mind [see question 110 below].

Remember the following:

- The total number of teeth changes only when superadded teeth erupt.

- Molars are the only superadded teeth.
- Molars erupt at 6, 12 and 18 years – a simple multiplication table to remember (the eruption of last is variable, but for the purposes of this question we can take the age as 18).
- Thus the total number of teeth changes only at 6, 12 and 18.
- Since one molar erupts in each quadrant at these ages, the total number of teeth will increase by 4.

Now remember that the child completes his primary dentition at two and a half years of age. The total number of teeth at this time is 20. Thus we can make the following table 3.4:

Table 3.4: Total number of teeth at various ages

Age	Total number of teeth
2.5-5 years	20
6-11 years	24 (addition of first molar in each quadrant)
12-17 years	28 (addition of second molar in each quadrant)
Above 18 years or possibly 24	32 (addition of third molar in each quadrant)

39. C. ***Related fact*:** This is a little more tricky question. Various permutations and combinations of this question have been asked in examinations. The student should realize that the total number of teeth here is 24 so the age of the child has to be between 6 and 11 years. This automatically ousts choice (D).

We are left with three choices now.

Let us study the Table 3.5 now.

It is clear from this table that between the ages of 6 and 11 years, with the passing of each year the number of temporary teeth decreases by 4 while permanent teeth increase by 4, total teeth remaining the same at 24. The period between 6 and 11 is known as *mixed dentition*, because teeth of both varieties are present.

During the period of mixed dentition, the age of a child could easily be calculated by this formula:

(Age in years – 5) × 4 = Number of permanent teeth in the mouth.

In the question above

(Age in years – 5) × 4 = 10.

From this formula, the age can easily be calculated.

40. C.

41. A. ***Related facts*:** As can be seen in the question above, third molars can erupt anytime between 18 to 24 years. Sometimes they fail to erupt even after 24. Thus they are quite unreliable in the determination of age.

42. C. ***Related facts*:** Third molars appear between 18 and 24 years – an age by which a person is supposed to have acquired "wisdom"—hence the name.

Table 3.5: A comprehensive table showing the relative number of temporary and permanent teeth at various ages

Age in yrs	Temporary teeth	Permanent teeth	Total teeth	Eruption of	Fall of
5	20	0	20	None	None
6	20	4	24	Permanent first molar	None
7	16	8	24	Permanent first incisor	Temporary first incisor
8	12	12	24	Permanent second incisor	Temporary second incisor
9	8	16	24	Permanent first premolar	Temporary first molar
10	4	20	24	Permanent second premolar	Temporary second molar
11	0	24	24	Permanent canine	Temporary canine
12	0	28	28	Permanent second molar	None
18-24	0	32	32	Permanent third molar	None

43. **D.** Galton system is another name for fingerprinting. Rule of Hasse is used to determine the intrauterine age of a fetus. Trotter and Glesser's formula is used to determine the stature of a human being from a single long bone. Gustafson's method was pioneered by Professor Gösta Gustafson of Sweden in 1950.

44. **C.**

45. **D.**

46. **A.** ***Additional info***: Since 1992, Lamendin method has come in vogue, which uses only two criteria (i) gingival recession (periodontosis) and (ii) transparency of the root. This is because the method is easy to apply, and it makes use of a single rooted tooth which needs no preparation. This is said to give a better result than Gustafson's method. It was advocated in 1992 by H. Lamendin.

47. **B.** ***Additional info***: This feature was first described in 1870, in Leipzig by Muhlreiter. Shovel shape is seen in upper central incisors in Mongoloid races. The posterior surfaces of these teeth have a depression centrally with two raised marginal bars. This feature makes them look like a coal shovel with turned up edges. This feature is most commonly seen in Mongoloid races (such as Eskimos, Japanese, Chinese and Mongols), but is also sometimes seen in other races, albeit in far lesser numbers.

BONES

General

48. **B.**

49. **A.**

50. **D.** ***Related facts***: The angle of mandible (the angle formed by the ramus with the body) is obtuse both in infancy and old age. In old age this angle is about 140°.

51. **C.** ***Additional facts***: At birth the mandible is in two separate halves united in the median plane by fibrous tissue. This union is known as symphysis menti. After birth, in the first year, the two halves of the bone begin to join *from below upwards*. A trace of separation may still be visible at the beginning of the second year. By the completion of two years, the two halves are completely joined.

52. **C.** ***Related facts***: In infancy the mental foramen is close to the lower border. In adult age it is midway, and in old age it is close to the alveolar border. Just keep in mind that the mental foramen is at its lowest position during infancy and as the age advances it "migrates upwards", till in the old age it reaches the alveolar border.

Ages of Ossification

53. **C.**

54. **D.**

55. **D.** ***Notes on ages of ossification***: Most students find it very confounding to remember ages of ossification. With a few mnemonics this can be done easily as follows:

A few facts regarding ossification ages must be borne in mind. Firstly the ages of ossification vary from place to place as they depend upon dietetic, hereditary and geographic factors. Secondly, the ossification takes place slightly earlier (by about a year) in females than in males. An important exception is skull sutures, which obliterate earlier in males than in females. And lastly ossification is seen earlier in tropical climates than in temperate ones. Unless otherwise stated, the ages mentioned here refer to Indian males.

We can have our first mnemonic now. Imagine a person reclining on a sand beach as shown in Figure 3.2. His elbows are sinking in the sand somewhat. Now draw four lines parallel to the horizontal plane. The lowest one passes through the elbow. The next one through the hip and ankle joints. The next one through the shoulder and knee joint, and the uppermost passes through the wrist joint. Epiphyses falling on a particular line fuse at a particular age. Thus all epiphyses around the elbow joint would complete fusion by 16 years, all epiphyses around hip and ankle joints by 17 years, all epiphyses around shoulder and knee by 18 years and all epiphyses around wrist by 19 years. It must however be stressed that this is a very general rule and probably its main utility is that it helps the mind to easily "latch" a joint to a particular age. Several important exceptions exist which must be borne in mind.

The above mnemonic gives us following 12 important ages of ossification:

- Medial epicondyle unites with the shaft at 16 years.
- Upper end of radius unites with the shaft at 16 years.
- Lower end of radius unites with the shaft at 16 years.

  (These three centres fall upon the lowest line – ossification centres around elbow joint).
- Head of femur unites with the shaft at 17 years.

  (This is the ossification center around hip joint – it falls on the second line from below)

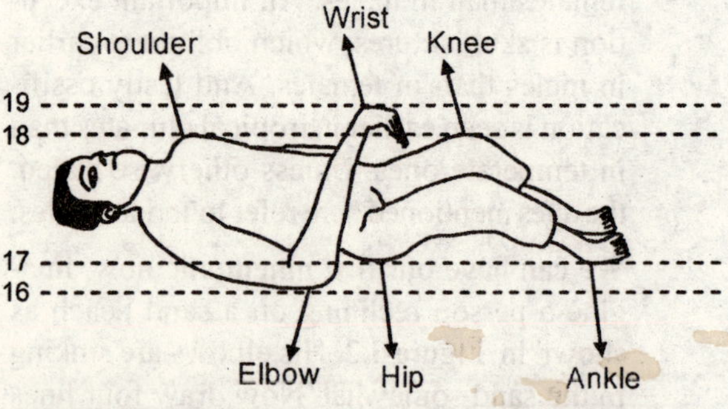

Fig. 3.2: A simple way to remember ages of fusion of some major epiphyses (refer text for details)

- Lower end of tibia unites with the shaft at 17 years.
- Lower end of fibula unites with the shaft at 17 years.

  (These two are the ossification centers around ankle joint – it falls on the second line from below)
- Head of humerus unites with the shaft at 18 years.

  (This is the ossification center around shoulder joint – it falls on the third line from below)
- Lower end of femur unites with the shaft at 18 years.
- Upper end of tibia unites with the shaft at 18 years.
- Upper end of fibula unites with the shaft at 18 years.

  (These three are the ossification centers around knee joint – it falls on the third line from below)
- Lower end of radius unites with the shaft at 19 years.
- Lower end of ulna unites with the shaft at 19 years.

  (These two are the ossification centers around wrist joint – it falls on the fourth line from below)

Regarding ages of appearances of various ossification centers, following mnemonics may be resorted to:

Upper end of humerus (Fig. 3.3)→ Remember the arithmetic series 1,3,5: Head of humerus appears at 1; Greater tuberosity at 3; Lesser tuberosity at 5. Remember that in English alphabet g comes before l, and in arithmetic 3 comes earlier than 5:

G→L

3→5

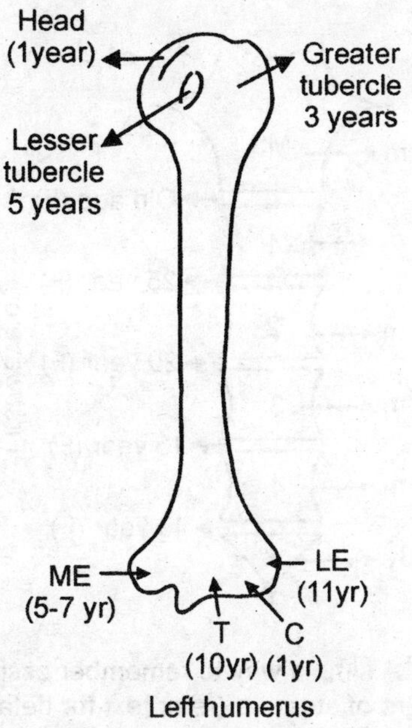

Fig. 3.3: Ossification centers of humerus

All three centers unite by 6 years, i.e. one year after the last centre comes.

Lower end of humerus (Fig. 3.3)→There are four major centers to remember here: Medical epicondyle, trochlea, capitulum and lateral epicondyle.

Capitulum appears at one (remember "c" for child. Children are younger so it comes very early, i.e. at 1).

Trochlea appears at Ten (remember "T").

Lateral Epicondyle appears at 11 (Remember "lateral". Both beginning and ending letters are "l". If we keep them together, they look like 11).

Medial epicondyle appears at 5-7. There is no good mnemonic for that. You would just have to remember it, as I have memorized it.

Union of lower end of humerus is very peculiar and must be remembered.

LTC (Lateral epicondyle, Trochlea and capitulum) join together to form a conjoint epiphysis, which then joins with the shaft.

Medial epicondyle joins the shaft of humerus separately. Remember Table 3.6.

Table 3.6: Ossification of lower end of humerus

Criteria	*Females*	*Males*
Conjoint epiphysis forms	12	13
Conjoint epiphysis unites with shaft	14	15
Medial epicondyle unites with shaft	15	16

For other long bones (radius, ulna, tibia, fibula) refer to figures 3.4 and 3.5.

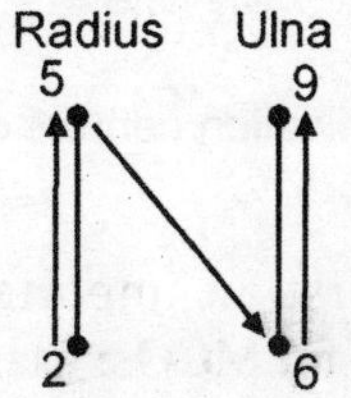

Fig. 3.4: A simple way to remember ossification centers of radius and ulna (refer text for details)

Radius and ulna: Make a representation of the two bones as shown in figure 3.4 and then make a capital "N" beginning from the lower end of radius as shown, and write numerals 2→5→6→9.

Lower end of radius appears at 2 years.
Upper end of radius appears at 5 years.
Lower end of ulna appears at 6 years.
Upper end of ulna appears at 9 years.

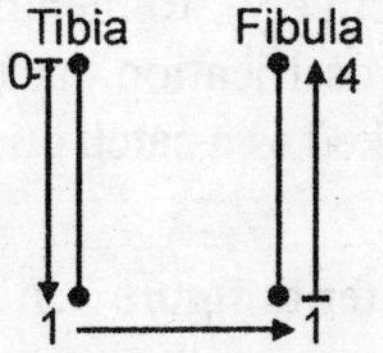

Fig. 3.5: A simple way to remember ossification centers of tibia and fibula (refer text for details)

Tibia and fibula (Fig. 3.5): Similarly make the bones and write a capital "U". Now write the numerals 0→1→1→4.

Upper end of tibia appears at 0 years, i.e. just at birth.

Lower end of tibia appears at 1 year.
Lower end of fibula appears at 1 year.
Upper end of fibula appears at 4 years.

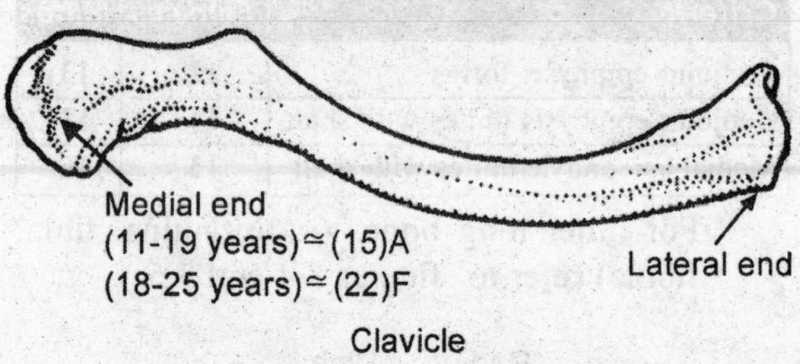

Fig. 3.6: Ossification centers of clavicle

Clavicle: First an important fact worth remembering for MCQs: Clavicle is the first bone to begin ossification.

Two centers appear in the shaft between the 5th and 6th weeks of Intrauterine life, and fuse about the 45th day. These are the primary centers.

For secondary centers refer to figure 3.6. Medial end appears between 11-19 years and unites with the shaft between 18-25 years. This is admittedly a very vast range. Students may want to remember the average: 15 years for appearance and 22 for union (there is a vast variation in what is accepted among experts. Some experts take the ages as 19 and 21 respectively). Remember there is no lateral end of ossification in clavicle. This is sometimes asked as a catch question in viva-voce.

Sternum: Refer to figure 3.7. Sternum consists of three parts—the manubrium sterni, the body of the sternum and the xiphoid process. The body of the sternum has four sternebrae. Thus the whole bone may be visualized as being composed of 6 parts (manubrium sterni + 4 sternebrae + xiphoid process).

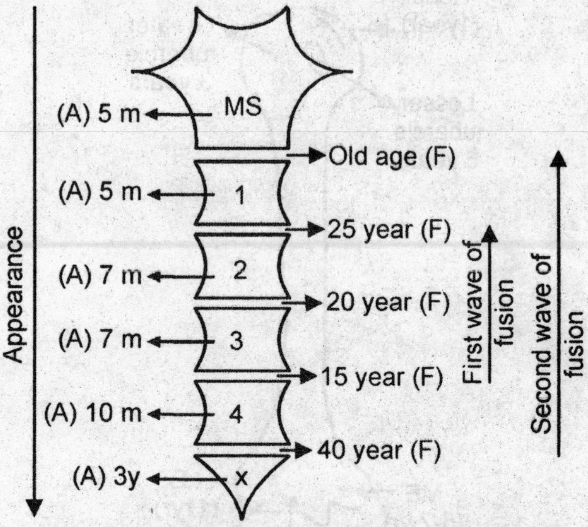

Fig. 3.7: A simple way to remember ossification centers of sternum (refer text for details)

Note the three arrows in the figure. Centers appear from above downwards, and unite from below upwards. The union occurs in two different "waves" so to say – hence the two upward arrows.

The centers for the manubrium sterni and the sternebrae appear during the IU life. Remember the figures 5m—5m—7m→7m→10m→3y.

All months refer to intrauterine period. The center for xiphisternum appears at 3 years of age.

In the first "wave" of union, the four sternebrae unite from below upwards. The figures are:

Union of 3rd and 4th sternebrae at **15** years.
Union of 2nd and 3rd sternebrae at **20** years.
Union of 1st and 2nd sternebrae at **25** years.

In the second "wave" of union:

Xiphisternum often unites with the body at **40** years.

Manubrium sterni unites with the body after **60** to **70** years, and quite often remains ununited.

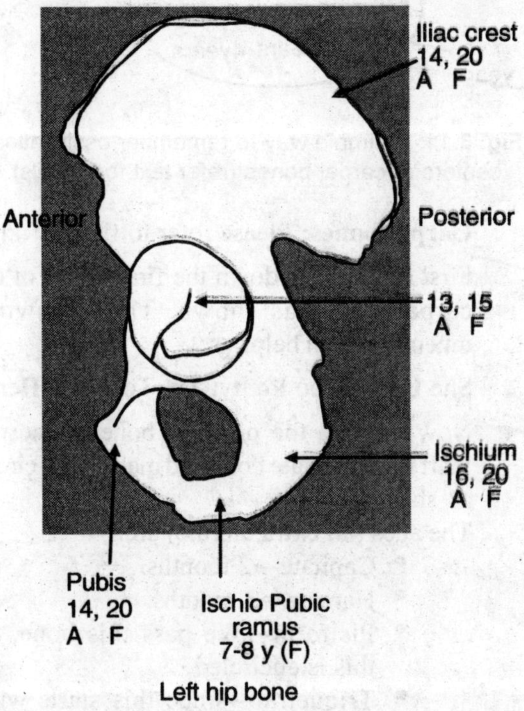

Fig. 3.8: Ossification of hip bone

Hip bone: Refer to figure 3.8. Ischio Pubic ramus unites by **7-8** years.

For iliac crest and pubis, remember **14→ 20** i.e. both iliac crest and pubis appear at 14 years of age and unite by 20 years. In the case of iliac crest, remember that the union occurs from before backwards, i.e. the crest begins uniting from the anterior side (from anterior superior iliac spine to be exact) and the union gradually proceeds backwards.

For ischium, remember **16→20**
i.e. ischium appears at 16 and unites at 20.

For acetabulum, remember **13→15**
i.e. the acetabular cup assumes the shape of a triradiate cartilage, which becomes noticeable in radiographs by 13 years. This is generally taken as the "age of appearance" of triradiate cartilage.

The triradiate cartilage disappears by **15** years.

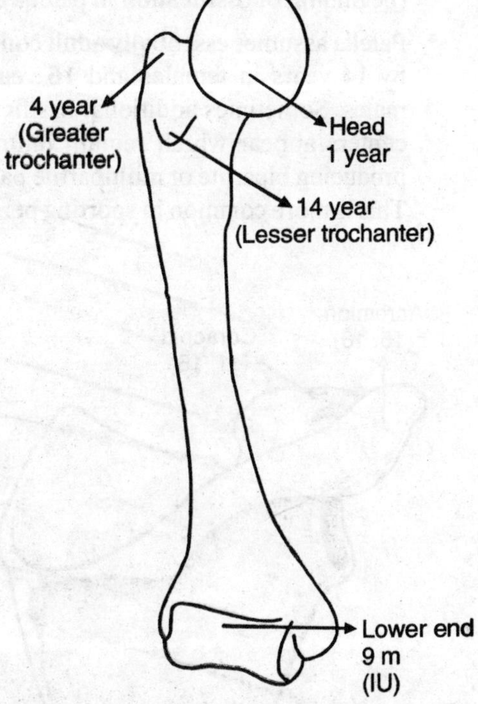

Fig. 3.9: Ossification centers in femur

Femur: Please refer to figure 3.9.

Remember **1→ 4→14** (formed by the first two digits)

i.e. head of femur appears by **1** year, greater trochanter by **4** years and lesser trochanter by **14** years.

Patella: Strangely sometimes questions are asked on this bone. The facts to remember are as below:

- Patella begins to ossify from several centers which appear between 3rd to 6th year. They coalesce quickly. Accessory marginal centers appear later. The centers appear in males between **1½ to 4** years, while in females between **2½ to 6** years (interestingly the centers appear later in females). Three years is generally the expected choice in MCQ questions (beginning of ossification in patella).

- Patella assumes essentially adult contours by **14** years in females and **16** years in males. Sometimes additional ossification centers appear which remain ununited, producing bipartite or multipartite patella. This is more common in sporting persons.

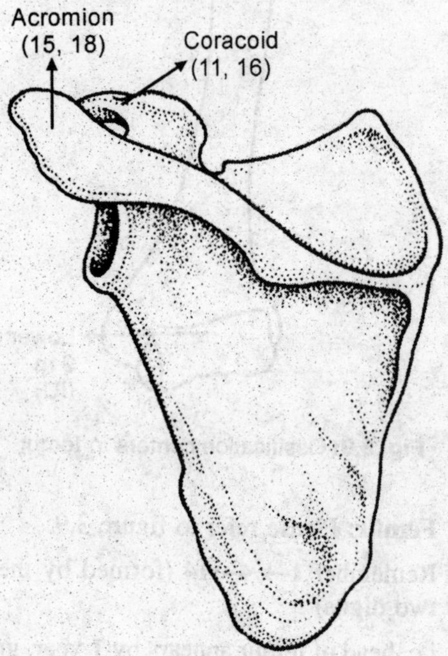

Fig. 3.10: Ossification centers in scapula

Scapula: Please refer to figure 3.10.

For coracoid, remember **11** (A)→**16** (F).
For acromion, remember **15** (A)→**18** (F).

There is no easy way to remember these figures. You just have to remember them by rote memory.

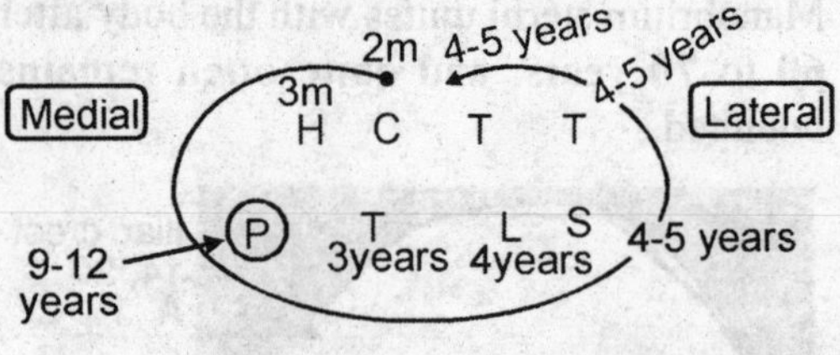

Fig. 3.11: A simple way to remember ossification centers of carpal bones (refer text for details)

Carpal bones: Please refer to figure 3.11

First of all write down the first letters of all carpal bones as shown. The following mnemonic will help:

She **L**ooks **T**oo **P**retty; **T**ry **T**o **C**atch **H**er.

Now encircle the pisiform bone as shown. Start from capitate bone and make a full circle as shown.

The ages (all extra uterine) are:

- Capitate→**2** months.
- Hamate→**3** months.
- Pisiform→We pass this bone, as this is encircled.
- Triquetral→since this starts with "tri" we can not assign the next number. It has to be "tri" or 3. So Triquetral appears at **3** months.
- Lunate→**4** months.
- Scaphoid→**4-5** months.
- Trapezium and trapezoid→**4-5** months (Trapezium comes slightly earlier than Trapezoid).
- Pisiform: We finally land on this bone. It appears between **9-12** years. It is the last carpal bone to appear.

Before going ahead, let us memorize some important centers of ossification which appear during intrauterine life.

We already learnt that the earliest bone to begin ossification is clavicle (**45 days**, or **1½ months**). The whole table of intrauterine ossifications is like this (Table 3.7):

Table 3.7: Ossification of some major bones in the intrauterine period

Bone	IU month
Clavicle	1½
Shaft of long bones	2
Ischium	3-4
Calcaneus	5
Manubrium sterni	6
Talus	7
Sacrum	8
Femur (lower end)	9
Cuboid	10

The ages of last 6 bones can be remembered by the following (rather meaningless) sentence:

CAST TAKES SAFE CUSHION

Ca→Calcaneus→**5.**

St→Sternum (manubrium)→**6** (remember that by a previous mnemonic, manubrium sterni is taken to come at 5. It is okay to consider it as **5-6** months now).

Ta→Talus→**7.**

Kes→It stands for nothing.

Sa→Sacrum→**8.**

Fe→Femur (lower end)→**9.**

Cu→Cuboid→10 (or just before birth).

Remember that Talus is important for us, since it appears at 7 months of IU life. This period is usually taken as the period of attainment of viability in this country.

Now let us memorize the ossification centers of the bones of foot.

This is the view of foot bones from above. We already know about ossifications of calcaneum (**5** months IU), Talus (**7** months IU) and Cuboid (**10** months IU).

For secondary centers of calcaneum remember 7 (A)→**16** (F).

Navicular appears at **3** years (just like xiphisternum in the upper half of the body).

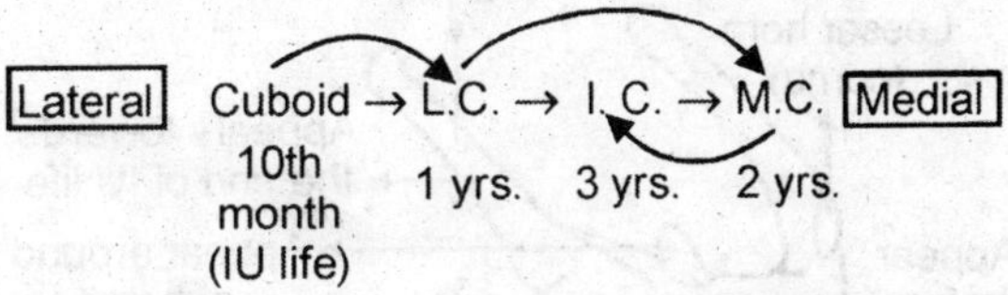

Fig. 3.13: A simple way to remember ossification centers of cuboid and the three cuneiforms (refer text for details)

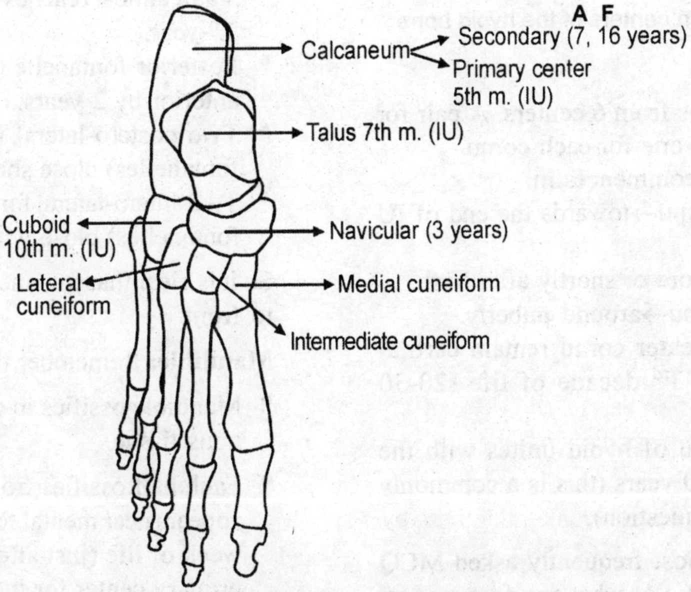

Fig. 3.12: Ossification centers of foot bones

For cuneiforms, refer to figure 3.13.

We have laid down (i) cuboid (ii) lateral cuneiform (iii) intermediate cuneiform and (iv) medial cuneiform in their anatomical fashion. Ossification centres in these bones appear from lateral to medial side. The years are **0, 1, 2, 3.**

First to appear is cuboid. We already know it appears at **10** months IU life, or just before birth (or zero years of life).

Next is Lateral cuneiform→**1** year.

Now we cheat a little and jump. Medial cuneiform→**2** years.

We come back to Intermediate cuneiform→3 years

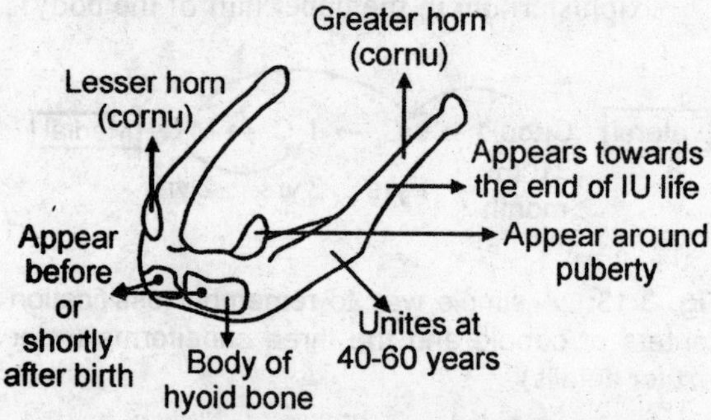

Fig. 3.14: Ossification centers of the hyoid bone

Hyoid:

- Hyoid ossifies from 6 centers. A pair for the body and one for each cornu.
- Ossification commences in:
  - o Greater cornu→towards the end of IU life.
  - o Body→before or shortly after birth.
  - o Lesser cornu→around puberty.
- Apices of greater cornu remain cartilaginous until 3rd decade of life (20-30 years).
- Greater cornu of hyoid unites with the body at 40-60 years (this is a commonly asked MCQ question).

Sacrum: The most frequently asked MCQ from this bone is→At what age does sacrum become one bone? The intended answer is **25** years, but look for any answer between 21-25 years, as this is the usual range cited by experts.

Other facts to remember about this bone:

- Bodies of sacral vertebrae begin to unite with one another after the 20th year of life at their adjacent margins, but the central area remains unossified. By 25th year, the sacrum is one bone, even though central area may remain unossified up to—or even after – middle age.
- The union occurs from below upwards.

Skull: Remember the following facts:

- Basi-occiput unites with the basi-sphenoid at 20 years (range 18-25 years). This is the most frequently asked question from this bone. There is no need for a mnemonic for this, as there is a very good natural reason why it happens at this age. It is related to continued expansion of the jaws to accommodate the erupting teeth; also to provide room for muscles of mastication and growth of nasopharynx.
- Vault almost reaches adult dimensions by 7th year.
- Posterior fontanelle closes by 2 months; anterior by 2 years.
- Two postero-lateral fontanelles (mastoid fontanelles) close shortly after birth.
- Two antero-lateral fontanelles (sphenoidal fontanelles) close within first 6 months.

So it is clear that fontanelles close from back to front.

Mandible: Remember the following facts:

- Mandible ossifies in dense fibromembranous tissue.
- Each half ossifies from one center which appears near mental foramen about the 6th week of life (just after the appearance of primary center for the clavicle).

- Two halves of mandible join from below upwards in the first year, but a trace of separation near the alveolar margin may still be visible at the beginning of 2nd year. An MCQ question which is often asked related to this information is: Two halves of mandible unite by (a) 6 months (b) 2 years (c) 6 years (d) 12 years. The expected answer is (b) **2 years.**
- Head of mandible completely ossifies by the 3rd decade (21-30 years).

Other Unions

56. D.

57. B.

58. D.

59. B. Ages of suture obliteration are commonly asked in MCQ exams and the student would do well to remember these. This is not so difficult as it appears.

First a few facts.

- Interestingly skull sutures obliterate earlier in males than in females. Generally all bones ossify earlier in females, so this is an important exception.
- Suture closure begins at the inner table and progresses outwards. Generally there is a gap of 5 years before outer table also obliterates. The ages given below are for outer table.

Closure of skull sutures takes place as below:

Table 3.8: Ages of closure of various skull sutures

Suture	Commencement	Halfway closed	Termination
Spheno-occipital synchondrosis	–	–	20
Coronal suture	25	30	40
Sagittal suture	25	30	40
Lambdoid suture	25	30	45
Pterion	40	–	65
Masto-occipital suture	45	–	80
Asterion	–	–	50

A few mnemonics may help here (Fig. 3.15):

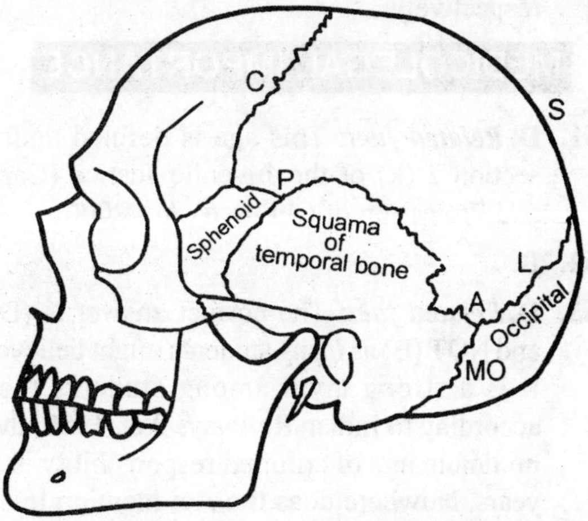

Fig. 3.15: Closure of skull sutures

- Spheno-occipital is the earliest to fuse (20 years).
- Coronal, sagittal and lambdoid start together at 25 years. The frontal ones (coronal and sagittal) finish at 40 years while posterior one (Lambdoid) finishes a little later – at 45 years (remember "back benchers").
- Two minor sutures are Pterion (at front) and Masto-occipital (at back).
- Front one (pterion) starts when front sutures close (40 years).
- Back one (Masto-occipital) starts when back sutures close (45 years).
- Pterion takes 25 years to close (65 years).
- Masto-occipital takes 35 years to close (80 years) [remember "back benchers" again].
- Asterion closes by 50 years.

SECONDARY SEXUAL CHARACTERS

60. C. Hair appear in the male on pubis, axilla and face at 14, 15 and 16 years respectively. Remember that hair appear on lower parts and "travel" up! In the female, hair begin to appear on pubis and axilla at 13 and 14 years respectively.

MEDICOLEGAL IMPORTANCE

61. **D.** ***Related fact***: This age is defined under section 2 (k) of the Juvenile Justice (Care and Protection of Children) Act 2000.

62. **B.**

63. **D.** ***Related fact***: The correct answer is (D) and NOT (B) as many students might believe. It is a strong myth among students that according to Indian Railways Act, 1989, the minimum age of criminal responsibility is 5 years. Nowhere does the Act mention this.

64. **C.** ***Related fact***: This is written in section 82 of Indian Penal Code.

65. **B.**

MISCELLANEOUS

66. **A.** According to this rule, the crown-heel (CH) length in cm bears a special relation to its age in lunar months. For the first five lunar months, the age of the fetus in lunar months is the square root of the CH length of the fetus in cms. Thus a fetus of 1 month is 1cm; 2 months = 4 cm; 3 months = 9 cms; 4 months = 16 cms and 5 months = 25 cms. After fifth month, the age is calculated by dividing the CH length by 5. Thus 6 month old fetus is 30 cm; 7 months = 35 cm; 8 months = 40 cm; 9 months = 45 cms and 10 months (or full term) is 50 cms.

Three facts need to be remembered. First is that the length is CH length and NOT Crown-Rump (CR) length. Secondly the age is measured in lunar months (1 lunar month = 28 days) and NOT in calender months and finally the length of the fetus is measured in cm and NOT in inches. A variant of this question is given below:

Variant of the above question→Rule of Haase is meant for (a) Estimation of age (b) Estimation of gestational age (c) Estimation of the height of the individual (d) Determination of sex. The answer is (b).

67. **D.** Let us analyse this interesting question. Remember what we said about the three facts to be remembered. These are (i) CH length and (ii) Lunar months (iii) inches. If one does not remember these three things, he may unnecessarily get confused sorting out the correct answer. A quick glance at the choices tells us that only two choices namely (B) and (D) talk about C-H lengths. Thus the correct answer has to be from among these two only. Out of these (B) talks of 7 lunar months. Since the age is greater than 5 months, it has to be multiplied by 5 to get the correct CH length. The C-H length comes to 35. So this is not the correct answer. The correct answer has to be (D).

68. **A.** In 1963, Boyde devised a method whereby age of a person could be determined by counting incremental lines in teeth in histological sections (just as one counts the age of a tree by counting its annual rings). At birth of every individual, an exceptionally well marked line is formed in all teeth. This is known as *neonatal line*. After this, daily increments of growth are represented by *incremental lines*, which can be counted on histological sections. Theoretically it is possible to count these incremental lines and opine upon the age of the individual.

Variant: A variant of this question is often asked like this→Boyde devised a method of accurate age estimation from (a) Finger tips (b) Foot prints (c) Changes in skull (d) Changes in teeth. The answer is (d) Changes in teeth.

STATURE

69. B. ***Related fact*****:** The body usually *lengthens* after death. The major reasons for lengthening are (i) complete loss of muscle tone in the first stage of flaccidity (ii) relaxation at large joints such as the hip and knee and (iii) Lost tensioning effect of the paraspinal muscles on intervertebral discs.

Some interesting developments in stature occur later which must be remembered by the student.

When rigor mortis develops later, the body actually shortens.

When decomposition sets in, joints become lax, and the body may lengthen once again.

70. B. ***Related fact*****:** Stature of a human being can often be calculated – rather accurately —if his entire skeleton or at least one complete long bone is available. In archaeological material it is rather rare for one to find complete long bones; fragmentary bones are found instead. In 1969, D. Gentry Steele and Thomas W. McKern of the University of Kansas, tried developing regression formulae for specified segments of the femur, humerus, and tibia to aid in the estimation of total long bone lengths from fragmentary remains. Once total length was determined, it was possible to calculate living stature of the individual with a reasonable degree of accuracy. For this study, they used a sample of 117 prehistoric Indians from various archeological sites in the southeastern United States. They published these findings in the prestigious *American Journal of Physical Anthropology*. These are now sometimes known as Steeles' formulae.

71. A. Multiplication factor is a number which when multiplied by the length of a long bone would give the height of the person. Thus if the police brings a femur bone to the forensic anthropologist and he finds that its length is, say 47 cm, he can multiply this length with the multiplication factor for the femur (3.6) to give a reasonably good estimate of the dead person's height (whom the police may be trying to identify). The height of the person in this hypothetical case comes to 47x3.6 or a little more than 169 cms.

Multiplication factors are available for all six long bones (femur, tibia, fibula, humerus, ulna and radius) and the students find them rather hard to memorize. These can be remembered by a small trick.

Start with the number 36. Go on adding 8 and generate 5 numbers as shown (Table 3.9):

Table 3.9: Method of generating numbers for derivation of multiplication factors

36
Add 8
44
Add 8
52
Add 8
60
Add 8
68

Now we have 5 numbers: 36, 44, 52, 60, 64.

Write them in a straight column. Modify third and fifth numbers as shown and then put a decimal point in between the two numerals.

Table 3.10: Multiplication factors finally derived (refer to Table 3.9)

Original number	*Modified number*	*Number after putting decimal point*
36		3.6
44		4.4
52	53	5.3
60		6.0
68	64	6.4

We get five numbers: 3.6, 4.4, 5.3, 6.0, and 6.4

These are the multiplication factors. Now we have to assign bones to them.

We know that out of the six bones mentioned above, femur is the largest bone, so it must have the smallest number. So the number 3.6 gets assigned to it.

If we arrange smaller bones in order of their decreasing length, we can go on assigning larger numbers to them, till the biggest number (6.4) gets assigned to the smallest bone, radius.

Table 3.11 can be made easily now:

Table 3.11: Assigning correct multiplication factors to bones (refer to Tables 3.9 and 3.10)

Bone	Multiplication factor
Femur	3.6
Tibia and fibula	4.4
Humerus	5.3
Ulna	6.0
Radius	6.4

With a little practice, this table can be remembered very easily and can easily be recalled during exams, because now we know how to generate this table.

ANTHROPOMETRY

72. **B.** ***More related facts***: Alphonse Bertillon (1853-1914) was a French national, who devised his method around 1879. He first put it in practice around 1882. His system had started shattering by 1896, when fingerprints began to be used in Argentina. The system was completely discarded in 1914, the year of Bertillon's death. So the system had its heydey for just about 14 years – from 1882 till 1896.

73. **D.** ***More related facts***: Indeed Bertillon system has been called a tripartite system, whereby three means of description were taken. Prisoner's physical description (descriptive data) was done with a characteristic rigor for which Bertillon even developed his own "morphological vocabulary". In the "Bertillon card" that he developed, there were spaces for the description of such things as prisoner's eyes, ears, lips, beard, hair color, skin color, ethnicity, forehead, nose, build, chin, general contour of head, hair growth pattern, eye brows, eyeball and orbit, mouth, physiognomic expression, neck, inclination of shoulders, attitute, general demeanour, voice, language and even habiliments. Special vocabulary was developed to describe these features. For instance lips might be "pouting", "thick" or "thin" or "upper prominent" or "lower prominent" and so on.

Under body marks, such marks as scars, cicatrices and tattoos were described very rigorously.

74. **C.** ***Additional facts to remember***: A Belgian statistician Adolphe Quételet (1796-1874) had once asserted that the chances of finding two persons of the same height were about 1:4 (Often known as Quételet's law). Bertillon reasoned that if he could add just one more measurement – say, the length of the trunk – he could increase the probability to 1:16 (4^2). If he took 14 measurements, he could increase the probability to 4^{14} or 1:268,435,546. He initially toyed with the idea of taking 14 measurements, but ultimately settled for 11. It still gave him a probability of 4^{11} or 4,194,304 (more than four million), which was quite reasonable to exclude or nail a suspect. The measurements he took were (i) Length of the head (ii) width of the head (iii) length of left middle finger (iv) length of left little finger (v) height (vi) sitting height (height of trunk) (vii) span of arms (viii) length of right ear (ix) width of right ear (x) length of left forearm (xi) length of left foot.

Note that of the bilateral things, generally all left measurements were taken except those of ear.

He first made three basic divisions for length of head – large, medium or small, and these were subdivided into large, medium and small width of head. Next came length of left middle finger and length of left little finger, whom he similarly divided into three categories. This gave him 81 different categories (3^4), and the probability of wrongly identifying a criminal to just 1:256 (4^4). He stored the cards of criminals in 81 separate drawers based on these four measurements only. Each card of course contained seven other measurements as well.

75. D. ***Related fact***: *Portrait parlé* is actually just another name for the Bertillon system. Other names are Bertillonage and anthropometry. *Portrait parlé* literally means "a spoken portrait". It is called so because in his system Bertillon insisted to have two photographs of the criminal – one full face and one in profile. This was the portrait. It became "spoken" because Bertillon added two additional things to it – body description and body marks.

DACTYLOGRAPHY

76. A.

77. C. Most forensic scientists divide fingerprints into three types: Arches, Whorls and Loops. Approximately 5% of the total population have arches, 35% have whorls and 60% have loops. This can perhaps best be remembered by the mnemonic **AWL→Arches, Whorls and Loops.**

Some workers recognize a fourth type also —Composite—which is a mixture of the above three types. If this is taken as a genuine separate class, then it becomes the rarest (it is supposed to be present in only 1-2% cases). The student must see if "composite" appears as a choice. If it does, then it is the intended correct choice.

Tombs is a fictitious class. No class exists with this name.

78. D. ***Additional information***: Galton worked out mathematically the number of possible variations, and he came up with the figure of 64 billion different fingerprints.

There are at least 80 characteristics in a fingerprint, but there may be more.

There is a difference of opinion amongst the world experts as to how many points of similarity should be there. The number of points vary from country to country. The full Table 3.12 is:

Table 3.12: Minimum number of points matched in different countries

Country	*Minimum number of points*
Austria	10-12
Australia	12
Belgium	8-12
Canada	10-16
Denmark	16
France	16
Great Britain	16
Interpol	12
Japan	12-14
Israel	10-12
New Zealand	8-12
Spain	10-12
Switzerland	No. of points not fixed
USA	7-12

The first All India Biennial Forensic Science Conference held at Srinagar (1973) passed the following resolution:

"The minimum number of points of establishing the identity beyond doubt in case of fingerprint identification was to be fixed at 8 points. However when there are 6 or 7 points of identity only, a qualified opinion can be offered by the expert on his responsibility.

The Supreme Court of India, in the case *Mohanlal v. Ajit Singh* (AIR 1978 SC 1183: 1978 Cri LJ 1107), has ruled as follows:

"A majority of fingerprints found at the Crime Scene or on a crime article are partially smudged and it is for the experienced Fingerprint Expert to say whether a mark is usable as finger-print evidence. Similarly it is for a competent technician to examine and give his opinion whether the identity can be established, and if so, whether that can be done on **eight** or identical characteristics in an appropriate manner."

In India, the number of points differ even from state to state:

Table 3.13: The minimum number of points matched in different states in our country (vis-à-vis the population of that state)

States	Minimum number of identical points	Population (2001 census)
Assam	7-12	26,638,407
Andhra	10-12	75,727,541
Bihar	7	82,878,796
Gujarat	12	50,596,992
Kerala	7	31,838,619
Tamil Nadu	8-10	62,110,839
Maharashtra	12	96,752,247
Madhya Pradesh	6	60,385,118
Karnataka	12	52,733,958
Orissa	5-7	36,706,920
Punjab	10-12	24,289,296
Rajasthan	10-12	25,724,142
Uttar Pradesh	7	166,052,859
West Bengal	6	80,221,171
Central Fingerprint Bureau (Calcutta)	9	—

From this table it appears that there is no fixed formula or parameter to make a decision on the number of points. **Population is no criteria.** The most populated state of UP takes 7 points, while least populated state (Punjab) takes 10-12 points!

Dr. E. Locard and Dr. Rechter have stated the following:

"A rare detail in an identification work is one hundred times more important than a whole series of forks. 4 to 5 details in the core of an unusual pattern have more evidentiary value than 12-15 forks in the periphery".

79. C. ***Related facts***: Edmond Locard (1877 - 1965) was a French criminalist, who is better known for his Locard's exchange principle. He discovered that there are about 9-18 sweat pores on each mm of the friction ridges over fingers. These pores have specific size and shape in each person. Furthermore they are permanent and immutable during life, making them excellent features for identification.

Poroscopy is supposed to be very useful when only fragmentary fingerprints are available. Locard first used this method in 1912 in France in the famous trial of Boudet and Simonin.

80. B. ***Additional facts***: These sweat pores range in size from 88 to 220 microns.

81. B. Fingerprint patters are made up of several friction ridges on tips of fingers. In 1962, it was discovered that the edges of these ridges had seven characteristic shapes. It was suggested that these characteristic shapes could also be used for identification. This is known as edgeoscopy. Some of the shapes described were convex, concave, peak, pocket and angle.

82. D. ***Related facts***: If fingerprints are invisible or barely visible, they are commonly referred to as latent prints. Fingerprints which have been made after the hand was contaminated with blood or some other staining material are known as visible prints. Prints made on soft surfaces such as soap, cheese, butter are known as plastic prints. These prints are caused by actual indentations made in the soft surface.

83. B. ***Related facts***: In July 1858, Sir William J. Herschel (1833-1917), who was at that time serving as the Chief Magistrate of the Hooghly district in Jungipoor, India, first used fingerprints on native contracts. He had observed that local Indians usually took palm prints on contracts. On a whim, and with no thought toward personal identification, Herschel had Rajyadhar Konai, a local businessman, impress his hand print on a contract. The idea was merely to frighten him so he may not repudiate his signature. Later Herschel recognized that taking fingerprints instead of palm prints could indeed serve as a sure means of identification. Sir Francis Galton (1822-1911) established that fingerprints of a person did not change with time. He also identified the characteristics by which fingerprints could be identified. These same characteristics (minutiae) are basically still in use today, and are often referred to as Galton's Details.

84. C. ***Related facts***: On 12 June 1897, the Council of the Governor General of India approved a committee report that fingerprints should be used for classification of criminal records. Later that year, the Calcutta (now Kolkata) Anthropometric Bureau became the world's first Fingerprint Bureau. Two well-known Indian fingerprint experts who worked in this bureau were Azizul Haque and Hem Chandra Bose. They are credited with primary development of the Henry System of fingerprint classification (named for their supervisor, Edward Richard Henry). The Henry classification system is still used in all English-speaking countries.

OTHER CRITERIA

85. D. ***Related facts***: From Gr. *Cheilos*, a margin, lip, brim. See question 5 above.

86. B.

87. D. The facts regarding the scar are: First the scar is vascular (bluish or reddish angry looking scar). Vascularity starts decreasing from 2 weeks onwards and the scar is completely avascular in 2 months. Then tenderness starts going, and it is completely non-tender by 6 months. Lastly the scar loses its softness, and it becomes tough. It is more than 6 months and may be upto years. Remember like this V→T→S.

88. D.

89. B. ***Related facts***: This case – also known as the shark-arm case – is an interesting case in which identification of a person was established by a tattoo on an arm. A 14 foot long tiger shark was caught by some fisherman on April 17, 1935 and given to the local Coogee Aquarium in Sydney, Australia. Eight days later – on April 25, when Australia was celebrating its annual Anzac (Australia and Newzealand Army Corps) day – the shark disgorged a single left arm of a human being, with a rope tied around. The arm had a tattoo depicting two sparring boxers. Fingerprints were prepared from the fingers of the arm, and it was discovered that the fingerprints belonged to a forger and petty thief James Smith. His wife was contacted who positively identified her husband from the tattoo. English forensic pathologist Sir Sydney Smith was contacted, who examined the arm and opined that the arm had been cut by a sharp instrument a few hours after the death. This set to rest doubts raised by many that the arm had been hacked off by the shark from the intact body of James Smith.

James Smith was involved in smuggling drugs in a boat named *Pathfinder*. The owner of the boat Reginald Holmes co-operated with the local police and said that he had indeed lent the boat to Smith, but was unaware of the smuggling activities going on. He however led the police to another man Patrick Brady, who might have killed Smith due to rivalry.

Reginald Holmes thus became a key witness for the police but he was murdered on 13 June 1935. With no key witness left in the case, the case was finally closed on 12 December 1935 – less than nine months after it had been opened. Another weak point in the case was that the whole dead body of James Smith was never found; just his left arm was found. Mr. Justice Hulse Rogers of the Australian Supreme Court ruled that, "A limb does not constitute a body". A complete body had traditionally always been essential for holding of an inquest!

There are some interesting co-incidences in the case too. The name of the victim was James Smith and the name of the pathologist Sir Sydney Smith. The case occurred in Sydney.

90. A.

91. D.

92. C.

93. B. Histological study of the regional lymph nodes may show the dye used for tattooing.

94. C.

95. A.

96. A.

97. C. ***Additional info*:** Cortex is the middle layer and consists of longitudinally arranged, elongated cells. These cells do not have nuclei, but contain pigment granules.

98. B. ***Additional info*:** Remember the following data about cross section of human hair:

Mongoloid →Circular. 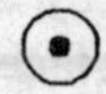

Caucasoid → Oval. 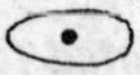

Negroid →Almost kidney shaped. 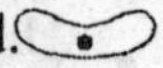

99. B.

100. D. ***Additional info*:** One of the ways human hair is differentiated from animal hair is by seeing the way pigmentation is distributed in the hair. Pigmentation is seen in middle layer (cortex). Within the cortex if the pigmentation is more evenly distributed, it is taken to be a human hair, while if the pigmentation is concentrated towards the inner medullary layer, it is taken to be animal hair.

Some anthropologists believe that distribution of pigmentation within humans show a variation characteristic of their race. It is the Mongoloid hair which is believed to show a real even distribution (of pigment granules) throughout the cortex. In both Caucasoid and Negroid head hair, the pigmentation tends to be localized around the outside.

To summarize:

1. Pigment granules are found within cortex. If they are concentrated outside→Human (Caucasoid or Negroid).
2. If they are more evenly distributed→Human (Mongoloid).
3. If they are concentrated on the inside (towards medulla)→Animal hair.

101. D. Some MCQ books would have us believe that race could be differentiated by observing the state of fragmentation of medulla. This is not true. If the medulla is fragmented the only thing that can be said is that the hair is likely from a human being. If the medulla is thick and continuous on the other hand, the hair could have come from an animal.

102. **C.** ***Additional info***: Mohammaden males often show callosities on the center of forehead, patella, tuberosity of left tibia and tip of left lateral (external) malleolus owing to special attitudes adopted during prayers. In an unidentified male body, it is useful to look for these callosities.

103. **D.** ***Related fact***: It is usual for jail authorities to obtain fingerprints at the time of admission in a jail, so the identity in this case could be established by dactylography. But the question is silent on whether fingerprints were obtained by jail authorities at the time of admission or not. Nor is this choice available in the answers. Blood grouping and DNA profiling would have been helpful if his blood or some other biological sample had been preserved, or if his relatives were available. That leaves us with Anthropometry. This system – as we have seen above – has been completely discarded since 1914, and now no one takes the 11 measurements that are required in this system. Thus there is no way his identify can be established now.

MULTIPLE ANSWER TYPE (PGI, CHANDIGARH PATTERN)

104. **A,B,D.** A, D are quite obvious and do not need much explanation. C is obviously a wrong choice and again does not need much explanation. The choices B and E are tricky, because one tends to intuitively associate all large things with male and smaller and rounded things with female. The exceptions in case of skull are (i) frontal eminences (ii) Parietal eminences and (iii) orbits all three of which are SMALLER IN MALES AND LARGER IN FEMALES. In addition, there is another "so-called anomaly" in the orbits in the males. The orbits in the males have rounded margins, while in females they have sharp margins. So the correct choices are A, B and D.

105. **A,B,D,E.** Fingerprints, the frontal sinus pattern is another major identification criteria, that is different even in identical twins. Other major facts to be remembered about frontal sinus patters are:

- The idea was first suggested way back in 1921 by Schuller. A decade later – in 1931 – Poole corroborated the idea by showing that the pattern was different even in identical twins.
- Frontal sinuses appear in 2nd year of life, and they keep growing in size during the first two decades. After they have stabilized, they make a very good criteria for identification, especially in cases where the bodies have been badly burnt or mutilated. In these cases, the antemortem X-rays may be obtained from the dead person's medical records/physicians.
- For identification by frontal sinus pattern, the scalloped upper margins of the sinuses are used. These are smaller and more numerous in the females. Several different techniques are used for comparison:
  - o Some workers simply trace out the patterns and compare.
  - o Some trace out the patterns on a card-board, cut it out and then weigh it. Weight derived from both antemortem and postmortem films must be same in order for a perfect match.
  - o Some advocate computed tomography of frontal sinuses.

106. **A,B,C,D,E.** All of the above dyes are used for tattooing. India ink gives rise to black colored tattoo, vermillion, red; and prussian blue, ultramarine and indigo, blue.

107. A,C,E. Medulla shows considerable variation in humans. However by and large, it is narrow, fragmented or sometimes even absent. If the medulla is very prominent, the hair is likely from an animal. Cuticular scales in humans are short and thin.

108. A. Correct facts about Barr bodies are as follows:

- They were first described by Mary Barr, and Ewart Bertram in 1949. They found that in the interphase nucleus of female cat neurons there were a significant number of cells that had one "darkly staining body" lying along the edge of the nucleus, but they never found a "darkly staining body" in the neurons of male cats. Similar "darkly staining bodies" are found in buccal epithelial cells of human females, although they could usually be found in only 30% to 40% of the cells. Compare this figure with Davidson bodies which is just about 3% of all female neutrophils.
- Mary Lyon in 1960 proposed that this was an inactivated X chromosome, and named it the Barr body. This is called the Lyon Hypothesis.
- At a critical point in development, one X chromosome in each cell of a female's body is randomly inactivated (it curls up into a little loop). In humans, this occurs 12 days after fertilization.
- The genes on the inactivated X chromosome are not transcribed or translated.
- Barr bodies are seen *inside* the nucleus near the nuclear wall.
- They are seen only in females.
- They represent the one inactive X chromosome (condensed form), which all females have. Males have only one X chromosome, so none is inactive. Hence no Barr bodies in males.
- Barr bodies are most readily visible in squamous cells of female vaginal mucus membrane or mucus membranes of the mouth.

109. B,D. ***Related facts***: Gustafson's method is used to determine the age of the individual and NOT the race. It can not be used in the living, because teeth have to be extracted. It is applicable in individuals above 15 years of age, because there are no appreciable changes in children below this age.

110. A,C,D. ***Related information***: Successional teeth are those permanent teeth which replace some other teeth. Thus their eruption does not change the total number of teeth of the individual. In contrast superadded teeth are those which are added to the existing set of teeth; they do not replace any teeth. Thus their eruption always increases the number of teeth. Incisors, canines and premolars are successional teeth while all molars are superadded teeth.

Remember the following:

Permanent incisors→replace temporary incisors.

Permanent canines→replace temporary canines.

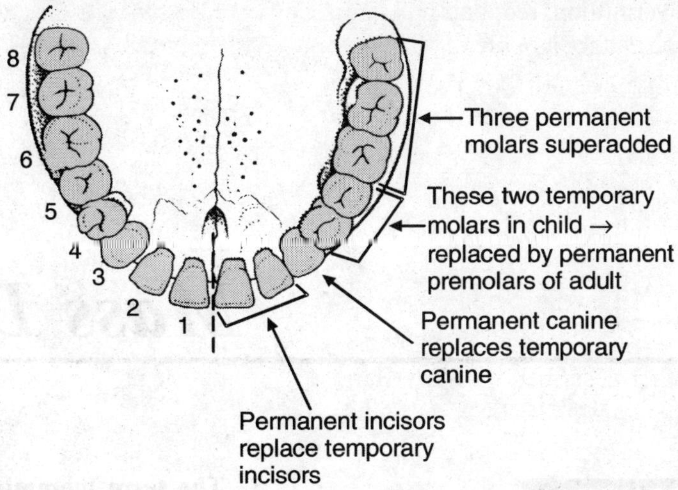

Fig. 3.16: Superadded and successional teeth

Permanent premolars→replace temporary molars.

111. B,E. Fingerprints are different even in identical twins. This is why fingerprinting is often regarded as the best system of identification.

4 Mass Disasters

GENERAL

1. **Which of the following best defines mass disaster?**
   - **A.** It is defined as the death of more than 12 victims in a single event
   - **B.** It is defined as the number of deaths which exceeds the capacity of the local death investigation system to handle it
   - **C.** It is defined as any number of deaths occurring in an unnatural event
   - **D.** It is defined as deaths occurring in an area greater than 10 km

2. **In cases of mass disaster, which of the following is true?**
   - **A.** If whole body is not available, and only parts such as arms and legs are available, the medical officer must delay the autopsy till the police recovers the whole body
   - **B.** The autopsy can not legally be conducted by a single doctor; it must be conducted by a board of three doctors
   - **C.** The doctor must conduct autopsy on whatever fragments are available
   - **D.** A single doctor can not legally conduct autopsies on more than 3 persons dying in a single incident

3. **The term 'commorientes' refers to:**
   - **A.** Simultaneous death of more than 100 persons in a mass disaster
   - **B.** Mass disaster due to a human mistake, such as fire in a building due to short circuiting
   - **C.** A special form of mass disaster when planes are crashed in buildings
   - **D.** Two or more people dying simultaneously or in circumstances rendering it uncertain which of them survived the other or others

4. **According to Indian law, if several close relatives die in a mass disaster, without having written a valid will, and the question is of inheritance and succession to property, what is the rule that is followed?**
   - **A.** Male survived the female
   - **B.** Younger survived the elder
   - **C.** Taller person survived the shorter
   - **D.** There is no law in India catering to this situation

5. **Triage is associated with:**
   - **A.** Warfare injuries
   - **B.** Road injuries
   - **C.** Gunshot injuries
   - **D.** Poisoning resuscitation

MULTIPLE ANSWER TYPE (PGI, CHANDIGARH PATTERN)

6. The objectives of forensic investigation in a mass disaster are:
A. To find the cause and manner of death of each individual
B. To obtain samples for toxicological analysis
C. To identify each individual properly
D. To arrange for the funeral of each individual
E. To find the cause of the disaster

7. Identification in a case of mass disaster can be achieved by:
A. Appearance
B. Fingerprints
C. Neck prints
D. Dental data
E. Occupation marks

8. Which of the following is NOT generally classified as a mass disaster by forensic pathologists?
A. Multiple deaths in a building collapse
B. Serial murder involving multiple victims
C. Multiple deaths during the course of a riot
D. Death of passengers in an aircraft accident
E. 2-3 deaths occurring at the same time in several districts, states and countries due to some common unnatural cause, all adding up to hundreds of victims

ANSWERS

GENERAL

1. **B.** Some authorities feel that the death of more than 12 victims in a single event may be called a mass disaster. However (B) is more widely accepted as the true definition of a mass disaster. In a way, mass disaster is said to occur when the *local infrastructure of death investigation is overwhelmed and is not capable of meeting the immediate requirements of the situation.* For instance, facilities may not be available to keep all bodies in local mortuaries (to keep them from rotting); there may not be enough staff to carry out investigations and deal with the concerned relatives; there may not be enough forensic pathologists to conduct the post-mortems on so many victims in a short time etc.

2. **C.**

3. **D.** ***Additional info*:** An example of "commorientes" is when a plane carrying hundreds of passengers crashes and everyone dies. In such a case, all people dying in the crash would be referred to as "commorientes".

   This is a situation having a special medicolegal significance, as the questions of inheritance etc would depend much on the knowledge of who died first. For instance if a wealthy childless couple, having not written their will, were travelling in a plane and it crashed, it would be important to know who died first. If the wife died first, the husband would have legally deemed to have passed on his wealth to his immediate relatives (such as his own brothers). But if he died first, his wife would be legally deemed to have acquired all his wealth just after his death. In that case the wealth would pass on to her relatives (e.g. her brothers). It can be appreciated from this situation that most countries have appropriate laws resolving such a situation.

4. **B.** ***Explanation and additional info*:** According to section 21 of *"The Hindu Succession Act, 1956"*, in such cases, the younger would be presumed to survive the elder, i.e. the younger person died later than the elder.

5. **A.** ***Related facts*:** Triage is a system used by medical or emergency personnel to ration limited medical resources (number of doctors, nurses, beds, medicines etc.) when the number of injured needing care exceeds the resources available to perform care so as to treat the greatest number of patients possible. When performed in accordance with accepted medical practices, triage is recognized and sanctioned by law in most countries.

   In warfare (and in several other situations involving mass disaster), there will always be some percentage of patients who will die regardless of medical care given to them, simply because their injuries are too extensive; they would perhaps live just for a few hours or days. Others will live given immediate medical care, but will die without it.

   In such extreme cases, any medical care given to people doomed to die is "care taken away" from people who might live if they had been given it. Triage involves sorting these patients out. Triage is used not just in warfare injuries. Any situation which gives rise to mass casualties (such as natural disasters, terroristic incidents etc.) will require an efficient triage system.

The word triage comes from the French word *trier*, which means "to sort". As we have seen above, triage indeed refers to sorting out wounded patients who can best be helped by the limited resources one has at hand. The concept of triage was begun by **Dominique Jean Larrey**, a famous French surgeon in Napoleon's army who devised a method to quickly evaluate and categorize the wounded in battle and then evacuate those requiring the most urgent medical attention. He instituted these practises while battle was in progress and triaged patients with no regard to rank.

MULTIPLE ANSWER TYPE (PGI, CHANDIGARH PATTERN)

6. **A,B,C,E.** ***Additional info*:** It is not the duty of forensic investigation to arrange for the funeral. Samples for toxicological analysis must be obtained, especially for alcohol and carbon monoxide.
7. **A,B,D,E.**
8. **B,E.** See the definition of mass disaster above. In a serial murder, typically the deaths occur at different times, so the question of overwhelming of local infrastructure does not arise. If 2-3 deaths are occurring in a local area, local infrastructure will be enough to meet the requirements of the situation, although the total number of deaths in a wide region may add up to hundreds. Choice (E) may be a mass disaster in a social or perhaps political sense, but NOT in the sense forensic pathologists understand.

5 Medicolegal Autopsy

GENERAL

1. The object of conducting a medicolegal autopsy is to find out:
A. The cause of death
B. The time since death
C. The manner of death
D. All of the above

2. Which of the following incisions is employed during a medicolegal autopsy?
A. Y-shaped
B. Modified Y-shaped
C. I-shaped
D. Any of the above

3. In Rokitansky technique of postmortem:
A. Organs are removed one by one
B. in-situ dissection is done
C. Thoracic and cervical organs, abdominal organs and the urogenital system are removed as separate organ blocks
D. Thoracic, cervical, abdominal and pelvic organs are removed as one large organ block

4. The actual dissection of the body during medicolegal autopsy should be carried out by:
A. The mortuary attendant
B. The mortuary technician
C. The forensic pathologist himself
D. Any of the above

5. To carry out a medicolegal autopsy, which one of the following is not an essential pre-requisite?
A. The consent of the relatives
B. The complete inquest report
C. Identification by the police officer accompanying the body
D. Identification by a relative or two accompanying the body

6. When a police officer or magistrate submits the dead body for postmortem to a doctor, generally it is implied that the autopsy would be done on:
A. The whole body
B. Only those parts which are injured
C. Only those parts which are not injured
D. Only those parts for which relatives give permission

7. After fixation in formalin, the weight of the brain:
A. Remains unchanged
B. Increases by about 5-10%
C. Decreased by about 5-10%
D. Increases in cases of males, and decreases in cases of females

8. Psychological autopsy is the name given to:
A. A detailed examination of brain, especially its limbic system

B. An attempt to reconstruct the dead person's psychological state prior to death
C. An autopsy at the scene of crime
D. Histological examination of the pineal gland

INTERNAL EXAMINATION

9. Which of the following valves has the largest circumference?
A. Tricuspid
B. Mitral
C. Aortic
D. Pulmonary

10. "Cardiac polyp" is a term used for postmortem:
A. Fibrinous clots in hearts
B. Aneurysms in heart
C. Infarcts in heart
D. Pale patches in heart

11. How best can you distinguish subarachnoid hemorrhage (SAH) from subdural hemorrhage (SDH)?
A. Subarachnoid hemorrhage is more clearly visible
B. Subdural hemorrhage is more clearly visible
C. Subdural hemorrhage can be washed off, while subarachnoid can not be
D. Subarachnoid hemorrhage can be washed off, while subdural can not be

12. On postmortem examination, metastases are most frequently encountered in:
A. Liver
B. Kidney
C. Brain
D. Bones

13. "Undertaker's fracture" is commonly seen in:
A. Skull
B. Cervical spine
C. Lumbar spine
D. Pelvis

PRESERVATION OF VISCERA IN POISONING

14. Saturated solution of common salt is not used as a preservative in
A. Corrosive poisoning
B. Organophosphorus poisoning
C. Arsenic poisoning
D. Lead poisoning

15. After postmortem examination, the body has to be handed over to the:
A. Investigating officer
B. Relatives
C. The authorities of the nearest crematorium or burial ground depending upon the religion of the dead person
D. Medical superintendent of the hospital in which the post mortem was conducted

16. About 6" of large bone is required to be preserved in:
A. Arsenic and antimony poisoning
B. Aconite poisoning
C. Datura poisoning
D. Smack poisoning

MULTIPLE ANSWER TYPE (PGI, CHANDIGARH PATTERN)

17. For fixation of brain for detailed study, which of the following steps are usually recommended?
A. The brain must be preserved in 10% formalin
B. Formalin should be injected in the substance of the brain through a 50 ml syringe from above, below and the two lateral sides
C. A long sagittal cut should be made through the corpus callosum
D. The brain should be suspended upside down, supported by a string passed under the basilar artery
E. The brain must be preserved in a mixture of acetone, ethylene glycol and zinc sulfate

ANSWERS

GENERAL

1. D.
2. D.
3. B. ***Related fact***: Remember the following four principal techniques:
   - **Technique of R. Virchow:** Organs are removed one by one.
   - **Technique of C. Rokitansky:** in-situ *dissection is done.*
   - **Technique of A. Ghon:** Thoracic and cervical organs, abdominal organs and the urogenital system are removed as separate organ blocks.
   - **Technique of M. Letulle:** Thoracic, cervical, abdominal and pelvic organs are removed as one large organ block.
4. C. ***Related facts:*** This is not a question of mere academic importance, and may carry severe legal repercussions. If the dissection is carried out by the mortuary attendant or the mortuary technician, and later the doctor tenders evidence in a court of law, he must specifically spell out to the court who carried out the actual dissection. Generally the doctor asserts on oath, that he conducted the post-mortem examination, which inherently means he himself carried out the dissection. If he did not actually carried out the dissection, it may amount to perjury.
5. A. ***Related fact***: Medicolegal autopsy is conducted to solve a specific question of law, and the consent of relatives is of no consequence. However in a different kind of autopsy—the hospital autopsy, or the pathological autopsy—which is done merely for research, the consent of relatives is a must.

   So before answering the question, do carefully read the question, and find out if the question is referring to a medicolegal autopsy or to a hospital autopsy.
6. A. ***Related facts***: By and large medicolegal autopsies are done on the whole body. In hospital autopsies, where autopsies are conducted only for academic reasons, limited autopsies may have to be done if relatives do not give consent for complete autopsies. Examples of limited autopsies are (i) Needle autopsy, where several tissues are sampled. This may be resorted to rarely even in medicolegal autopsies, when the body is highly infectious and proper infection precautions can not be taken (ii) endoscopic autopsies, where information about internal organs is obtained through an endoscope.
7. B.
8. B. ***Related facts:*** In many suspicious deaths it is essential to assess the mental state of the deceased prior to death. This is done by several methods, most important of which is to interview people who were known to him, such as his relatives, friends, employers and others. This is known as "psychological autopsy" or "psychiatric autopsy". Another name given to this technique is "reconstructive psychological evaluation". This technique is not yet popular in India, but quite popular in the US.

   Psychological autopsy is helpful to law enforcement agencies in several ways. For instance in the much publicized case of *State v Jones 1978*, a woman who killed her sleeping husband got away with a verdict of involuntary manslaughter (a much less serious charge than murder). A psychiatric autopsy done by an expert on her dead husband revealed that he used to batter his wife (the defendant) and on the night of the killing, her husband had even announced to her that he was going to kill their children before she woke up. The results of this psychological autopsy went in favor of the woman who got away with a much lesser sentence.

If a person has tried to commit suicide on a number of occasions before and his dead body is found in suspicious circumstances, it would be useful to know that he had suicidal tendencies.

INTERNAL EXAMINATION

9. **A.** ***Mnemonic***: Remember the word **TaMPA**, which is a place in Florida. **T**ricuspid, **M**itral, **P**ulmonary and **A**ortic valves have circumferences in this order. Actual circumferences:

Tricuspid →12 cm
Mitral →10 cm
Pulmonary →8.5 cm
Aortic →7.5 cm

Note that the differences are 2.0, 1.5 and 1.0 cm respectively. This is an easy series to remember because it is in Arithmetic Progression. The only figure to remember is the first one, i.e. 12 cm.

This question is relevant in forensic pathology, because by measuring the circumferences of the valves, we can say if the deceased was suffering from stenosis or regurgitation.

10. **A.** Cardiac polyp is the name given to two things: either a ball thrombus or a tumor attached by a pedicle to the inside of the heart.

11. **C.** ***Related fact***: This is so, because subarachnoid is covered with arachnoid membrane. Subdural is exposed after removal of skull and dura.

12. **A.** ***Related facts***: Liver is uniquely vulnerable to invasion by tumor cells. The reasons are (i) its big size (ii) its high rate of blood flow (iii) its double perfusion by hepatic artery and portal vein (iv) local tissue factors and endothelial membrane characteristics enhance metastatic implants.

Other related facts to remember are:

- Hepatic metastases have been reported at autopsy in 30-50% of patients dying from malignant disease.
- Metastatic malignant tumors of the liver are common in clinical practice, ranking second only to cirrhosis as a cause of fatal liver disease.
- In the United States, the incidence of clinically significant metastatic hepatic carcinoma is at least 20 times greater than that of primary carcinoma.
- Liver is the most common site of metastases (except for lymph nodes).
- Virtually all types of neoplasms except primaries in the brain may metastasize to the liver.

13. **B.** Undertaker's fracture is basically a post-mortem fracture, and occurs due to careless handling of the dead body by undertakers; in fact this fracture can be produced by anyone who has to do anything with the dead body. Pathologists are known to extend the head to make the removal of the neck structures easier. To do this, they usually insert a block about 10-15 cm high under the shoulders. If this is done carelessly, the neck may fall forcibly backwards, producing this fracture. It involves subluxation of the lower cervical spine due to tearing of the intervertebral disc at about C6-C7.

PRESERVATION OF VISCERA IN POISONING

14. A. ***Related facts***: Regarding preservation of viscera in cases of poisoning remember the following quick pointers:

- If analysis of viscera can be done within 48 hours, no preservative is needed at all.
- If analysis is expected to take longer time than this, samples may be sent in an insulated ice box with sufficient crushed ice, or alternatively preservatives may be used.
- Formalin should never be used as a preservative→Makes the extraction of poisons difficult, especially non-volatile organic compounds.
- Most common preservative (for viscera) used in India→Saturated solution of common salt.
- Saturated solution of common salt not used in→Acids (except carbolic acid where it can be used). In acid poisonings, use rectified spirit.
- In which poisonings you can not use rectified spirit as a preservative for viscera→Alcohol, phosphorus, acetic acid, phenol and paraldehyde.
- Should you send samples of preservatives separately? Yes. Why?→To rule out contamination.
- Preservative used for toxicological analysis of blood (10 ml)→30 mg potassium oxalate (anticoagulant) and 100 mg sodium fluoride (enzyme inhibitor). Remember that the preservative used when blood is taken for grouping is→equal quantity of 5% w/v solution of sodium citrate in water and 0.25% v/v formalin.
- In which poisonings you can not use the above preservative, i.e. potassium oxalate and sodium fluoride→(i) oxalic acid (ii) ethylene glycol (iii) fluoride (iv) carbon monoxide.
- Preservative used in oxalic acid and ethylene glycol→Use 30 mg sodium citrate in place of potassium oxalate.
- In cases of fluoride poisoning→use 10 gm of sodium nitrite in place of sodium fluoride.
- Why Heparin and EDTA should never be used as anticoagulants?→They interfere with the detection of methanol.
- How do you preserve blood in CO poisoning→Add a layer of 1-2 cm liquid paraffin (to avoid exposure to atmospheric oxygen).
- Blood for analysis should **never** be taken directly from the heart or scooped out of thoracic or abdominal cavities, since some poisons such as alcohol and barbiturate can diffuse passively from stomach and intestines into adjacent organs.
- Best site to collect blood for toxicological analysis is from→peripheral vein such as those in neck or limbs (femoral vein).
- Do not "milk" the limb while collecting the blood, since it can produce significant alterations in drug concentrations in the expressed blood.
- How much quantity of blood to be taken for toxicological analysis→10-20 ml.
- How much quantity of blood to be taken for grouping→2-3 ml.
- How to be taken (this 2-3 ml for grouping)→Prepare two blood stains with a diameter of about 5 cm each, on a sterile cloth and dry.

- What to take from putrefying bodies →CSF or vitreous humor.
- Why can't you take blood for toxicological analysis from putrefying bodies?→(i) difficult to collect (ii) post-mortem generation of alcohol as a result of putrefaction.
- How to know post-mortem synthesis of alcohol has occurred? → Alcohol is detected in blood but not in urine and vitreous humor (for more pointers, please see chapter 41–"Inebriant poisons").
- Synovial fluid from joints such as the knee can provide reliable estimates of alcohol concentrations in blood.
- In which poisonings do you preserve:
    - o CSF→Alcohol (how much to be preserved→As much as can be withdrawn).
    - o Brain→Alcohol, anaesthetics, barbiturates, CO, cyanides, opiates, strychnine (how much to be preserved → Half i.e. one hemisphere).
    - o Spinal cord→Gelsemine, strychnine (how much to be preserved→ Entire length).
    - o Lung→Inhaled poisons (how much to be preserved→One lung).
    - o Skin with underlying tissues→ Corrosives, injected poisons.
    - o Long bones (femur)—Heavy metals (how much to be preserved →10 cm length).
    - o Scalp hair→Heavy metals (how much to be preserved→15-20 strands).
- How do you preserve urine for toxicological analysis→Use any of these (i) add an equal quantity of saturated solution of common salt (ii) equal quantity of rectified spirit (iii) some fine grains of thymol (iv) one gm of sodium benzoate (v) 5 ml concentrated HCl (the last two for about 200-500 ml of urine).

15. A. It is important to remember that the doctor hands over the body to the investigating officer only (to the police in cases of police inquest and to the magistrate in cases of magisterial inquest). It is the investigating officer who passes on the body to the relatives. The relatives then take the body to the crematorium or burial ground.

Frequently—especially in bride burning deaths—the parties of both sides (maternal as well as in-laws) claim the dead body of the bride. The doctor does not decide whom to pass on the body to. He simply hands over the body to the investigating officer, and it is the I.O.'s problem to pass on the body further.

16. A. ***Related facts:*** This is because heavy metals are deposited in bones, especially long bones.

MULTIPLE ANSWER TYPE (PGI, CHANDIGARH PATTERN)

17. A,C,D. Formalin is NEVER injected in the brain for fixation. Sagittal cut should be made through the corpus callosum, as it facilitates the entry of formalin into the lateral ventricles. If it is not done, the brain starts putrefying from the inside, and presents a dark pinkish color on dissection. The solution mentioned in choice (E) is completely fictitious.

6 Examination of Decomposed and Mutilated Bodies, Fragmentary Remains, Bones, Etc.

GENERAL

1. Which of the following facts regarding identification of a putrefied and decomposed body is false?

A. Remnants of genital organs help to determine sex because they resist putrefaction

B. Peeled off skin cannot be used for fingerprinting

C. Hair, its color and dyeing when present can be used for identification

D. Body and dental X-rays are useful in identification

2. If a decomposed body has been brought by the police, which has earth and clothes stuck to it, with lots of maggots crawling around, what should the pathologist preferably do?

A. Put the body on flame to burn all maggots

B. Put the body in cold room and come back next day to dissect, so that all maggots crawl away

C. Put the body in a tank of weak carbolic acid for a day or two and then start dissection

D. Put the body in boiling water to kill the maggots

3. If the police brings only the peeled off skin of an individual, can the fingerprints be taken from it?

A. Yes

B. No

C. Yes but only in women

D. Yes but only if the skin was from the right hand

4. Lower end of femur can help to determine the:

A. Age and sex

B. Height and sex

C. Weight and sex

D. Only age

MULTIPLE ANSWER TYPE (PGI, CHANDIGARH PATTERN)

5. In a badly decomposed body, which of the following features would help in its identification?

A. Bones

B. Color of the iris

C. Hair

D. Teeth

E. Contours of cerebrum

6. Which of the following techniques can be used for determining the time of death of a badly decomposed/skeletonized body for medicolegal purposes?

A. Carbon-14 dating

B. Rigor mortis

C. Lead-210 dating

D. Cooling of the body

E. Polonium-210 dating

ANSWERS

GENERAL

1. **B.** Peeled off skin CAN be used for finger-printing
2. **C.** In such cases, the pathologist would preferably first take samples of maggots and insect eggs, and then put the body away in a tank containing weak carbolic acid (lysol) to soften the earth and get the clothing away without disintegration. A day of weak carbolic acid bath also kills the maggots making the subsequent dissection a lot easier.
3. **A.**
4. **A.** It is common knowledge that lower end of femur can help in age determination (e.g. by seeing whether the epiphysis has appeared or not, and whether it has united with the shaft or not). What is not commonly known is that it can be used to determine sex also. In fact four different features of femur can be used to determine sex. These are (i) Vertical diameter of the head (ii) Popliteal length (iii) Bicondylar width and (iv) Trochanteric oblique length as shown in the Table 6.1

Table 6.1: Major differences between female and a male femur

Criteria	Female	Male
Vertical diameter of head	<41.5 mm	>45.5 mm
Popliteal length	<106 mm	>145 mm
Bicondylar width	<72 mm	>78 mm
Trochanteric oblique length	<390 mm	>450 mm

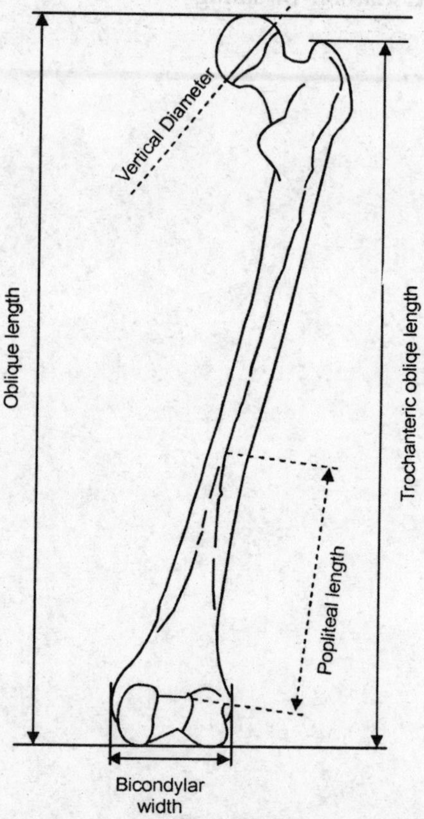

Fig. 6.1: Femur and its various forensically important dimensions

MULTIPLE ANSWER TYPE (PGI, CHANDIGARH PATTERN)

5. **A,C,D.** Color of the iris is not very helpful in identification in any case, least of all in decomposed bodies. Hair, their length, and their color, especially if they were dyed are helpful in identification. Bones can help in identification of sex, stature etc. Teeth are unique in each individual and are extremely valuable in identification.
6. **C,E.** C^{14} has a half life of 5,730 ± 40 years, which is very long as far as medicolegal cases are concerned (note that the question asks for dating *for medicolegal purposes*). Generally the police all over the world tend to use 75 years as cut-off point in murder

cases, after which it is unlikely the killer would still be alive. Thus a body which has been dead for more than 75 years is generally not important from a medico legal standpoint. With C^{14} dating having such a long half life, the minimum time of death that can be correctly determined is 500 years, which is hardly important in a medico legal sense. Radiocarbon dating is more useful in determining the age of archaeological specimens.

For medico legal purposes, isotopes with a far lesser half life are useful. Lead 210 has a half life of 22 years, and Polonium-210, just 138 days. Lead-210 is universally scattered in the human food chain and therefore all people have more or less constant quantities of lead-210 in their bodies. When a person stops eating (as after death), lead-210 starts to disintegrate and diminish. Polonium-210 too is universally scattered in the environment and is found in equal quantities in all humans. With Polonium-210, the forensic pathologist can fine-tune the date of death to within a fortnight.

7 Exhumation

1. **Which of the following is the correct definition of exhumation?**
   - **A.** Digging out of the body by the police after a criminal has murdered and buried it
   - **B.** Authorized removal of a dead person from his grave
   - **C.** Digging out of the body by grave diggers to sell it to anatomists
   - **D.** Both (A) and (B)
2. **An order for exhumation can be given by:**
   - **A.** District Magistrate
   - **B.** Inspector General of Police
   - **C.** Nearest relative of the deceased
   - **D.** Any of the above
3. **Which of the following regarding exhumation is correct?**
   - **A.** It is done in the presence of a police officer
   - **B.** It is done under the supervision of a medical officer
   - **C.** It can be done after a written order from a District Magistrate
   - **D.** All of the above
4. **For which of the following reasons can an exhumation be done?**
   - **A.** For establishing the identity of the deceased
   - **B.** To reestablish the cause of death, if some doubt occurs later
   - **C.** For civil purposes, such as compensation
   - **D.** For any of the above
5. **What is the time limit of exhumation in India?**
   - **A.** 10 years
   - **B.** 30 years
   - **C.** 35 years
   - **D.** No time limit
6. **The best time for exhumation is:**
   - **A.** Early morning
   - **B.** Late in the evening
   - **C.** Early night
   - **D.** Midnight
7. **Before exhumation, the grave is formally identified by:**
   - **A.** The police officer
   - **B.** The medical officer
   - **C.** The coroner
   - **D.** Warden of the cemetery

MULTIPLE ANSWER TYPE (PGI, CHANDIGARH PATTERN)

8. **Which of the following are genuine recognized artefacts produced due to exhumation?**

A. Fungal growth in and around body orifices—removal of this fungal growth leaves a discolored area, which may simulate bruising
B. Gastric hemorrhages produced due to long burial
C. Digging tools producing postmortem fractures
D. Retinal hemorrhages
E. Kidney stones

9. Exhumation may be done under which of the following circumstances?
A. Reestablishing the cause of his death
B. For paying annual homage to the deceased
C. For correct identification of the deceased
D. To allow friends to view the body
E. To rebury the remains at a different location

10. In all exhumations what should the doctor normally do?
A. He should never collect earth from around the coffin as it is considered a sacred site
B. He should collect earth from above and below the coffin
C. He should collect earth from all four sides of the coffin
D. He should collect earth from some distance away from the coffin as control samples
E. If the grave is waterlogged, he should take samples of water

ANSWERS

1. **B.** The correct definition of exhumation is choice (B) only. Choice (A) is not a correct choice, because in this case, the body was never given a proper legal burial in the first place. It is simply a case of digging out of the body by the police for investigation.
2. **A.** ***Related fact:*** **Other right choices in place of District Magistrate can be**: (i) Sub-divisional magistrate, (ii) Any executive magistrate especially empowered in this behalf by the State Government or the District Magistrate

   Other wrong choices: (i) A police officer (ii) SHO (iii) Civil Surgeon (iv) Villagers of the locality (v) Sarpanch of the locality
3. **D.**
4. **D.**
5. **D.**
6. **A.** Although law does not specify any time for exhumation, it is preferable to conduct exhumation early morning, so the whole process of digging, and autopsy if required, can be completed during the day.
7. **D.**

MULTIPLE ANSWER TYPE (PGI, CHANDIGARH PATTERN)

8. **A,C.** ***Additional info:*** Postmortem fractures produced by digging tools may be very difficult to differentiate from genuine antemortem fractures.
9. **A,C,E.** ***Related facts:*** Reestablishing the cause of death may become necessary, when at the time of death foul play was not suspected, but later new facts come to light that point to some foul play. Besides choices (A), (C) and (E), exhumation may sometimes also be ordered at the request of the family to recover an object placed inadvertently with the remains.
10. **B,C,D,E.** ***Related facts***: If some toxic substance such as arsenic is found in the body on subsequent autopsy, it may be alleged that it leached in the body from the surrounding ground. To disprove such allegations samples of earth from around the coffin must be taken. If the toxic substance is absent in the soil or is present in lesser concentration than in the body, such allegations can be discarded. Soil should also be taken from some distance away from the coffin as control samples.

8 The Pathophysiology of Death (Including Sudden and Unexpected Death)

THANATOLOGY

1. **Forensic thanatology deals with:**
   A. Study of maggots swarming the body after death
   B. Study of cooling of the body after death
   C. Medico legal study of death
   D. Suspended animation
2. **The traditional "tripod of life" dealt with functions of:**
   A. Brain, heart and lungs
   B. Brainstem, heart and lungs
   C. Brain, left heart and both lungs
   D. Heart, lungs and kidneys
3. **Magnus test was used in the 19th Century to detect the stoppage of function of:**
   A. Lungs
   B. Heart
   C. Brain
   D. Both brain and heart
4. **Icard's test was once used to detect the stoppage of function of:**
   A. Brain
   B. Lungs
   C. Diaphragm
   D. Heart
5. **Winslow's test was once used to detect the stoppage of:**
   A. Brain function
   B. Liver function
   C. Respiration
   D. Circulation
6. **Which of the following is NOT a test of circulation?**
   A. Magnus test
   B. Icard's test
   C. Winslow test
   D. Diaphanous test
7. **"Tower of silence" is used by .... to dispose off dead body:**
   A. Muslims
   B. Parsees
   C. Buddhists
   D. Nagas
8. **Somatic death is said to occur when:**
   A. All individual cells of the person die
   B. The person is dead clinically, although many of his individual cells may still be functional
   C. The heart stops beating permanently
   D. The person is on artificial life support system

9. Zsako's phenomenon is the name given to:
- **A.** Dilation of pupils just after somatic death
- **B.** Growing of hair after death
- **C.** Contraction of the quadriceps femoris muscle on mechanical stimulation just after somatic death
- **D.** Cheyne-Stokes respiration observed just before death in many cases

10. What is the surest sign of death?
- **A.** Cadaveric lividity
- **B.** Cadaveric spasm
- **C.** Adipocere
- **D.** Putrefaction

SUSPENDED ANIMATION

11. Which of the following is the correct definition of suspended animation?
- **A.** It is the period of first 2 hours after death, i.e. when somatic death has occurred, but molecular death has not occurred
- **B.** It is a state when signs of life are not found, although the person is alive
- **C.** It is the name given to the position of the dead body in cases of hanging
- **D.** It is the name given to the time period during which a doctor is not allowed to conduct autopsies because of some temporary disability

MODERN CONCEPT OF THE MOMENT OF DEATH

12. According to the modern concept of the moment of death, death is said to occur ONLY when there is complete stoppage of the function of:
- **A.** Tripod of life
- **B.** Brain cortex and thalamus
- **C.** Brain stem
- **D.** Heart

13. Which of the following modes of death is duly recognized by *The Transplantation of Human Organs Act, 1994*?
- **A.** Whole brain death
- **B.** Brain stem death
- **C.** Extinction of the tripod of life
- **D.** Complete cessation of respiration

NEGATIVE AND OBSCURE AUTOPSY

14. Which of the following is called a negative autopsy?
- **A.** When the relatives of the deceased refuse to allow postmortem examination
- **B.** When the relatives of the deceased want a postmortem examination but the magistrate finds nothing wrong in his inquest and so does not order an autopsy
- **C.** When gross and microscopic examination, toxicological analysis and laboratory investigations fail to reveal a cause of death
- **D.** When the autopsy is conducted in the presence of the defense lawyer

15. What is the usual percentage of negative autopsies?
- **A.** <0.01%
- **B.** 2-5%
- **C.** 10-15%
- **D.** 20-30%

SUDDEN AND UNEXPECTED DEATH

16. The most frequent site of coronary occlusion is:
- **A.** Left anterior descending
- **B.** Right main coronary
- **C.** Left circumflex
- **D.** Left main coronary

17. A patient with myocardial infarction, after death, underwent autopsy. Microscopic examination of the cardiac tissue as part of autopsy revealed granulation tissue. The time from infarction till death is most likely to be:

A. < 24 hrs
B. < 2 hrs
C. < 10 days
D. < 1 month

18. Most common cause of sudden death due to CNS lesions is:

A. Subarachnoid or intracerebral haemorrhage
B. Meningitis
C. Encephalitis
D. Tumors of the fourth ventricle

MULTIPLE ANSWER TYPE (PGI, CHANDIGARH PATTERN)

19. Which of the following tests were once used to detect stoppage of circulation?

A. Diaphanous test
B. Feather test
C. Fingernail pressure test
D. Mirror test
E. Icard's test

20. Which of the following tests were once used to detect the stoppage of respiration?

A. Feather test
B. Diaphanous test
C. Mirror test
D. Magnus test
E. Icard's test

21. A negative autopsy may be due to the following reasons:

A. Lack of training of the doctor
B. When the body is that of a very young child
C. Inadequate history taking
D. When the body is of a eunuch
E. Inadequate external examination

ANSWERS

THANATOLOGY

1. C.
2. A. Classically it was believed that a person can be considered dead only when his three vital organs had stopped working. These were brain, heart and lungs. Life was considered in a way "standing" on these three vital organs. So they came to be known as the "tripod of life".
3. B. *Related fact*: Magnus test was suggested by an Italian Ugo Magnus in 1879. It was a test to see the stoppage of circulation. The test consisted of tying a string around one of the fingers of the supposedly dead man. The pressure applied had to be just above that in venous channels, but just below that in arterial channels. This would occlude the venous channels but not the arterial channels. If the circulation was still maintained the finger distal to the ligature would swell.

   Although stethoscope had been discovered by Laënnec in 1816, it was still very basic in design, and it could not be used reliably to listen to heart sounds, especially if it was beating very feebly. Magnus test was in vogue for sometime, but is now completely outdated.
4. D. *Related facts*: Icard's test was suggested by Dr. Séverin Icard of France in 1895. It was another test of circulation. It consisted of subcutaneous injection of a strongly fluorescent compound. If the circulation was still going on, the whole skin would turn a vivid yellow. This phenomenon would last until the compound had been completely metabolized. It was suggested that the test should be conducted only in daylight, as the yellow color was difficult to appreciate in the artificial light. The fluorescent compound which was usually employed was fluorescein with sodium bicarbonate.

   If the person was already dead, no such change would be seen. This test is completely outdated now.
5. C. *Related facts*: This test was suggested by the Danish physician Jacques-Bénigne Winslow. It consisted of keeping a small pot containing water or mercury over the thoraco-abdominal region (usually just at or below xiphisternum). A ray of light was allowed to fall over the liquid. If the respiration was taking place, the ray of light (over the surface of the liquid) would appear to move. This test is also outdated.

   The three tests—Magnus, Icard and Winslow—however weird they may appear today, were once widely accepted. They gained prominence because the stethoscope had not been developed fully and in cases of suspended animation, one could easily mistake a living person for dead.
6. C. For explanations, see answers to questions above.
7. B. *Related facts*: Known also as "*dakhma*", the "tower of silence" is a Parsi funerary tower erected on a hill for the disposal of the dead according to the Zoroastrian rite. Such towers are about 25 feet (8 m) high, built of brick or stone, and contain gratings on which the corpses are exposed. After vultures have picked the bones clean, they fall into a pit below. This fulfils their belief that a corpse must not suffer contact with either fire or earth.

8. **B.** ***Related facts*****:** Somatic death is also known as systemic or clinical death. Many of his individual cells may still be functional. For instance many WBCs in his blood may still display phagocytic activity or many spermatozoa in his seminal vesicles may still be motile. 2-3 hours after somatic death, all cells of the deceased stop functioning. This stage is known as *cellular* or *molecular death.* The period between somatic death and molecular death is known as *supravital period.*

9. **C.** ***Related facts*****:** Just after somatic death and before molecular death (i.e. within the supravital period), it is possible to show in a number of ways that individual cells are still functional. One of these ways was first described by Zsako and is known after him as Zsako's phenomenon (also known as Tendon reaction). It is elicited as follows: the lower third of the quadriceps femoris muscle is struck with a reflex hammer about 4-5 fingerbreadths (about 10 cms) above the patella. The patella moves upwards because of the contraction of the quadriceps femoris muscle. Another similar test is *idiomuscular contraction* (bulge). It was first described by Dotzauer and Prokop. The biceps brachii muscle is struck with the back of a knife. It causes a muscular bulge at the point of contact due to local contracture of the muscle.

10. **D.** This is the generally accepted answer from the student, but at the outset, it may be mentioned that it is a highly controversial question, its only *raison d'etre* being it has been asked so many times in examinations. The answer is equally controversial (even absurd!) and a little background may be in order. From 16th till 18th centuries, there had been a number of instances when seemingly dead people had come back to life, often during their journey to the graveyard. The reasons can only be surmised now, but some plausible reasons could be (i) they were rich people and their greedy nephews and nieces were only too eager to bury them without ensuring they were really dead (ii) in those times medical profession was not fully regulated, and the death was pronounced by medically unqualified people, and finally (iii) they were cases of suspended animation.

So common had these instances become that people were very afraid of premature burial [The American short-story writer and poet Edgar Allan Poe (1809-1849) wrote a classic story entitled "The Premature Burial" based on this theme in 1844]. In order to bring about burial reforms, the Danish anatomist Jacques-Bénigne Winslow (1669-1760) [of "foramen of Winslow" and "Winslow's test" fame] published a thesis (in Latin) in 1740. Entitled *Morte incertae signa*, it argued that the traditional signs of death (such as stoppage of heart beat and respiration) were not infallible, and the only surest sign of death was putrefaction! (It is significant that earlier he himself had prescribed the so called Winslow's test for differentiating life from death; this is a test of respiration). His work was later translated in French by Jean-Jacques Bruhier d'Ablaincourt (1685-1756). He carried the reasoning of Winslow further and even suggested that Jesus Christ would never have been capable of raising Lazarus from the dead, if the onset of putrefaction had been awaited before the man was declared dead. In 1745, he presented before Louis XV, the then king of France, an audacious proposal of building a system of morgues, or receiving houses for the dead, where each corpse would be watched by competent physicians for at least 72 hours, till they putrefied! If there was "life" in any of those corpses, they would come to life well before this period. Although King Louis XV did not implement this system in France, it did find favour in several other European countries, where such systems of "waiting mortuaries" were indeed built.

Needless to say, this method has no place in modern medicine. This question appears to be a relic from the remote past. There is no reason why other choices, say, adipocere can not be a sure sign of death. But the intended choice is "putrefaction" and hopefully with this background the student can understand why.

SUSPENDED ANIMATION

11. B.

MODERN CONCEPT OF THE MOMENT OF DEATH

12. C.

13. B. ***Related facts***: *The Transplantation of Human Organs Act* 1994, recognized the latest concept of the moment of death, i.e. the death of the brain stem. Section 2(d) of this Act defines "brain-stem death" as "the stage at which all functions of the brain-stem have permanently and irreversibly ceased". According to section 3(5) of the same Act, before removal of organs for transplantation, the doctor must satisfy himself that brain-stem death had occurred. Furthermore the brain-stem death has to be certified by a team of doctors under section 3(6).

NEGATIVE AND OBSCURE AUTOPSY

14. C.

15. B.

SUDDEN AND UNEXPECTED DEATH

16. A. ***Related Fact***: Actual incidences are LAD→45-64%; Right main coronary→24-46%; left circumflex→3-10%, and Left main coronary→0-10%. It has been said that the incidence at left anterior descending (also called anterior interventricular artery) is more than the combined incidence in all other parts of the coronary system.

17. C. ***Related fact***: The changes are:

3-6 hours: Visibly not differentiable. Depletion of oxidative enzymes. Dip the slice of heart in Triphenyl-tetrazolium chloride (TTC), normal area red brown, infarcted areas unstained pale zone.

6-12 hours: Slight pallor. By and large undifferentiable to the naked eye.

18-24 hours: Appears gray-brown to the naked eye, contrasting with the surrounding normal red-brown myocardium.

2-4 days: Necrotic focus is sharply defined. Hyperemic, quite irregular border. This irregularity of the border is because of the interdigitating pattern of vascular supply. Central portion is distinctly yellow-brown and soft, owing to the onset of fatty change.

4-10 days: Infarct is clearly distinguishable. Varies from yellow-gray to bright yellow, with the progression of fatty change. The central necrotic tissue is maximally soft and often contains areas of hemorrhage. Margins intensely red and highly vascularized.

10th day onwards: Progressive replacement of the necrotic muscle by the ingrowth of fibrous, vascularized scar tissue.

6th week (end of): Scarring is well advanced. Time for total replacement depends on the size of the original infarct.

18. A.

MULTIPLE ANSWER TYPE (PGI, CHANDIGARH PATTERN)

19. A,C,E. ***Related facts***: Diaphanous test consisted of bringing before bright light the hand of a supposedly dead person. The fingers were outstretched, and the bright light allowed to fall over the webs between the fingers. If the person was alive, the circulation would still be continuing; consequently the webs would appear translucent and reddish in appearance. If the person was dead and his circulation had stopped, the webs would appear opaque and yellowish.

Fingernail pressure test consisted of applying firm pressure over the fingernails. If circulation was continuing, the fingernails would become pale on application of pressure, but would resume normal reddish appearance on release of pressure. No such changes would be visible in a dead man.

All these tests are obsolete now.

20. A,C. ***Related facts*****:** Feather test was as straightforward test consisting of holding before the nostrils a fine feather or a fine cotton fibre. If respiration was continuing, the feather would be seen to flicker. Mirror test consisted of placing a mirror over the front of the nose or mouth of the supposedly dead person. If the person was still alive the mirror would turn hazy due to deposition of moisture on the mirror. No such change would be seen in a dead man.

Both these tests are obsolete now.

21. A,C,E. ***Related facts*****:** Lack of a proper training of the doctor is an obvious reason for negative autopsy. In some cases such as deaths due to extreme emotion (such as sudden fright), death may occur as a result of vagal inhibition. Such cases may not show any pathological finding whatsoever, and unless an adequate history was taken, the case would be reported a case of negative autopsy. Similarly in cases of deaths due to insect bites (especially if they were at odd places) a lack of an adequate external examination may result in a negative autopsy.

9 Postmortem Changes and Time Since Death (Including Presumption of Death and Survivorship)

CHANGES AFTER DEATH

General

1. **"Rail-roading", an immediate sign of death is seen in:**
   A. Retina
   B. The region of the heart
   C. Cornea
   D. Anterior capsule of the lens

2. **Suggilation is a term synonymous with:**
   A. Cooling of the body
   B. Postmortem staining
   C. Rigor mortis
   D. Cadaveric spasm

3. ***Tache noir de la sclérotiques* are seen within .... of death on ....**
   A. 1 hour, nasal septum
   B. 3 hours, sclera
   C. 6 hours, lungs
   D. 24 hours, gastric mucosa

4. **Honeycombing is seen in liver in cases of:**
   A. Cirrhosis
   B. Early development of postmortem staining
   C. Putrefaction
   D. Hydatid disease

Cooling of the Body

5. **Cooling of the body is also known as:**
   A. Rigor mortis
   B. Livor mortis
   C. Algor mortis
   D. Colliquative putrefaction

6. **Rate of cooling helps in determining:**
   A. Time of death
   B. Manner of death
   C. Place of death
   D. Cause of death

7. **Postmortem caloricity is:**
   A. Temperature remaining constant after death
   B. Temperature decreasing after death
   C. Temperature increasing after death
   D. Temperature first sharply falling and then sharply rising after death

8. **In which of the following conditions post-mortem caloricity may be seen?**
   A. Massive haemorrhage in the liver
   B. Cyanide poisoning
   C. Corrosive poisoning
   D. Septicemia

9. **A dead body of a male is found lying in a courtyard on 25 June at 5.30 am. Its rectal**

temperature is 91.0^{0}F. What is the approximate time of death?
A. 8.30 pm on 23 June
B. 4.00 pm on 24 June
C. 7.30 pm on 24 June
D. 1.00 am on 25 June

Livor Mortis

10. **Red brown p.m. staining is seen in**
A. Dhatura
B. Cyanide
C. CO
D. Aniline dyes

11. **Which of the following names is given to tiny, spot-like, oval-to-round, bluish black hemorrhages of postmortem origin?**
A. Vibices
B. Postmortem ecchymoses
C. Death spots
D. All of the above

12. **Postmortem lividity is unlikely to develop in a case of**
A. Drowning in a well
B. Drowning in a fast flowing river
C. Postmortem submersion
D. Drowning in a chlorinated swimming pool

Rigor Mortis / Allied Conditions

13. **Primary relaxation occurs:**
A. After rigor mortis has fully set in
B. Just after death
C. After putrefaction
D. After postmortem staining has fully appeared and established itself

14. **Rigor mortis first starts in:**
A. Eyelids
B. Gluteus maximus
C. Neck muscles
D. Trapezius

15. **Rigor is initiated when the ATP concentration falls to:**
A. 15% of the normal
B. 45% of the normal
C. 65% of the normal
D. 85% of the normal

16. **Which of the following facts about Cadaveric spasm is NOT CORRECT?**
A. It is instantaneous in onset
B. It is confined to a small group of muscles
C. It occurs only in voluntary muscles
D. It shows that the person was sleeping at the time of his death

17. **Rigidity of the muscles is at maximum when the level declines to:**
A. 15% of the normal
B. 45% of the normal
C. 65% of the normal
D. 70% of the normal

18. **During rigor mortis, the reaction of the muscle changes from:**
A. Slightly acidic to distinctly alkaline
B. Slightly alkaline to distinctly acidic
C. Strongly acidic to weakly acidic
D. Strongly alkaline to weakly alkaline

19. **In rigor mortis, the muscle:**
A. Just stiffens but does not shorten
B. Shortens but does not stiffen
C. Both stiffens and shortens
D. Stiffens and lengthens

20. **Which of the following is the Nysten's law?**
A. Cadaveric rigidity does not appear in living people
B. Cadaveric rigidity appears faster in older and the young than in the middle age
C. Cadaveric rigidity occurs in men earlier than in the women
D. Cadaveric rigidity affects successively the masticatory muscles, those of the face

and the neck, those of the trunk and arms and finally those of the lower limbs

21. **In electrocution, rigor mortis:**
    - **A.** Appears late but passes quickly
    - **B.** Appears late and passes late
    - **C.** Appears early and passes early
    - **D.** Never appears

22. **Sommer's movements are:**
    - **A.** Involuntary tetanic movements of muscles just before death
    - **B.** Continuation of beating of the heart for about 5 minutes after death
    - **C.** Changing of position of limbs after death allegedly due to contraction of muscles due to rigor mortis
    - **D.** Involuntary tetanic movements of muscles just after death

23. **Which of the following statements about rigor mortis in a fetus is correct?**
    - **A.** It does not appear in a fetus less than seven months of age
    - **B.** It does appear but may be so feeble as to be unappreciable
    - **C.** It appears in upper limbs but not in lower limbs
    - **D.** It appears in lower limbs but not in upper limbs

24. **Breaking of rigor mortis usually occurs during:**
    - **A.** Routine inspection of the body
    - **B.** Transportation of the body
    - **C.** Preservation of the body in cold chamber
    - **D.** Opening of the skull

25. **Immediate rigidity of a group of muscles without passing into a stage of primary relaxation is called:**
    - **A.** Cadaveric spasm
    - **B.** Instantaneous rigor
    - **C.** Rigor mortis
    - **D.** Both a and b above

Putrefaction

26. **Color changes of putrefaction are first observed in:**
    - **A.** Right iliac fossa
    - **B.** Left iliac fossa
    - **C.** Popliteal fossa
    - **D.** Cubital fossa

27. **Which of the following facts regarding putrefaction of internal organs is NOT correct?**
    - **A.** Softer organs putrefy earlier
    - **B.** Organs which contain more blood putrefy earlier
    - **C.** Organs nearer to the source of bacteria putrefy earlier
    - **D.** Organs composed of less muscular and fibrous tissue putrefy earlier

28. **Which of the following facts regarding putrefaction is NOT correct?**
    - **A.** Putrefaction is arrested below 0°C
    - **B.** Putrefaction is arrested above 48°C
    - **C.** Rate of decomposition is about twice as rapid in summer as in winter
    - **D.** Bodies of males putrefy faster than that of females

29. **Putrefaction is delayed in:**
    - **A.** Organophosphorus poisoning
    - **B.** HCl
    - **C.** Carbolic acid
    - **D.** Oxalic acid

30. **Marbling appears .... after death:**
    - **A.** 4-6 hours
    - **B.** 36-48 hours
    - **C.** 3-4 days
    - **D.** One week

31. **Which of the following is the Casper's dictum?**
    - **A.** Time taken for same amount of putrefaction to occur when the body is

in air, water and buried in earth is in the ratio of 1:2:8
B. Body putrefies fastest when buried in earth
C. Postmortem lividity does not appear when the body is buried immediately after birth
D. Rigor mortis does not appear in water

32. The correct sequence of putrefaction (earliest to last) of the internal organs is:
A. Brain-Heart-Spleen-Kidney
B. Heart-Spleen-Uterus-Brain
C. Heart-Trachea-Bone-Uterus
D. Stomach-Brain-Kidney-tendons

33. Which of the following organs is the last to putrefy in males?
A. Seminal vesicles
B. Prostate
C. Testes
D. Liver

34. Which of the following organs is the last to putrefy in females?
A. Spleen
B. Ovary
C. Fallopian tubes
D. Uterus

35. Mummification refers to:
A. Hardening of muscles after death
B. Colliquative putrefaction
C. Saponification of subcutaneous fat
D. Desiccation of the dead body

36. Mummification is likely to occur in which of the following environment?
A. Cold and dry
B. Warm and dry, with hot air blowing constantly
C. Cold and humid, with icy cold winds blowing
D. Warm and humid, with humid air blowing

37. In favorable circumstances, how much time will be taken by a body to mummify completely?
A. 1-2 days
B. 1-2 weeks
C. 3 months to a year
D. 3 years to 10 years

38. In India, colliquative putrefaction is seen after about:
A. 10-15 minutes
B. 24 hours
C. 72 hours
D. 1 week

39. Adipocere is likely to occur in:
A. Warm humid climate
B. Dry hot climate
C. Subzero humid climate
D. Bodies buried in sandy soil

40. Which of the following is NOT an optimal condition for the formation of adipocere?
A. Abundance of moisture
B. Absence of bacteria
C. Warm temperature
D. Abundance of adipose tissue

41. Entomology of cadaver helps best in determining:
A. Time since death
B. Mode of death
C. Manner of death
D. Identity of the deceased

42. Which of the following statements is true about adipocere?
A. It is due to dehydration of subcutaneous tissues
B. It is due to hydogenation of subcutaneous fat
C. It is formed first in the epidermal tissues
D. It is retarded by heat and accelerated by cold

Other Changes

43. Sturner's formula to calculate the time since death takes into account which of the following parameters?

A. Sodium concentration in the vitreous humor
B. Potassium concentration in the vitreous humor
C. Chloride concentration in the vitreous humor
D. Potassium concentration in the pericardial fluid

Presumption of Death and Survivorship

44. If a person is not seen for some time, the law presumes that he is alive, if it is shown that he was alive within a certain number of years, and the burden of proving that he is dead shifts on the person who affirms it. He must be shown alive within how many years?
A. 4 years
B. 7 years
C. 15 years
D. 30 years

45. If a person is not heard of for a certain number of years by those who would naturally have heard of him, he is supposed to have been dead, and the burden of proving that he is alive shifts on the person who affirms it. For how many years, he should not have been heard of?
A. 4 years
B. 7 years
C. 15 years
D. 30 years

MULTIPLE ANSWER TYPE (PGI, CHANDIGARH PATTERN)

46. From the color of postmortem staining, one can usually know the poison involved if it is:
A. Carbon monoxide
B. Hydrocyanic acid
C. Arsenic
D. Marking nut
E. Nitrobenzene

47. Postmortem luminescence in a decaying body is due to:
A. Photobacterium fischeri
B. Entamoeba coli
C. Armillaria mellea
D. Clostridium welchii
E. Formation of methane

48. Which of the following facts are NOT correct?
A. Onset of rigor is accelerated and its duration shortened when the environmental temperature is high
B. Rigor mortis is late in onset and is of longer duration after prolonged muscular activity
C. Onset is relatively more rapid in children and the aged than in muscular young adults
D. It develops early and passes quickly in deaths from septicaemia or from wasting diseases
E. It is delayed in asphyxial deaths, notably by hanging or carbon monoxide poisoning, and also when death has been immediately preceded by severe haemorrhage

ANSWERS

CHANGES AFTER DEATH

General

1. **A.** ***Related facts*:** Many workers believe that just after brain death, if one examines the retina with an ophthalmoscope, one can see segmentation of the retinal blood columns. Groups of red cells within retinal vessels are seen to move in either direction at random and collide with each other. Since this movement has been likened to the movement of unbraked wagons of a goods train when it stops, it is known as rail-roading (or trucking).

2. **B.** The term "suggilate" in English means "to beat black and blue". Since postmortem staining has a similar color, the term "suggilation" is sometimes used to denote it. Other terms synonymous with postmortem staining are: (i) postmortem hypostasis (ii) subcutaneous hypostasis (iii) livor mortis (iv) cadaveric lividity and (v) darkening of death. Vibices are tiny spots often seen within the area of postmortem staining. These form because of postmortem mechanical rupture of subcutaneous capillaries and smaller vessels—predominantly veins. For a related question, see below.

3. **B.** *Tache noir de la sclérotique* are nothing but two yellow triangles of desiccated discoloration. These appear on each side of the cornea, with their bases resting on the circumference and apices jutting into the inner and outer canthi (Fig. 9.1). Later these become brown and then black. They indicate that the eyes were open after death.

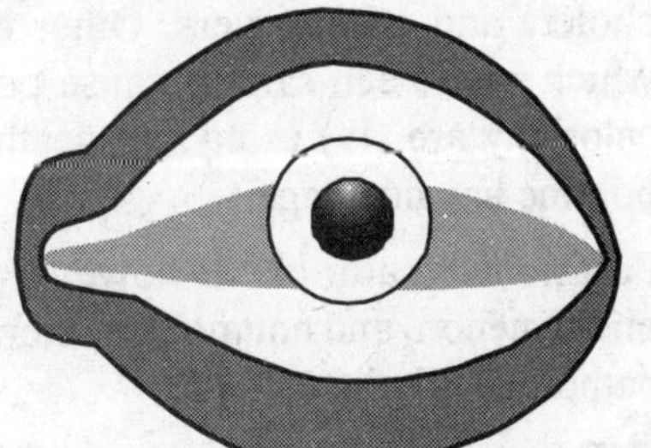

Fig. 9.1: *Tache noir de la schérotique.* These are seen as light brown triangular dried up areas on both sides of the cornea. They are usually seen when eyes remain open after death

4. **C.** During putrefaction, there is production of minute gas bubbles within the substance of the liver. This causes an appearance popularly known as honeycombing of the liver. Sometimes also referred to as "foamy liver". In fact same question has been asked in this form→ Foamy liver is seen in (a) Putrefaction (b) Drowning (c) Mummification (d) Adipocere. The answer is (a).

Cooling of the Body

5. **C.**
6. **A.**
7. **C.** ***Related facts*:** It has been classically asserted—albeit without much undisputed evidence—that in some cases the temperature of the body *increases* for the first two hours after death instead of decreasing. The classical conditions which have been said to cause postmortem caloricity are (i) disorders where regulation of heat production has been severely disturbed before death, e.g.

sunstroke (ii) when there was great increase in heat production during life due to convulsions, e.g. tetanus and strychnine poisoning and (iii) when there was great bacterial activity such as in septicaemia, cholera and other fevers. Other conditions which have been said to cause postmortem caloricity are (iv) asphyxial deaths and (v) pontine haemorrhage.

Postmortem caloricity is however a debated phenomenon, and not many modern forensic pathologists believe in it.

8. **D. For details, see answer to Q.7.**

Variant: A variant is often asked like this: The following situations are associated with rise of temperature after death except (a) Burns (b) Heat stroke (c) Pontine haemorrhage (d) Septicaemia. The expected answer is (a). It has been traditionally believed that the temperature of the body should increase after death in other three conditions, although a convincing scientific reason has never been offered. The authenticity of this fact is very much doubtful.

9. **C.** This is a rather tricky question. In such types of questions, first of all the student must see the date given in the question. This will tell us the season. In the given question, we know that it is summer. Had it been, say, 25 December, we would know it is winter.

In India, generally the fall in rectal temperature occurs like this:

In summers→0.75°F/hour.

In winters→1.5°F/hour.

In the given case, since it is the summer season, the body would cool 0.75°F/hour.

We would assume that the rectal temperature at the time of death was 98.5°F (To be exact it is 98.4°F, but assuming it to be 98.5°F will make matters simpler for us, without compromising too much on accuracy).

The loss of rectal temperature is 98.5°F–91.0°F→7.5°F.

Since in summers the body cools 0.75°F/hour, the body must be lying dead for 7.5°F/0.75°F or 10 hours.

The time of discovery of body is 25 June at 5.30 am. We subtract 10 hours from this, and we get 7.30 pm on 24 June.

Additional facts: After death, the body cools obeying the Newton's law of cooling, which states, "For a body cooling in a draft (i.e., by forced convection), the rate of heat loss is proportional to the difference in temperatures between the body and its surroundings."

> It is worth noting that this method can be used not only to determine time of death of an individual, but to determine the time period of virtually *any system* that cools.
>
> One can easily use this method to determine, say, when a cup of coffee was prepared. This method can similarly be used on systems that cool much more slowly (such as a body of lava or magma, which may take years to cool). In fact, Lord Kelvin attempted to use this method to date the age of the earth! However, because many of his assumptions were incorrect, he found an age of 24,000,000 years, which falls far short of the currently-accepted value.

Livor Mortis

10. **D.** ***Related fact*:** It is due to the formation of methemoglobin. Other poisons causing similar color are nitrites, nitrates, chlorates, potassium bicarbonate and nitrobenzene. Other colors of postmortem staining and their associated conditions are:

Table 9.1: Colors of postmortem staining in various poisonings

Color	Death by
Cherry red	Carbon monoxide
Bright red, pink	Cyanide

Most books taught in this country would have us believe that postmortem staining is dark brown in phosphorus, bluish green in hydrogen sulphide and almost black in opiates. This is erroneous.

11. **D.** All the three names mentioned above have been given to these tiny spots, which form because of postmortem mechanical rupture of subcutaneous capillaries and smaller vessels–predominantly veins. After death, blood pools up in the most dependent parts of the body, causing increased intravascular pressure in the capillaries of these regions. This is the main cause of the rupture. Vibices are thus formed in most dependent parts of the body.

12. **B.** For postmortem lividity to develop, the dead body must be in a fixed position for some length of time. Since in a fast flowing river, the body would keep turning about, it is difficult for postmortem lividity to develop.

Rigor Mortis / Allied Conditions

13. **B.** ***Additional info:*** Just after death all muscles are relaxed (primary relaxation). Soon they pass into rigor mortis. When the rigor mortis passes off, the muscles are relaxed once again. This is known as the stage of *secondary relaxation.*

14. **A.** ***Related fact***: Rigor mortis appears first in involuntary muscles followed by voluntary muscles. The first organ traditionally thought to undergo rigor mortis is heart. Within voluntary muscles, rigor mortis typically has a proximo-distal progression, i.e. it starts in the facial muscles and then spreads down – to neck, upper limbs and lower limbs in that order. Some questions will give "upper eyelids" and "lower eyelids" as two separate choices. These can not be regarded as ideal questions (because the rigor mortis starts in both eyelids almost simultaneously), but if they are encountered, the intended choice is "upper eyelids".

    Variant: A variant is often asked like this— Rigor mortis first starts in (a) Right iliac fossa (b) Left iliac fossa (c) Brain (d) Heart. The correct answer to this question is (d) Heart.

15. **D.**

16. **D.**

17. **A.**

18. **B.** ***Related facts***: This is owing to the local formation of pyruvic and lactic acids:

    - Lactic acid content of resting muscle during life is→0.03%.
    - Lactic acid content when rigor mortis occurs is→0.5% (more than 10 times).

    It is said that the cellular pH falls to around 6 after death. According to some authorities, this fall in pH actually causes rigor mortis by causing coagulation of the actinomyosin.

19. **C.** ***Related fact***: The stiffening is the more prominent change. Shortening is there but is not very prominent. Shortening in various organs can cause different phenomena. It is useful to remember them:

    - Rigor in iris→causes pupil to change in size, making its postmortem position an unreliable indicator of toxic or neurological conditions during life.
    - Rigor in heart→may be mistaken for ventricular hypertrophy (can be resolved by measuring total weight of the heart).
    - Rigor in dartos, seminal vesicles, prostate →postmortem extrusion of semen from urethral meatus.
    - Rigor in erector pili muscles→pimpling or "goose-flesh" appearance of the skin. May also give a false impression that the beard grows after death.

- Rigor in pregnant uterus→may cause postmortem delivery.

20. **D.** ***Related fact***: Pierre-Hubert Nysten (1774-1817), a French pediatrician/pathologist, was the first to investigate rigor mortis, in 1811. His Law (or Rule) states that rigor mortis begins in the head area, and slowly descends down the body.

21. **C.**

22. **C.** ***Related fact:*** There have been semi-apocryphal tales of dead changing the position of their limbs after death. In 1833, this was attributed by Sommer to contraction of muscles after death due to rigor mortis. Since then these movements have been known as Sommer's movements.

23. **B.** ***Additional info:*** Many books in the past have suggested that rigor mortis does not appear in a fetus below seven months of age. This is a complete myth, and there is absolutely no reason, why it shouldn't. Rigor mortis is due to the formation of actinomyosin and it can form in a fetus as completely and efficiently as in an adult. Perhaps the only reason this myth gained ground is that the rigor mortis in infants is very feeble and difficult to appreciate. Another reason could be that rigor mortis in a fetus appears and passes off very early.

24. **B.**

25. **D.**

Putrefaction

26. **A.** ***Related fact***: Right iliac fossa is affected first, as caecum is located there. Putrefactive bacteria form hydrogen sulfide there, which converts haemoglobin into sulphmethemoglobin, which is greenish in color. Thus the first change is greenish discoloration of right iliac fossa.

27. **D.** Organs composed of muscular tissue and those containing large amount of fibrous tissue resist putrefaction longer than the parenchymatous organs.

28. **D.**

29. **C.**

30. **B.** ***Related fact***: After death, putrefactive bacteria tend to colonize the venous system. The blood in the superficial veins over thighs and sides of abdomen hemolyses as a result. The released pigment not only stains the blood vessel walls, but also infiltrates into the surrounding tissues. This gives a somewhat marbled appearance to these regions of the body. This appearance is known as marbling.

31. **A.** ***Related fact***: Remember the mnemonic is AWE (Air, Water, Earth, with putrefaction occurring fastest in air and slowest in earth). In water and earth, atmosphere is not available for putrefaction. In water, moisture may cause faster putrefaction than when the body is in earth.

    Variant: A variant is often asked like this →Casper's dictum regarding the time taken for equal amount of putrefaction to occur in air:water:buried bodies is (a) 8:1:2 (b)1:4:16 (c)1:2:8 (d)1:2:4. The correct answer is (c) 1:2:8.

32. **D.** ***Related fact***: The internal organs putrefy in the following order (i) Larynx and trachea (ii) Stomach, intestines, spleen (iii) Liver, lungs (iv) Brain (v) Heart (vi) Kidney, Bladder, Uterus (vii) Skin, muscle, tendons (viii) Bones.

    Hint to tackle such questions: If you can't remember the whole sequence, just try to remember the first and last organs. If you don't see them in their proper place, that choice is most probably wrong. Also remember that "watery" organs putrefy earlier. "Drier" organs like tendons and bones putrefy latter.

33. B.

34. D. *Related fact*: Gravid uterus decomposes earlier than a non-gravid uterus. Virgin uterus is the last organ to putrefy.

35. D.

36. B.

37. C.

38. D. *Related facts*: Colliquative putrefaction is the name given to a very late stage of putrefaction, when the walls of abdomen soften and burst due to pressure of gases formed inside.

39. A.

40. B. Presence of bacteria, especially *Clostridium welchii* helps to accelerate the formation of adipocere.

41. A.

42. B.

Other Changes

43. B. *Related facts*: During life, potassium concentration is low in the vitreous humor but much higher in peripheral tissues such as retina. After death potassium from peripheral tissues starts diffusing in the vitreous raising its concentration. This occurs in a linear fashion so regularly that a relationship between it and the time since death can be established. Two formulae most popular in this regard are:

Time since death = $7.14 \times [K^+] - 39.1$ (Sturner's formula).

Time since death = $5.26 \times [K^+] - 30.9$ (Madea's formula).

Presumption of Death and Survivorship

44. D. This is according to section 107 of the *Indian Evidence Act (IEA)*. This is generally known as *Presumption of continuance of life*. Here is the full statement of Sec 107 of IEA.

S 107. Burden of proving death of person known to have been alive within thirty years

When the question is whether a man is alive or dead, and it is shown that he was alive within thirty years, the burden of proving that he is dead is on the person who affirms it.

45. B. This is according to section 108 of the IEA. This is known as *Presumption of Death*. Here is the full statement of Sec 108 of IEA

S 108. Burden of proving that person is alive who has not been heard of for seven years

[Provided that when] the question is whether a man is alive or dead, and it is proved that he has not been heard of for seven years by those who would naturally have heard of him if he had been alive, the burden of proving that he is alive is [shifted to] the person who affirms it.

[For discussion on all related IEA sections, please see, chapter 25 (sexual offences and sexual perversions), where s114A is discussed].

Illustration of the above two sections: Imagine a very rich man "A" living with his wife and an adolescent son. He has a brother and mother, who are neither living with him, nor sharing his property. He has written a will saying that in the event of his death, his property would be equally divided among his wife, son, mother and brother. One day he goes out to swim in a fast moving river, and never returns. His body is not found in the river despite all attempts. His wife and son assume control of the property and start enjoying it. She does not allow access of the property to the mother and brother of her husband. Since death is not proved, A's will cannot be executed. This is a situation where

A's mother and brother are interested in proving that A is dead (so his will can be executed and they get a share), while A's wife and son are interested in proving that A is still alive (so they continue to have a hold over the property). The question is whether A is really dead or alive in a legal sense.

After say, 3 years the brother moves the court saying that his brother is dead and the property should be equally divided. Now the situation can be analysed as follows:

- It is an undisputable fact that the person was alive 3 years back. According to s107 of IEA, the court assumes he is alive (because he was alive within last 30 years), and it is the brother's responsibility to prove that he is dead. He has to produce the dead body of "A" (or bones or some such other indisputable fact of A's death), which he can not. So his will can not be executed.

  Now suppose 8 years pass, and again the brother files a suit. Now the situation is like this.

- It is again an undisputable fact that "A" was alive 8 years back. According to s107 of IEA, the court still assumes he is alive (because he was alive within last 30 years), and it is the brother's responsibility to prove that he is dead. He has to produce the dead body of his brother, which he cannot.
- But now he can invoke section 108 of IEA. During last 7 years "A" should have met his wife, son, brother, mother, his business associates etc, which he has not. So the court now assumes that "A" is dead. Now the responsibility of proving that he is alive shifts to the wife and son of "A".

Case from real life: Australian Prime Minister Harold Holt (1908-1967), a devoted water sportsman, disappeared (on Dec. 17, 1967) while swimming off Cheviot Beach in Bass Strait about 60 miles south of Melbourne. His body was never found. He had to be presumed dead to prevent a constitutional crisis, and an acting Prime Minister was sworn in office on Dec 19 (Sir John McEwen). In normal circumstances (according to Indian law), one would have to wait for 7 years to establish legally that he was dead.

MULTIPLE ANSWER TYPE (PGI, CHANDIGARH PATTERN)

46. A,B,E. The color of postmortem staining in CO is cherry-red and in Hydrocyanic acid bright-red. So choices A and B are quite obvious. The tricky choice could be E. Remember that all OXIDISING AGENTS would cause methaemoglobinemia (which is nothing but an oxidised form of hemoglobin; Fe having three plus charges in methemoglobin, while it has just two plus charges in hemoglobin), which imparts a red-brown or brown color to the postmortem staining. The oxidising agents which cause red-brown or brown postmortem staining (in addition to nitrobenzene) are (i) Nitrates (ii) Potassium chlorate (iii) Potassium bicarbonate and (iv) Aniline. No postmortem staining colors are associated with arsenic and marking nut. Marking nut or *Semecarpus anacardium* is associated with false bruises, and NOT with any particular kind of post-mortem staining.

47. A,C. Post-mortem luminescence or shining of a decaying dead body especially in dark is a legendary supernatural phenomena, that has often been described, but never explained fully. However it is believed that a decaying corpse can be contaminated by certain light emitting bacteria such as *Photobacterium fischeri* and luminous fungi such as *Armillaria mellea* (Ramsbottom).

48. **B.** All other facts are correct. Rigor mortis is *rapid in onset* and of *shorter duration* after prolonged muscular activity, e.g. after exhaustion in battle, and following convulsions (strychnine poisoning, tetanus). Conversely there is a late onset of rigor in many sudden deaths. It might be explained by the lack of muscular activity immediately prior to death.

Onset of rigor is accelerated and its duration shortened when the environmental temperature is high. If the temperature is below 10ºC it is said to be exceptional for rigor mortis to develop, but if the environmental temperature is then raised, rigor mortis is said to develop in a normal manner.

3 INJURIES AND THEIR SIGNIFICANCE

10 *Injuries: Classification and Medicolegal Aspects*

DEFINITIONS

1. **Grievous hurt includes which of the following injuries?**
   A. Injury which keeps the patient away from work for 10 days
   B. Fracture of radius
   C. Abdominal trauma
   D. Laceration on the thigh
2. **All of the following are examples of grievous hurt *except*:**
   A. Fracture tooth
   B. Avulsion of a single nail
   C. Facial burns
   D. Emasculation
3. **Grievous hurt includes all of the following *except*:**
   A. Emasculation
   B. Permanent privation of hearing
   C. Privation of any member or joint
   D. Inability to follow one's ordinary pursuits for a period of a week
4. **A 25-year-old person sustained injury in right eye. He developed right corneal opacity following the injury. Left eye was already having poor vision. Corneoplasty of right eye was done and vision was restored. Medicolegally such injury is labelled as:**
   A. Simple
   B. Grievous
   C. Dangerous
   D. Serious
5. **Which of the following sections defines dangerous weapons?**
   A. Section 320 I.P.C.
   B. Section 324 I.P.C.
   C. Section 326 I.P.C.
   D. Both (B) and (C)
6. **The punishment for voluntarily causing grievous hurt by dangerous weapons or means is given in:**
   A. Section 320 I.P.C.
   B. Section 320 Cr.P.C.
   C. Section 324 I.P.C.
   D. Section 326 I.P.C.
7. **Section 320 of I.P.C. deals with:**
   A. Assault
   B. Hurt
   C. Grievous hurt
   D. Causing grievous hurt by a dangerous weapon
8. **Culpable homicide has been defined in:**
   A. Section 299 I.P.C.
   B. Section 299 Cr. P.C.
   C. Section 304 I.P.C.
   D. Section 304 Cr. P.C.

9. Murder has been defined in:
A. Section 300 I.P.C.
B. Section 302 I.P.C.
C. Section 304 I.P.C.
D. Section 300 Cr.P.C.

10. If a sentence for imprisonment for life has been passed on a convict, the appropriate Government may do one of the following things:
A. Increase it to death sentence
B. Commute it to imprisonment for a term not exceeding 14 years
C. Exile the offender
D. Ask the offender to work on barren lands for life

11. Legally speaking, any offer, threat, or attempt to apply criminal force to the body of another in a hostile manner is called:
A. Injury
B. Grievous hurt
C. Assault
D. Hurt

12. Dowry death is defined under:
A. S. 498A I.P.C.
B. S. 304A I.P.C.
C. S. 304B I.P.C.
D. S. 302 I.P.C.

13. All of the following are true about "dowry death" ***except:***
A. The death of a woman occurs within 7 years of marriage
B. The death must occur either by hanging or burns
C. The minimum punishment is 7 years
D. The maximum punishment is imprisonment for life, and not death sentence

14. What is the punishment for dowry death?
A. A minimum of 7 years, but which may extend to imprisonment for life
B. A maximum of 7 years
C. Maximum 7 years and a fine of Rs. 100,000
D. Capital punishment

15. Section 113B of ***Indian Evidence Act*** **deals with:**
A. Presumption of death of a person if he has not been heard for last 7 years
B. Abetment of suicide of a woman within 7 years of marriage
C. Absence of consent in case of rape, if female asserts she did not consent
D. Presumption of dowry death

16. Attempt to commit suicide is defined under:
A. Section 306 IPC
B. Section 307 IPC
C. Section 308 IPC
D. Section 309 IPC

CAUSES OF DEATHS FROM WOUNDS

17. The minimum amount of air usually accepted to be able to cause fatal air embolism in adults is:
A. 5 ml
B. 100 ml
C. 250 ml
D. 500 ml

18. The minimum amount of fat necessary to cause fat embolism is:
A. 5-10 ml
B. 12-120 ml
C. 220-300 ml
D. 320-440 ml

19. The fat in fat embolism is derived from:
A. The bone marrow after trauma
B. From the plasma by agglutination of chylomicrons
C. Infusion of exogenous fat
D. All of the above

20. Mortality rate in Fat Embolism Syndrome (FES) is:
A. 0.5-1.0%
B. 4-6%
C. 10-20%
D. >80%

MULTIPLE ANSWER TYPE (PGI, CHANDIGARH PATTERN)

21. Fat embolism may be seen in:
A. Skeletal trauma
B. Diabetes mellitus
C. Chronic pancreatitis
D. Sickle cell disease
E. Acute decompression syndrome

22. Which of the following facts are correct about *felony*?
A. This term is not used in Indian law anywhere
B. It is the term for a "very serious" crime
C. This term is used for theft
D. This term is identical with dowry death
E. This term is synonymous with infanticide

23. Major diagnostic criteria of fat embolism syndrome are:
A. A petechial rash
B. Spastic paraplegia
C. Respiratory distress
D. Gangrene of lower legs especially the great toe
E. Cerebral signs such as stupor, seizures, or coma

24. Which of the following are examples of justifiable homicide?
A. A police officer killing an escaped armed convict, while attempting to recapture him and the convict was going to shoot at him to avoid recapture
B. A jailer hanging a condemned criminal
C. A person killing another in self defense
D. Homicide committed by an insane person
E. Police officer accidentally killing a person due to firing to suppress riots

ANSWERS

DEFINITIONS

1. B. ***Related fact***: Grievous hurt includes the following eight clauses:

First—Emasculation.

Secondly—Permanent privation of the sight of either eye.

Thirdly—Permanent privation of the hearing of either ear.

Fourthly—Privation of any member or joint.

Fifthly—Destruction or permanent impairing of the powers of any member or joint.

Sixthly—Permanent disfiguration of the head or face.

Seventhly—Fracture or dislocation of a bone or tooth.

Eighthly—Any hurt which endangers life or which causes the sufferer to be during the space of twenty days in severe bodily pain, or unable to follow his ordinary pursuits.

A number of questions are encountered in MCQs on Grievous hurt. To solve them, please note the following points:

- First and foremost, in Indian law, nowhere does the phrase "simple injury" exist (although this phrase is talked about a lot in emergency and casualty wards). Indian law only mentions "Hurt", which is described in section 319 of I.P.C. and "Grievous Hurt", which is described in section 320. For the same reason it is fallacious to speak of grievous injury; one should instead speak of grievous hurt, as it is the latter term which is defined in law. However by common usage, simple injury has come to refer to "hurt" (section 319 I.P.C.); similarly the term "grievous injury" too is often used synonymously with "grievous hurt".
- Emasculation is confined to males only. It means depriving a man of his virility or of his masculine vigour, i.e. of his power to have intercourse. Castration – which means removal of testicles - is not same as emasculation. However castration is also a case of grievous hurt, because it comes under fourth clause. If in a female, clitoridectomy (as in Female Genital Mutilation, FGM) is done, it too comes under fourth clause and not under emasculation.
- It is of no consequence that after surgery/treatment, the patient was alright. The rule of the thumb is *what would have happened to the patient in the natural course of events, i.e. without treatment.* A question is frequently asked where a patient sustains an injury to the cornea, but after corneoplasty he can see clearly. Though the patient is able to see clearly, this is a case of grievous hurt, as his vision would have been impaired without treatment.
- The meaning of the word "privation" is not clear to many students. It only means some "compromise" of function; thus only a partial loss of eye or ear function would qualify for being a grievous hurt. Note that the word "deprivation" is not used in this section, which would have meant complete loss.
- The meaning of the word "member" must also be clarified. "Member" usually means an organ or a limb. However it could also

be taken to mean an organ with a specific and distinct function. Hair is not considered "member" in the usual sense of the word. Regarding nails the situation is somewhat trickier. Avulsion of a single nail has been considered grievous many authorities, while many others regard it as simple. But it is difficult to regard avulsion of, say, all ten nails as simple. So avulsion of just one nail may be taken is simple, while of all ten nails, it may be grievous.

- What constitutes "head" or "face"? It is not clear if the scalp comes within this definition. However in a practical sense, incised or lacerated wounds of the scalp are treated as simple, until and unless they can fit in some other clause.
- Look at clause seven. Some confusions exist here too. Fracture of a bone through and through is of course grievous, but a cut on the bone is generally not taken to be as grievous. The cut must reach the medullary cavity to be taken as grievous. Greenstick fractures, which do not result in complete separation of the two ends are grievous as well. Fracture of just one table of skull – either inner or outer – is generally taken as grievous. Dislocation of a temporary tooth is grievous too.
- A question is often asked, "Name a grievous hurt which can be corrected within minutes". The usually expected answer in such cases is "dislocation of shoulder". Dislocation of shoulder (in fact any joint) is a grievous hurt, and it can be corrected within minutes.
- Look at clause eight. The person must be unable to pursue his ordinary pursuits during the space of 20 days. The ordinary pursuits are brushing teeth, going to toilet, taking bath etc. If the person was bedridden for 20 days or more, the injury could qualify as grievous. A mere hospital stay for 20 days may not necessarily be grievous. What has to be proved is that the patient was in severe bodily pain during this period or he was unable to do his ordinary pursuits. Please note that the law does not insist that these twenty days *have to be continuous.*
- Thrusting of a *lathi* in the anus of a person is grievous, because it endangers life.
- A person is stabbed in the abdomen. It is a grievous hurt, even if his hospitalization was less than 20 days, because any stab injury to abdomen (and for that matter to chest) is a dangerous injury.
- All dangerous injuries are grievous hurt, but all grievous hurt are not dangerous injuries. If a hurt is dangerous (e.g. a stab in the abdomen), it is upto the doctor to label it as dangerous or grievous. If the injury is labelled as dangerous, the Investigating Officer (I.O.) will charge the accused under section 307 I.P.C. (attempt to murder). If the injury is labelled as grievous, the I.O. will charge the accused under section 326 I.P.C. (Voluntarily causing hurt by dangerous weapons or means). The punishment for both is ten years and fine.
- A person is hospitalized for 18 days, but his life was in danger for one day only during this period. This is a case of grievous hurt.
- A contusion of bone is *not* a grievous hurt.
- A single contusion or even a few contusions do not constitute grievous hurt. However multiple contusions all over the body (as may occur in police beating) may endanger life, and thus may collectively constitute grievous hurt.
- Burns covering one-third of the body surface may endanger life and may thus be classified as grievous hurt.

- Coma for twenty days due to head injury of course is a grievous hurt.
- Forearm laceration requiring stitches is simple in nature.

2. **B. *Related fact*:** Many authorities do not take avulsion of a single nail as grievous. However avulsion of all ten nails definitely appears to be grievous. Thus the choice (B) in the above question appears best. The only other confusing choice is (C). Facial burns however are likely to cause disfiguration of face, which will be covered under clause six.
3. **D.** The correct period for choice (D) would be 20 days.
4. **B. *Related fact*:** The answer of course is "Grievous", and not "simple" as many students might believe.

   The only confusing aspect here is that corneoplasty restored the vision. The poor vision in the left eye is immaterial, and that fact has been introduced only to cause some confusion. The age – 25 years – is also of no consequence.

   The legal philosophy in this case is "WHAT WOULD HAVE HAPPENED IN THE NATURAL COURSE OF EVENTS". And it is clear that in the natural course of events the corneal opacity would not have dissolved.

   Take another example. A teacher hits a student on the temple with the result that his tympanic membrane ruptures. Despite the fact that a myringoplasty can restore the tympanic membrane – and his hearing —it is a grievous hurt.
5. **D. *Related fact*:** These sections attempt to give guidelines on what a dangerous weapon is. A dangerous weapon is said to be *any instrument for shooting, stabbing or cutting, or any instrument which used as a weapon of offence, is likely to cause death.*
6. **D. *Related fact*:** The answer is NOT (A) as many students might believe. Section 320 I.P.C. *defines* grievous hurt, but *does not* give punishment for it. Similarly Section 319 I.P.C. *defines* hurt, but *does not* give punishment for it. The punishment for hurt and grievous hurt are given in Sections 323, 324, 325 and 326 I.P.C. The punishments are:

   Section 323 I.P.C: Punishment for voluntarily causing hurt→1 year or Rs 1000 or both.

   Section 324 I.P.C: Punishment for voluntarily causing hurt by dangerous weapons or means→3 years or fine or both.

   Section 325 I.P.C: Punishment for voluntarily causing grievous hurt→7 years *and* fine.

   Section 326 I.P.C: Punishment for voluntarily causing grievous hurt by dangerous weapons or means →10 years *and* fine.
7. **C.**
8. **A.**
9. **A. *Related fact*:** This is a common "catch" question. Most students think murder is defined in section 302 I.P.C. Remember, section 302 I.P.C. defines *punishment for murder, but not murder itself.* Murder is defined in Section 300 I.P.C.
10. **B.** Section 55 of the Indian Penal Code clearly states, "In every case in which sentence of imprisonment for life shall have been passed the appropriate Government may, without the consent of the offender, commute the punishment for imprisonment of either description for a term not exceeding fourteen years". Section 433 (b) of Cr.P.C. also says the same thing.

    In September, 2005 a Supreme Court Bench comprising Justice KG Balakrishnan and Justice BN Srikrishna has clarified that it is not the *right* of the prisoner (convicted of life imprisonment) to be released after 14 years. *Only* in cases where there has been a formal revision of the sentence under the above sections, can a prisoner be released after 14 years. According to the court, imprisonment for life is a class of punishment different from ordinary punishment which could be of two descriptions namely, "rigorous" or "simple". The Supreme Court bench was of the view that imprisonment for life is to be treated as rigorous imprisonment for life. This means there can be no simple imprisonment for life.

11. C. ***Related fact***: Note that the interesting thing here is just offer, threat or attempt. ACTUAL FORCE IS NOT USED. If actual force is used, it becomes a different offence altogether; it is then called use of **criminal force**. While assault is defined in section 351 of I.P.C., criminal force is defined in section 350 of I.P.C.. In English law these terms are known as **assault** and **battery** respectively. If the assault is consummated by the unlawful application of force, the crime is called **battery** (as a mnemonic, remember "battered baby syndrome"). The term **battery** is nowhere used in Indian law.

12. **C.**

13. **B.** The death may be caused by burns, or bodily injury, or occurs otherwise than under normal circumstances. If a woman kills herself, say, by a firearm, section 304B can still be invoked if all other components are present.

    Note: 304B is NOT at par with 302. 304B will only be invoked when 302 can not be, for instance, when a woman has committed suicide. Death sentence is NOT prescribed in 304B.

14. **A.** The law is silent on whether the imprisonment will be simple or rigorous. Strangely, no fine has been prescribed for this crime. Students must be on the lookout for this distractor. The punishment is prescribed in Section 304 B (2), which can form the basis of yet another possible question.

    More on Minimum punishments: There are very few crimes for which a minimum punishment has been prescribed. These are:

    i. Section 304 B (2)–Dowry Death→A minimum of 7 years, but which may extend to imprisonment for life. No mention about simple or rigorous.
    ii. Section 376 (1)–Rape→A minimum of 7 years (of either description), but which may extend to imprisonment for life.
    iii. Section 376 (2)–Rape under special circumstances (such as custodial rape, gang rape, rape of a child below 12 years, rape on a pregnant woman)→Minimum 10 years rigorous. May extend upto life imprisonment. Also liable to fine.
    iv. Section 398 (not concerning forensic specialists though)–Attempt to commit robbery or dacoity when armed with deadly weapon→The imprisonment shall not be less than seven years (no mention about simple or rigorous here as well).

15. **D.** [*For discussion on all related IEA sections, please see, chapter 25 (sexual offences and sexual perversions), where s114A is discussed*].

16. **D.** ***Additional facts:*** When the British framed the Indian Penal Code in 1860, the English law at the time regarded suicide as a felony. So they kept section 309 in Indian Penal Code too as a crime. However with the passage of time, viewpoints changed. It was increasingly felt that it was not just to punish a person who was already under so much suffering that he had contemplated suicide. Henry Romilly Fedden, author of "Suicide: A Social and Historical Study" (London, 1938) wrote, "it seems a monstrous procedure to inflict further suffering on an individual who has already found life so unbearable, his chances of happiness so slender, that he has been willing to face pain and death in order to cease living". Subsequently the UK in its *Suicide*

Act, 1961 specifically decriminalised suicide and attempt to suicide. In India however the situation remained unchanged. In 1971, ten years after the Suicide Act was passed in the UK, the Law Commission in India recommended repeal of section 309. Interestingly it quoted Romilly Fedden in its recommendation. Subsequently the Indian Penal Code (Amendment) Bill to repeal section 309 was passed in the Rajya Sabha in 1978. It was pending in the Sixth Lok Sabha when it was dissolved in 1979. Attempts to repeal section 309 were forgotten afterwards.

In 1986, P Rathinam assailed the constitutional validity of section 309 IPC in the Supreme Court. The court (a two-judge bench comprising Mr. Justice R.M. Sahai and Mr. Justice B.L. Hansaria) took into consideration issues of religion and morality in arriving at a decision. They declared section 309 unconstitutional and struck it down. Following reasonings were offered:

i. Examples were cited from mythology of Lord Rama taking *Jal Samadhi* in Saryu to Buddha and Mahavira achieving death by seeking it. The court declared that suicide could not be termed as an irreligious act.
ii. Furthermore it observed that suicide-prone persons need soft words and wise counselling, not "stony dealing by a jailor following harsh treatment meted out by a heartless prosecutor".
iii. The court listed several circumstances in which people may wish to end their lives, including disease, cruel or unbearable condition of life, and a sense of shame or disenchantment with life. It was held that everyone should have the freedom to dispose of his life as and when he desires.
iv. Fundamental rights were held to have positive as well as negative aspects. For instance, the freedom to speech and expression included the freedom not to speak. Similarly, freedom of association and movement included freedom not to join any association or move. On a parity of reasoning, the freedom to live was held to include the freedom not to live. The court delivered its judgment in April 1994 (*P. Rathinam v. Union of India [(1994) 3 SCC 394]*), observing that penalising an attempt to suicide was unconstitutional and violative of the right to life under Article 21.

However section 309 remained struck off only for about two years. In March 1996, it was reinstated in the case of *Gian Kaur v. State of Punjab [(1996) 2 SCC 648]*, where a five-judge Constitution Bench of the court overruled the P. Rathinam's case and held that 'Right to Life,' under Article 21 of the Constitution, does not include 'Right to Die' or 'Right to be Killed'. It was held that the Right to Die is inherently inconsistent with the Right to Life. It was held that in the earlier judgment the issues of euthanasia were not considered, and the "legal sanction" given to suicide could be used by criminal elements to cover cases of euthanasia (killing old and disabled parents for instance) and even dowry death.

CAUSES OF DEATHS FROM WOUNDS

17. B. ***Related fact*:** The volume of air needed to cause fatal embolism has been hotly debated for years, but no real consensus has emerged. The figures vary from 10 to 480 ml. If the volume of the right side of the heart is accepted as the minimum space that has to be filled, about 100 ml would appear to be reasonable volume.

18. B. ***Related facts*:** Two related facts which may be of use in other MCQs are (i) Fat Emboli were first noted by F.A. Zenker in 1861 in a railroad worker with a thoraco-lumbar crush injury (ii) The Fat Embolism Syndrome (FES) was first described by Von Bergman in 1873 in a diagnosis confirmed by post mortem examination. This patient had a fractured femur.

19. D. Two theories mainly explain the pathogenesis of fat embolism. First is the **mechanical theory**, which is quite straightforward. Fat cells and venous sinuses are disrupted after a bony trauma or injury to adipose tissue. The liberated fat globules enter the circulation by means of lacerated veins in the traumatized area. Fat droplets of between 20-40 micron diameter block the smallest branches of the pulmonary vasculature whereas smaller fat droplets may pass through the capillaries and enter the systemic circulation.

Mechanical theory is not able to explain convincingly how bigger fat droplets (>20-40 microns) can be found in the brain. Two mechanisms have however been suggested (i) They may pass through arteriovenous shunts in the lungs (ii) They may pass through patent foramen ovale. The paradox of how fat can pass from lower pressure right atrium to higher pressure left atrium (even if there were a patent foramen ovale) is explained like this. In the initial phase pulmonary emboli with fat droplets less than 20-40 microns in size occur. Pulmonary-artery and right-heart pressures increase in response to multiple episodes of pulmonary embolization. The increased pressure in the right heart causes the bigger emboli to pass into the left side of the heart. From here they get distributed to the brain. Shunting across a patent foramen ovale can also occur during coughing, after the release phase of the Valsalva maneuver, and during mechanical ventilation. It is important to note that 20 to 34 percent of people have a patent foramen ovale. Since fat is readily deformable, it accounts for the passage of masses *larger* than the diameter of the patent foramen ovale.

Second is the **biochemical theory**. According to this theory, embolic fat is derived NOT from bone marrow or traumatized adipose tissue, but from circulating blood lipids in a diverse series of nontraumatic conditions (e.g. diabetes mellitus, chronic pancreatitis, alcoholism, sickle cell disease and acute decompression syndrome).

According to this theory, trauma and/or subsequent sepsis causes hormonal changes (most notably catecholamine release). This causes mobilization of lipids. The increased blood levels of neutral fats and free fatty acids may then induce the formation of more and larger chylomicrons. Acute phase reactants, such as *C-reactive proteins* (CRP), cause these chylomicrons to coalesce into still bigger droplets. CRP is synthesised in the liver in association with a variety of inflammatory and malignant processes. It is also formed in association with trauma. Chylomicrons are known to undergo calcium dependant agglutination by CRP. These droplets then travel to lungs, brain and skin and cause fat embolism.

The biochemical theory helps explain several features of fat embolism not properly explained by mechanical theory. For instance (i) why fat embolism is sometimes seen in non traumatic cases, such as diabetes (ii) how fat emboli greater than 20-40 microns in diameter escape the lung capillaries to get lodged in brain.

20. C. ***Related facts:*** About 1-2% cases of fat embolism develop Fat Embolism Syndrome (FES), a clinical disorder with respiratory, cerebral and dermal manifestations (respiratory failure, diffuse or focal cerebral disturbance and petechiae). Rarely, fat embolism produces a fulminant fat embolism syndrome due to mechanical obstruction within the pulmonary circulation causing a severe right heart failure.

The fat embolism syndrome is believed to be caused by the toxic effects of free fatty acids (FFAs) liberated at the endothelial layer. The sequence is like this: (i) Subsequent to trauma, fat collects in the pulmonary or systemic capillary network (ii) it is acted upon by lipoprotein lipases which are activated by catecholamine release (iii) this liberates high concentrations of toxic FFAs locally (iv) the toxic effect of FFAs results in platelet aggregation, capillary disruption, perivascular haemorrhage, a mild disseminated intravascular coagulation, disruption of the pulmonary and cerebral capillary walls and oedema.

The syndrome is largely self limiting with treatment being symptomatic. Mortality is 10-20%. Therapy is directed at maintaining respiratory function and largely follows the same principles of management used in patients who have the acute respiratory distress syndrome. Early immobilization of fractures and methods to reduce the intramedullary pressure during total hip arthroplasty have reduced the incidence of operative fat embolisation. Corticosteroids either before or after the development of respiratory or cerebral symptoms are not of any benefit.

Fulminant fat embolism syndrome is caused by a sudden intravascular liberation of a large amount of fat causing pulmonary vascular obstruction, severe right heart failure, shock and often death within the first 1-12 hours of injury.

MULTIPLE ANSWER TYPE (PGI, CHANDIGARH PATTERN)

21. **A,B,C,D,E.** Fat embolism is seen in all conditions where either skeletal trauma is produced (causing extrusion of fat from bone marrow), or where physico-chemical environment of the body causes coalescence of smaller chylomicrons in bigger droplets. While skeletal trauma causes extrusion of fats in the blood, all other conditions cause fusion of smaller chylomicrons into bigger droplets causing fat embolism.

    Other major conditions where fat embolism may be seen are burns, joint reconstruction, liposuction, cardiopulmonary bypass and parenteral lipid infusion.

    It is important to note however that in 90 percent of instances, the fat embolism syndrome occurs after blunt trauma complicated by long-bone fractures.

22. **A,B.** The term "*felony*" does not appear in Indian law anywhere, but in many legal systems (US, Australia), it is the term for a "very serious" crime; *misdemeanors* are considered to be less serious.

    Crimes which are commonly considered to be felonies include: aggravated assault, arson, burglary, murder, and rape. Examples of misdemeanors include petty theft, prostitution, simple assault, trespass and vandalism.

    Those who are convicted of a felony are known as *felons*; those who are convicted of a misdemeanor are known as *misdemeanants*.

    Originally, felonies were crimes for which the punishment was either death or forfeiture of property. Nowadays, felons receive lesser punishments too. In the United States felons often receive additional punishments such as the loss of voting rights, exclusion from certain lines of work, are prohibited from obtaining certain licenses, may not purchase/possess firearms or bullet-resistant armor, and are not eligible to run for nor be elected to public office. In addition, some states (of US) consider a felony conviction to be grounds for an uncontested divorce, i.e. the spouse of a felon can get a divorce without any opposition.

23. **A,C,E.** The three classical major diagnostic criteria of fat embolism syndrome are:

i. **Pulmonary signs:** These are usually seen first. These comprise of respiratory distress (patient becomes tachypneic, dyspneic, and hypoxic). These signs result from the embolic fat being hydrolyzed by lung lipase with the release of lung-toxic Free Fatty Acids (FFAs). These FFAs induce an acute lung injury and subsequent ARDS. This process accounts for the time period between injury and onset of clinical signs of fat embolism syndrome (often known as lucid interval). This time period is normally 24 to 72 hours.

ii. **A petechial rash:** These are reddish-brown nonpalpable petechiae developing over the upper body, particularly in the axillae, within 24-36 hours of insult or injury. These petechiae occur in about 20-50% of patients and resolve quickly, but they are virtually diagnostic in the right clinical setting.

iii. **Cerebral signs:** Patient is agitated, delirious and may progress to stupor, seizures, or coma. Correction of hypoxia is generally of no avail. There may be retinal hemorrhages with intra-arterial fat globules which may be visible upon funduscopic examination.

24. **A,B,E.** ***Related facts:*** First and foremost thing to remember is that the words "justifiable homicide" and "excusable homicides" DO NOT appear in Indian law anywhere. They are essentially foreign terms.

Secondly, the meanings of justifiable and excusable homicides are not watertight. In different countries and even in different states of the same country (USA), the meanings are different with frequent overlappings.

In a most general sense however, *Justifiable homicide* is one which is commanded or authorized by law, such as the act of a police officer killing an armed suspect who is shooting at him or a jailer hanging a condemned criminal. Remember that in Justifiable homicide, usually there is a legal officer involved who commits the homicide in order to carry out a perfectly legal task. Persons committing justifiable homicide are at NO fault in a legal sense.

Excusable homicide differs from justifiable homicide in that one who commits an excusable homicide is to some degree at fault, but the degree of fault is not enough to constitute a criminal homicide. It is a homicide done by persons other than law and justice officers (mostly members of general public).

It includes homicides, where the person committing the homicide had no other option but to kill. It also includes homicides where there was no guilt on the part of the killer such as an insane person or a child below 7 years.

Some examples of excusable homicide are (i) a person shooting an armed intruder in his own home (ii) a person dying on the operation table during an extremely difficult operation, with no fault of the surgeon, and (iii) death caused by an insane person.

Finally, it may be helpful to quote the *California State Penal Code (state law)* that covers justifiable homicide. Section 196 states as follows:

S 196. Homicide is justifiable when committed by public officers and those acting by their command in their aid and assistance, either—

1. In obedience to any judgment of a competent Court; or
2. When necessarily committed in overcoming actual resistance to the execution of some legal process, or in the discharge of any other legal duty; or
3. When necessarily committed in retaking felons who have been rescued or have escaped, or when necessarily committed in arresting persons charged with felony, and who are fleeing from justice or resisting such arrest.

11 Mechanical Injuries (Including Torture)

GENERAL

1. A clean incised wound heals by:
- **A.** Primary intention
- **B.** Secondary intention
- **C.** Excessive scarring
- **D.** None of the above

2. Which of the following is an open wound?
- **A.** Contusion
- **B.** Abrasion
- **C.** Laceration
- **D.** Concussion

3. Which of the following is a characteristic feature of healing by second intention?
- **A.** Inflammatory reaction is more intense
- **B.** Much larger amounts of granulation tissue are formed
- **C.** There is significant amount of contraction
- **D.** All of the above

ABRASIONS

4. Which of the following best defines abrasion?
- **A.** It is a superficial injury involving only the superficial layers of the skin
- **B.** It is an injury involving epidermis and dermis, but not the muscles
- **C.** It is an injury from which blood does not ooze
- **D.** It is any injury which is caused by a sharp edged weapon

5. Brush burns are due to:
- **A.** Friction
- **B.** Electric shock
- **C.** Moist heat
- **D.** Bullet injury

6. Crescentic abrasions are caused by:
- **A.** Blunt knife
- **B.** Nails
- **C.** Wooden sticks
- **D.** Scissors

CONTUSIONS

7. Contusions are synonymous with:
- **A.** Abrasions
- **B.** Bruises
- **C.** Lacerated wounds
- **D.** Incised wounds

8. A bruise becomes brownish in about:
- **A.** 2-4 hours
- **B.** 2 days
- **C.** 4 days
- **D.** 10 days

9. Greenish color in a contusion is due to:
- **A.** Haemosiderin
- **B.** Haematoidin
- **C.** Sulphmethemoglobin
- **D.** Methaemoglobin

10. In a large bruise, color changes begin:
- **A.** From the center
- **B.** From the periphery
- **C.** From an area somewhere in the middle of centre and periphery
- **D.** At the same time everywhere

11. Artificial bruise can be produced by:
- **A.** Marking nut
- **B.** Whipping
- **C.** Dhatura
- **D.** Opium

12. A motor car running over the thigh, leaving tire marks over it is a good example of:
- **A.** Ectopic bruise
- **B.** Fictitious bruise
- **C.** Gravitating bruise
- **D.** Patterned bruise

INCISED WOUNDS

13. Tentative cuts are seen in:
- **A.** Homicide
- **B.** Suicide
- **C.** Drowning
- **D.** Hanging

STAB WOUNDS

14. Which of the following is true about a stab wound?
- **A.** Its breadth is maximum
- **B.** Its length is maximum
- **C.** Its depth is maximum
- **D.** It has a wound of entry and exit

15. When a wound enters a body cavity such as chest or abdomen, it is usually referred to as a:
- **A.** Near fatal wound
- **B.** Langerhans wound
- **C.** Perforating wound
- **D.** Penetrating wound

16. When a weapon enters the body on one side and come out through the other, it is usually referred to as?
- **A.** Double sided wound
- **B.** Perforating wound
- **C.** Entry-exit wound
- **D.** Penetrating wound

17. Stab wounds with a "fish tail" appearance are seen when the stab is made by:
- **A.** A knife which is single edged
- **B.** A knife which is double edged
- **C.** A knife generally used to cut fishes
- **D.** A bayonet

18. "Hilt bruise" or "Hilt abrasion" can be seen around the stab wound when:
- **A.** The knife has been partially plunged in the victim with relatively lighter force
- **B.** The knife has been fully plunged in the victim with great force
- **C.** The knife has been obliquely plunged
- **D.** Stab is made by a lance

19. A stab wound produced by a double edged weapon is:
- **A.** Tear drop shaped
- **B.** Spindle shaped
- **C.** Fish-tail shaped
- **D.** Chimney shaped

LACERATED WOUNDS

20. Where does a lacerated wound appear like an incised wound?
- **A.** Abdomen

B. Thorax
C. Hand
D. Forehead

21. **A heavy-edged weapon such as chopper, axe or hatchet can produce:**
A. Tears
B. Split lacerations
C. Stretch lacerations
D. Cut lacerations

22. **Small superficial lacerations on the back caused by whipping with a cycle chain, roughly reflecting its shape may best be described as:**
A. Patterned lacerations
B. Avulsion
C. Stretch lacerations
D. Split lacerations

TORTURE

23. **"*Dry submarino*" in relation to torture refers to:**
A. Beating on soles of the feet
B. Covering the face of victims with a plastic bag
C. Immersing head in contaminated water
D. Suspending the accused by the ankles

24. **Forced standing is known as:**
A. Planton
B. Picana
C. Parrilla
D. Pau de arara

25. ***Picana* in relation of torture refers to:**
A. Forced sitting in an uncomfortable position
B. Water torture
C. Beating on the palms
D. Electrical torture

26. **Falanga refers to:**
A. Pushing moist cloth up the nostrils
B. Forcing the victim to walk on broken glass
C. Beating of the soles of the feet with canes or rods
D. Tying of legs and forcing the victim to walk

27. **Telefono as a method of torture refers to:**
A. Repeated slapping of the sides of the head of the victim by the open palms of the assailant
B. Inserting a telephone receiver in the anus of the victim
C. Inserting a hot rod in the rectum of the victim
D. Both (B) and (C)

ANSWERS

GENERAL

1. **A.** Healing by first intention occurs when there is (i) Minimal loss of tissue (ii) Minimal or no bacterial contamination. When these are present (as in lacerations), healing is by second intention.
2. **C.**
3. **D.** ***Related fact:*** A defect of about 40 sq cm in the skin of a rabbit is reduced in approximately 6 weeks to 5-10% of its original size, largely by contraction (to about 2-4 sq cm).

ABRASIONS

4. **A.**
5. **A.** ***Related fact*:** Brush burn is nothing but name given to an abrasion which is produced by violent rubbing against a surface, as in dragging over the ground.
6. **B.** ***Related facts*:** These are often seen on the victim's neck in throttling. See a related question in chapter 18 (Deaths from asphyxia).

CONTUSIONS

7. **B.**
8. C. ***Related fact*:** Color changes in a bruise depends on a number of factors, including the size of bruise (large bruises take longer to heal) and age of the individual (bruises heal slower in older people). However the general dates that are accepted are as follows:

   Immediately: Red
   Few hours to 3 days: Blue.
   4th day: Bluish black to brown (formation of iron containing haemosiderin).
   5-6 days: Greenish (formation of haematoidin).
   7-12 days: Yellowish (formation of bilirubin).
   2 weeks: Normal.

   Variant: **Which of the following is NOT true regarding color of bruise?** (a) 4th day–Bluish black to brown (b)7-12 days–Green (c) 1st day–Red (d) 2 weeks– Normal.
   The correct answer is (b) 7-12 days– Green.

9. **B.** ***Related facts*:** Haematoidin is a loose term formerly applied to the crystals of bilirubin or biliverdin. Besides occurring in old contusions it also sometimes occurs in faeces after intestinal haemorrhage. When present in the corpora lutea it is called **haemolutein.** Important thing to remember is that while haemosiderin contains iron, haematoidin is iron free.
10. **B.** ***Related facts*:** A large bruise takes longer time to heal than a smaller bruise. The color changes begin at the periphery first. A large old bruise may contain all possible colors seen in a bruise – from purple in the centre to yellow at the edges.
11. **A.** Whipping will produce a true bruise. Dhatura and Opium do not produce any bruise. Marking nut is botanically known as *Semecarpus anacardium*.
12. **D.** Patterned bruise are important from a medicolegal point of view, because they can give a fairly good idea of the striking surface. Among the most commonly encountered patterned injuries are patterned abrasions, patterned bruises and patterned lacerations. These are so called because these injuries reflect the pattern of the striking surface. Beating with whips having patterned thongs and kicking with boots may leave patterned

bruises on the body. Whip with patterned thongs may even cause superficial patterned lacerations.

INCISED WOUNDS

13. B.

STAB WOUNDS

14. C. ***Related facts*:** A stab wound is often known as a *punctured wound* too, especially if it is produced by a pointed object such as an ice pick, needle or screw driver.

15. D.

16. B. ***Variant*:** This question has alternately been asked as follows: A perforating injury is one which (a) perforates the eye (b) is circular in shape (c) penetrates a body cavity (d) has an entry and exit wound. The answer is (d) has an entry and exit wound.

The concept of punctured, penetrating and perforating wounds is best understood with the following diagram (Fig. 11.1):

Wound number 1 goes into the gluteus muscle without entering into any body cavity.

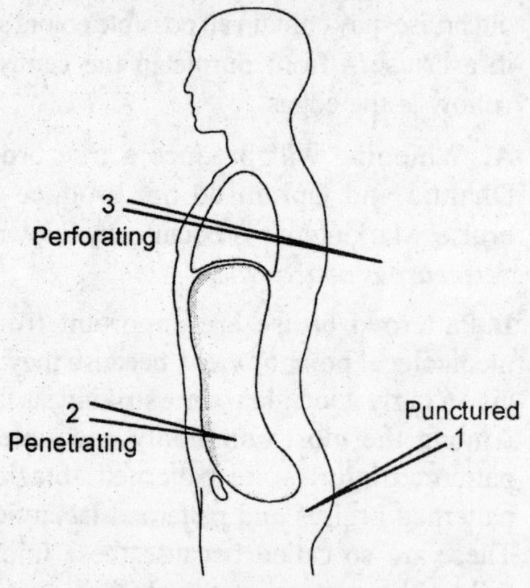

Fig. 11.1: The concept of punctured, perforating and penetrating wounds

Since its depth is greater than its width, technically it is a stab wound. A stab wound caused typically by an "ice pick" shaped object is called a punctured wound.

Wound number 2 enters into abdominal cavity, without coming out of it. This is a penetrating wound, since it "penetrates" a body cavity. Major body cavities are chest, abdomen and skull (penetrating wounds of skull are exceedingly rare though). Other body cavities, upon entering which the wound would qualify as a penetrating wound are eye balls and major joints such as knee joint.

Wound number 3 enters the chest cavity and comes out. It is technically a "perforating wound". Like the perforations in a large "stamp sheet", these wounds are "through and through" wounds, having an entry and an exit wound.

An MCQ question is often asked about the size of entry and exit wounds in firearm wounds and perforating wounds. Remember, in a firearm wound, exit is bigger than entry, while in a perforating wound, entry is bigger than exit, as shown in the figure 11.2:

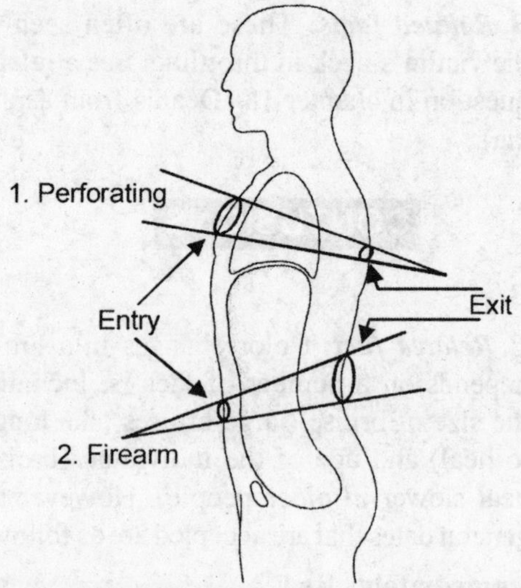

Fig. 11.2: In a perforating wound, entry wound is bigger than the exit; in a firearm wound, it is the other way round

17. **A.** Many students do not really understand the concept of fish-tailing. A look at the accompanying diagram will clarify this concept. This is a typical fish-tail produced by a single edged stabbing weapon. The edge "a" of the wound is produced by the sharp edge of the stabbing weapon, while the other edge of the wound represented by the triangle "bcd" is produced by the blunt edge of the weapon. Note that "bcd" is actually a small triangular flap of skin. The "base" of this triangle ("bd") mirrors the other (blunt) edge of the stabbing weapon.

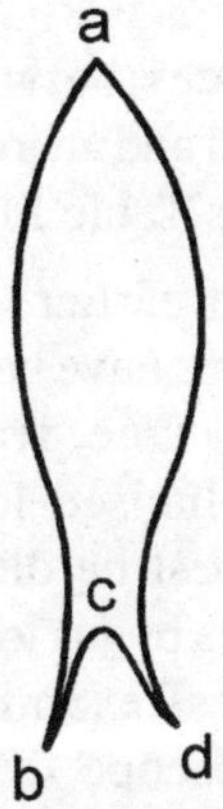

Fig. 11.3: A fish tail wound produced by a single edged stabbing weapon. [Refer text for details]

If one removes this small triangular wedge of tissue, one would be left with the typical wedge shaped wound seen in stabs by single edged weapons. Fish-tailing is thus nothing but the usual wedge shaped wound, where a small triangular piece of skin remains attached to the blunt edge, giving the appearance of a fish-tail.

18. **B.**

19. **B.** As shown in the figure, stab wounds produced by single edged weapons are typically tear drop or wedge shaped. Stab wounds produced by double edged weapons are spindle shaped.

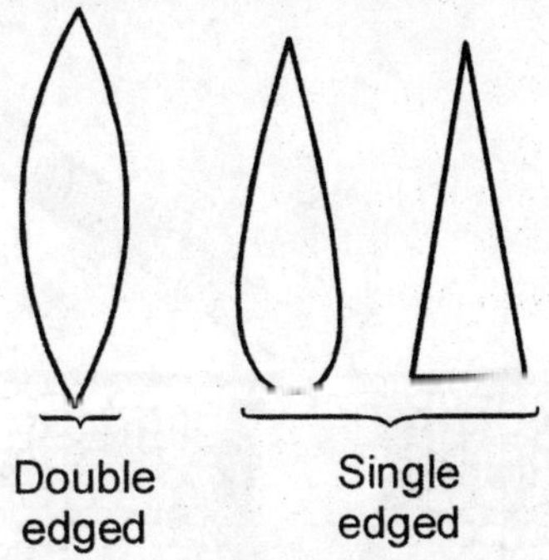

Fig. 11.4: Stab wounds produced by double edged weapons are spindle shaped; those produced by single edged weapons are typically tear drop shaped or wedge shaped

LACERATED WOUNDS

20. **D.** Whereever in the body, the skin lies directly over the bone, with a scanty layer of fat in between, lacerated wounds appear like incised wounds. These are known as *incised looking lacerated wounds*. Other areas where lacerated wounds would appear like an incised wound are scalp, chin, eyebrows, lower jaw, iliac crest and shin.

21. **D.** This is a commonly asked question. To solve this and related questions, the student should have a clear concept of various types of lacerations.

Forensic pathologists usually encounter five different types of lacerations:

1. **Tear:** The most common and frequently encountered is the **tear**. This is the most general kind of laceration. It has ragged and bruised margins and is caused by a heavy blunt weapon such as a cricket bat, a hockey stick or a *lathi* acting upon an area of a body where there is sufficient amount of underlying fat and muscle, as on a thigh (Fig. 11.5).

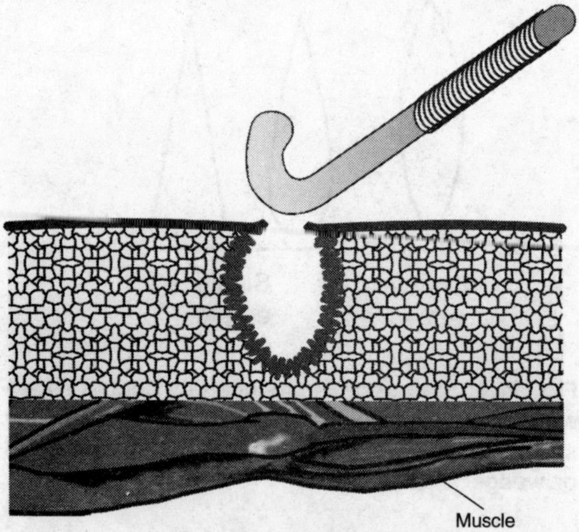

Fig. 11.5: Tear, the most general kind of laceration ***(See also Colour Plate 1)***

2. **Split laceration:** If the same weapon hit upon an area of the body where there was scanty layer of tissue underneath (such as the scalp), the skin would be split between the weapon and the underlying bone. This results in a **split laceration** which appears very much like an incised wound – so much so that it is often called an *incised looking lacerated wound*. There are ways to differentiate between the two however (the student must try to learn these as many MCQs are based on this information). The edges are ragged in laceration but to naked eye the raggedness may not be readily apparent. An examination with a hand lens can immediately reveal the raggedness of the edges. Furthermore the edges are bruised in a true lacerated wound but not in a true incised wound. The blood vessels and other structures such as muscles, nerves and tendons at the base of the wound are crushed in a true lacerated wound but cleanly cut in a true incised wound. If the area is hairy (as in scalp), the hair are crushed in a true lacerated wound (Fig. 11.6) but clean cut in a true incised wound.

   The differences between an incised-looking wound and an incised wound may be tabulated as Table 11.1:

   As mentioned earlier, several multiple choice questions have been framed on this information. One frequently asked question is→Incised looking lacerated wounds can best be differentiated from incised wounds by (a) toluidine blue stain (b) histological examination (c) comparison microscope (d) hand lens. The answer is (d) hand lens.

3. **Stretch laceration:** If the force is applied in such a manner that a portion of the skin is overstretched, as in a glancing kick by a shod foot (foot wearing a shoe), it would result in a large flap on one side. This is the **stretch laceration**. The mechanism

Table 11.1: Criteria to differentiate between an incised and incised looking lacerated wound

S. No	*Criteria*	*Incised wound*	*Incised looking lacerated wound*
1.	Margins, when seen under a hand lens	Clean cut	Ragged and bruised
2.	Edges	No, or minimal bruising	Heavily bruised
3.	Blood vessels at the base of the wound	Blood vessels at the base are clean cut	Blood vessels at the base are crushed
4.	Other tissues at the base of the wound	Tissues such as fascial bands and nerves are clean cut	Fascial bands and nerves are either crushed or seen intact. They show continuity
5.	Hair around the wound	Clean cut	Crushed

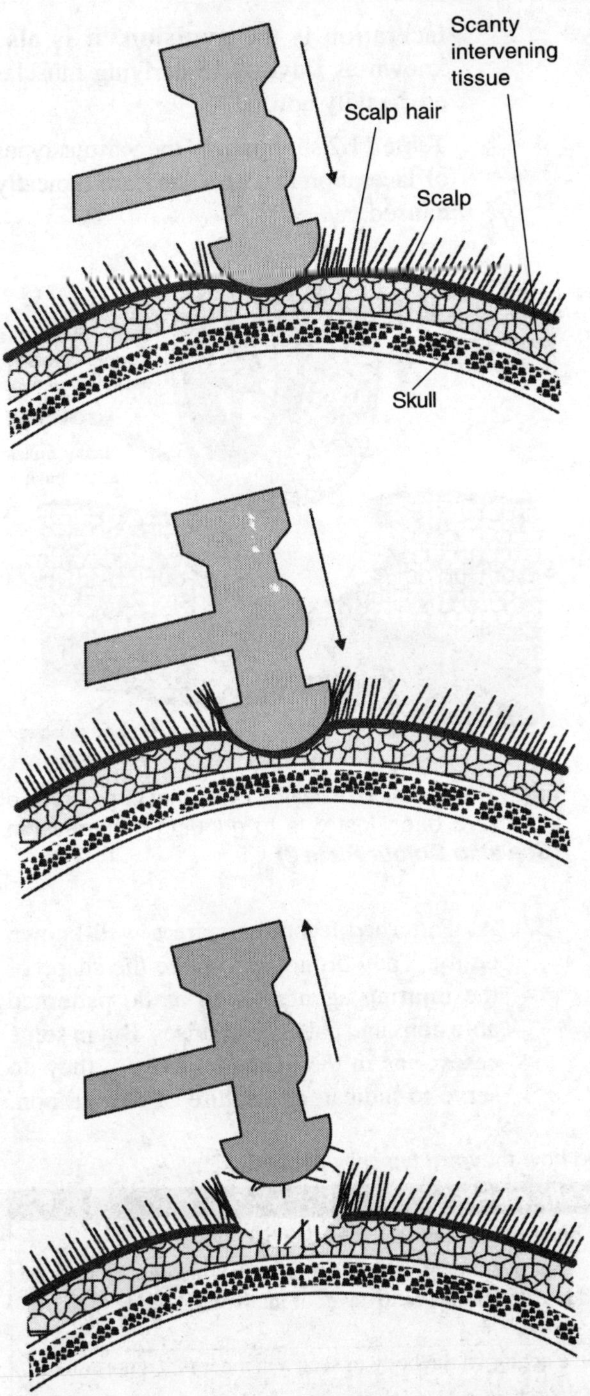

Fig. 11.6: Split laceration caused by a heavy weapon hitting on scalp *(See also Colour Plate 1)*

can best be understood by studying figure 11.7.

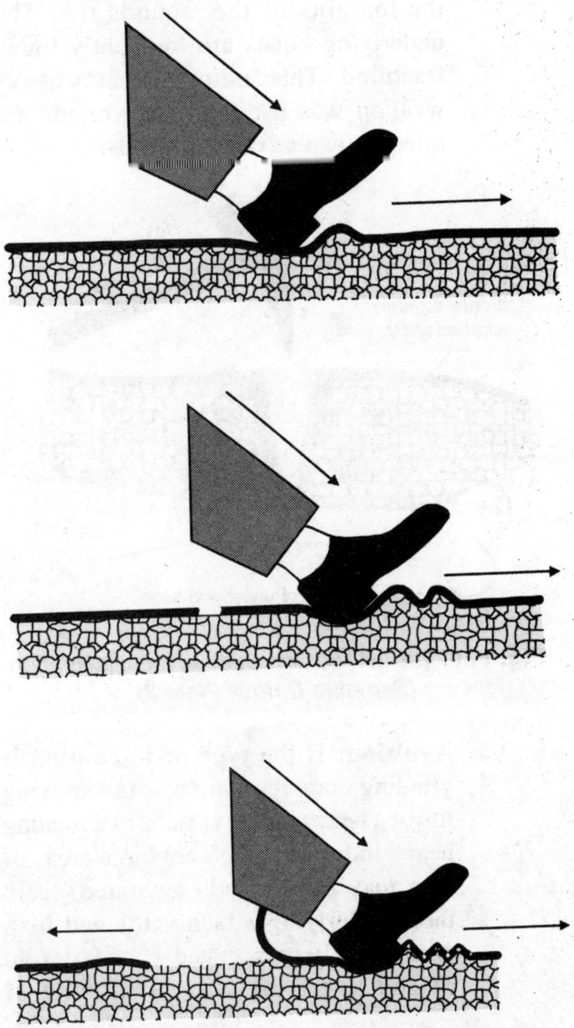

Fig. 11.7: Mechanism of a stretch laceration. Note that a large flap of skin is formed on one side *(See also Colour Plate 2)*

4. **Cut laceration:** This type of laceration is produced by heavy cutting weapons, such as a chopper, axe, hatchet or meat cleaver. This wound may be visualized as a "cross" between a true laceration and a true incised wound. The edges of

the weapon do cut the skin, but since the edges are heavy, they crush and bruise the margins of the wounds too. The underlying bones are frequently found fractured. This indicates that a heavy weapon was used. These wounds are often known as **chop wounds**.

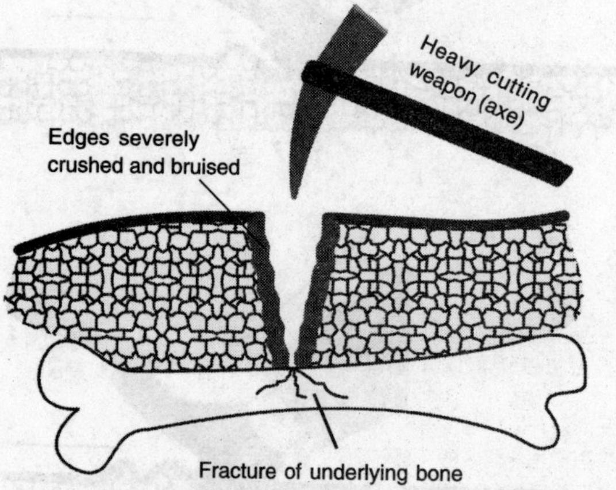

Fig. 11.8: Typical features seen in a cut laceration ***(See also Colour Plate 2)***

5. **Avulsion:** If the type of force used is grinding compression (as a fast moving tire of a heavy motor vehicle, or a rotating heavy industrial machine) large areas of skin may be avulsed (separated) from their underlying attachments and lost, resulting in large lacerated wounds devoid of any overlying skin. This type of laceration is the **avulsion**. It is also known as **flaying**. Underlying muscles are heavily bruised.

Table 11.2 summarizes the various types of laceration and how they are typically caused.

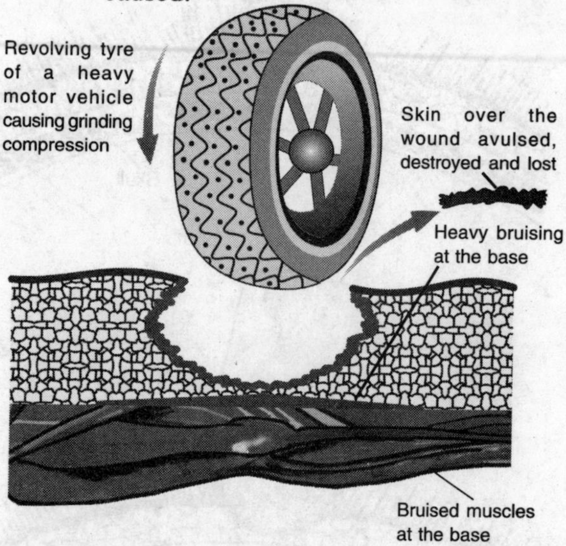

Fig. 11.9: Avulsion or flaying. Note that large areas of skin have been lost due to grinding compression. ***(See also Colour Plate 2)***

22. **A.** Patterned lacerations are a well-known entity. They do not reproduce the shape of the injuring agent as well as do patterned abrasions and patterned bruises. But in some cases – as in the example above – they do serve to indicate the nature of the weapon.

Table 11.2: Different types of lacerations and how they are typically caused

S.No	*Type of laceration*	*How typically caused*
1.	Tear	Any heavy blunt instrument (e.g. a cricket bat)
2.	Split laceration	Any heavy blunt instrument, on an area of body which has some bone directly underneath with a scanty layer of intervening tissue (e.g. scalp)
3.	Stretch laceration	A heavy force acting on the body in such a manner that a portion of skin is overstretched
4.	Cut laceration	Heavy cutting weapon with an edge which may not be too sharp
5.	Avulsion	Heavy weights (e.g. a truck) passing over the body, causing large areas of skin to be avulsed and lost. Also called “flaying”

Lacerations caused by a bicycle chain is perhaps the best example of a patterned laceration (Fig. 11.10). A hammer blow on the head may occasionally cause a circular laceration outlining the periphery of the striking surface. This is also a fairly good example of a patterned laceration.

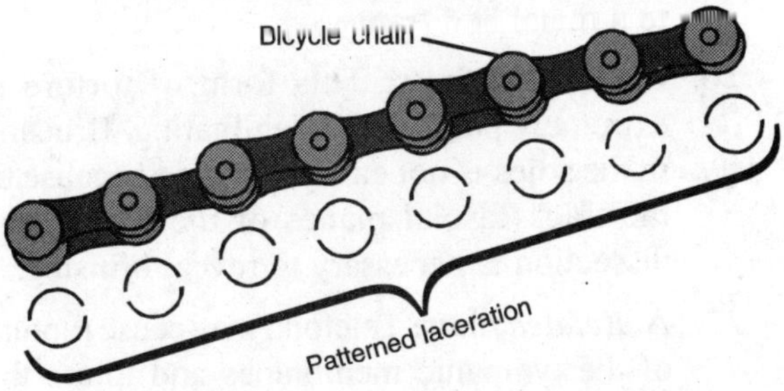

Fig. 11.10: Patterned laceration produced by a bicycle chain

Many students ask, where do patterned lacerations fit in our scheme of classification of lacerations (see answer to previous question). Patterned lacerations are actually small tears which are arranged in a pattern reflecting the shape of the weapon.

TORTURE

23. B. ***Related facts*:** Two varieties of "submarino" are usually applied for torture. One is the "dry submarino" (or *Submarino seco* in Spanish), which is near-suffocation by pulling a plastic bag over the head and face. This is usually a shopping bag sometimes containing chillies and/or petrol.

The other is "wet submarino" (or *Submarino mojado* in Spanish), where the face of the victim is forced under water usually contaminated with excrement, urine, vomit or blood. These victims may die of drowning. Feces in lungs may be an autopsy feature in such cases.

24. A. ***Related facts*:** Forced standing is a standard form of torture. It is called the *planton* (*Planton* in Spanish means "Long wait") in Latin America and the *stoika* in the Soviet Union. *Planton* is an attractive option for torturers because like water torture, it leaves no marks.

Effects of forced standing are (i) Swelling of the ankles and feet to twice their size within 24 hours (ii) Moving becomes agonizing (iii) Development of large blisters (iv) Increasing of the heart rate and fainting.

In the early 20th century, forced standing was a prescribed field punishment for soldiers in West European armies. Soldiers in the British Army referred to it as the "crucifixion", and French legionnaires called it the silo.

By the 1920s, forced standing was a routine police torture in America. In 1931, the National Commission on Lawless Enforcement of the Law found numerous American police departments using forced standing to coerce confessions. In the 1930s, Joseph Stalin's NKVD used forced standing to coerce seemingly voluntary confessions for show trials.

The British used forced standing as early as 1937-1939 on Arab and Jewish prisoners in Mandatory Palestine. The Gestapo routinely used it as a punishment in concentration camps, sometimes creating tiny, narrow cells where prisoners had to stand all night.

In the mid-20th century, torturers learned how to use the swelling and blistering to cause more pain. The Chinese wrapped the feet in gauze, which squeezed painfully as the feet swelled. Brazilian police made prisoners stand on the edges of cans or bricks, causing excruciating pain to the feet. During apartheid in South Africa, forced standing was the third most common torture technique after beating and electricity.

25. D. ***Related facts***: The *"picana"* is a type of electric torture in which an electrically charged needle is applied to areas of heightened sensitivity such as the nipples, genitals, eyes, tongue and teeth. Electric shocks to the gums and teeth, may result in the loss or fracture of teeth.

    In this form of torture, victims are strapped to a wooden table and wetted to aid the flow of current. The prod operator applies the wand to sensitive parts of the body (head, temples, mouth, genitalia, breasts) while the machine operator works the bobbin, raising and reducing voltage. Usually, a doctor is present to make sure that the victim has no heart problems and can survive the interrogation. The picana operates on direct current. It is transported in a suitcase and usually powered by an automobile battery.

    A variation of electrical torture is known as *la parrilla*, (or the metal grill). It consists of electric shocks on the most sensitive parts of the victim's body while the victim is tied to a metal bed frame.

26. C. ***Related facts***: This form of torture is extremely painful and debilitating. Bruising in the soles is not easily revealed because of the thick fascial planes of the foot. Deep dissection is necessary to reveal bruising.

27. A. ***Related facts***: Telefono may cause rupture of the tympanic membranes and injure the inner ear.

12 Firearm Injuries

GENERAL

1. A thermodynamic machine in which the potential energy of the gun-powder is transformed into the kinetic energy of the projectile is known as:
- A. A shot gun
- B. A rifle
- C. A revolver
- D. A firearm

2. The science which deals with the motion of projectiles, is known as:
- A. Ballistics
- B. Internal ballistics
- C. External ballistics
- D. Forensic ballistics

3. The branch of ballistics that deals with what happens to a cartridge and its bullet from the time the trigger of the gun is pulled until the bullet exits from the gun barrel is known as:
- A. Terminal ballistics
- B. Trigger ballistics
- C. Internal ballistics
- D. Cartridge and bullet ballistics

4. The branch of ballistics that deals with what happens to a bullet or projectile from the moment it leaves the gun barrel to the moment of impact on a target or object is known as:
- A. Terminal ballistics
- B. External ballistics
- C. Projectile ballistics
- D. Impact ballistics

5. Any scientific investigation of firearms evidence in a criminal or civil matter of litigation is known as:
- A. Forensic ballistics
- B. Criminal ballistics
- C. Civil ballistics
- D. Both (B) and (C) above

6. Black powder consists of:
- A. 50% Potassium nitrite, 25% charcoal and 25% sulphur
- B. 50% Potassium chlorate, 20% charcoal and 30% sulphur
- C. 50% Potassium nitrate, 10% charcoal and 15% sulphur
- D. 75% Potassium nitrate, 15% charcoal and 10% sulphur

7. Smokeless gunpowder is composed of:
- A. $KMnO_4$
- B. HCN
- C. Nitrocellulose
- D. Sulphur

8. Mercury fulminate is used in firearm ammunition as:
- A. Primer
- B. Smokeless powder

C. Black powder
D. Mixed powder

9. If "M" be the mass of a bullet, "i" its form factor and "d" its diameter, its ballistics co-efficient is given by:

A. $\frac{M}{id^2}$ B. $\frac{Mi}{d^2}$

C. $\frac{id^2}{M}$ D. $\frac{Md^2}{i}$

10. Which of the following bullets contains a powder in their base that burns very brightly during their flight?

A. Dum dum bullet
B. Tracer bullet
C. Tandem bullet
D. Ricochet bullet

11. Which of the following bullets has an exposed lead nose which undergoes rapid expansion on impact thus increasing the amount of destruction?

A. Tracer bullet
B. Incendiary bullet
C. Tandem bullet
D. Dum dum bullet

12. Which of the following cartridges are fired from launchers called rocket hand guns?

A. Tracer bullets
B. Gyrojets
C. Dum dum
D. Ricochet

13. One bullet is impacted at the tip of the gun barrel. It is expelled with another bullet. This is known as:

A. Ricochet bullet
B. Tandem bullet
C. Dum-dum bullet
D. Gyrojet

FIREARMS–TYPES

14. A musket is a:

A. Smooth bore weapon
B. Rifled weapon
C. Special type of shotgun in which the bore has been rifled
D. Smooth bore weapon which can be converted to a rifled one at the touch of a button

15. 12 bore gun technically means that a sphere of:

A. 1/6 pound of lead will exactly fit the bore of the gun
B. 1/12 pound of iron will exactly fit the bore of the gun
C. 1/12 pound of lead will exactly fit the bore of the gun
D. 1/24 pound of lead will exactly fit the bore of the gun

16. Which of the following facts about a carbine are correct?

A. It is a short barreled firearm
B. It can either be a musket or a rifle
C. It was once chiefly a cavalry weapon
D. All of the above

17. In which of the following weapons empty cartridge case is NOT ejected after firing?

A. Shotgun
B. Revolver
C. Pistol
D. Rifle

18. Markings on a projectile occur when it is fired from:

A. A double barrel shot gun
B. A single barrel shot gun
C. Pistol
D. Both single and double barrel shot guns

19. **During operative procedures on a victim of firearm injury, the bullet should preferably be taken out of the body with:**
A. Toothed forceps
B. Hands
C. Scissors
D. Needle

20. **Which of the following is associated with shotgun alone?**
A. Gunpowder
B. Primer
C. Projectile
D. Wads

21. **The effective range of shotgun is:**
A. 10-15 yards
B. 20-30 yards
C. 30-40 yards
D. 60-80 yards

22. **Helixometer is used for:**
A. Finding the effective range of a gun
B. Finding the gauge or bore of a gun
C. Examining the interior of the barrel
D. Calculating the amount of gunpowder placed in a cartridge, so spurious cartridges could be separated

23. **The principal residues formed after burning of the black powder are:**
A. Potassium permanganate
B. Potassium sulfate
C. Potassium carbonate
D. Both (B) and (C)

24. **The terms "FFFFg", "FFFg", "FFg", and "Fg" are used in relation to:**
A. Cartridge
B. Black powder
C. Bore of a gun
D. Wadding of the shot gun

25. **Gunshot residue on hands can be detected by:**
A. Phenolphthalein test
B. Dermal nitrate test
C. Benzidine test
D. Hydrogen Activation Analysis

FIREARM INJURIES

26. **Dirt collar is seen in:**
A. Firearm entry wound
B. Firearm exit wound
C. Both of the above
D. None of the above

27. **Stellate wound is produced with firearm in:**
A. Contact wound
B. Close shot
C. Range within 60 cms
D. Distant shot

28. **A bullet, which strikes some intervening object, and after rebounding from this intervening object, strikes the target is known as:**
A. Secondary bullet
B. Facetious bullet
C. Intervening bullet
D. Ricochet bullet

29. **A wound produced by a ricochet bullet shows which of the following features:**
A. It is small and round
B. It is large, irregular and elongated
C. Abrasion collar is very prominent
D. Burning and blackening at the margins is more than that seen in normal entry wounds

30. **Blackening and tattooing of skin and clothing can best be demonstrated by:**
A. Luminol spray
B. Infra red photography
C. UV light
D. Magnifying lens

31. Puppe's rule is used to determine:

A. The gun from which the shot was fired

B. The distance from which the shot was fired

C. The sequence in which the shots were fired

D. Whether the shots were accidental, homicidal or suicidal in nature

32. Blackening in an entry wound produced by a shot gun is typically seen upto:

A. 6"

B. 12"

C. 24"

D. 36"

MULTIPLE ANSWER TYPE (PGI, CHANDIGARH PATTERN)

33. Primers may consist of:

A. Calcium carbonate

B. Lead styphnate

C. Tetrazene

D. Barium nitrate

E. Antimony sulfide

ANSWERS

GENERAL

1. **D.**
2. **A.**
3. **C.** ***Related fact*:** The other name for this branch is *Interior ballistics*. It can be easily remembered by recalling that it deals with those things that happen in the interior of the gun barrel and chamber. Also remember that it deals with primers, primer ignition, gunpowders, burn rate, rifling, rate of rifling twist, chamber and barrel dimensions and breech pressure. The question can be cleverly changed to include these things.
4. **B.** ***Related fact*:** The other name for this branch is *Exterior ballistics*. It can be easily remembered by recalling that it deals with what happens to the bullet or projectile *exterior* or *external* to the firearm. It deals with such things as flight of the bullet, bullet trajectory, air resistance, bullet drop and gravity, bullet drift and bullet stability.
5. **A.** ***Related fact*:** Watch out for these other definitions of forensic ballistics. It is a branch which deals with the examination of fired bullets and cartridge cases and their identification as having been fired from a particular gun to the exclusion of all others. It also relates to distance determinations made from an examination of shot pellet patterns and firearms combustion residue patterns.
6. **D.** ***Related facts*:** These percentages are by weight, not volume. The charcoal serves as the fuel, sulfur is the binding agent, and the potassium nitrate (saltpeter) is the oxidizer.

   As an oxidizer, any nitrate salt can be used, but KNO_3 works best as it is least hygroscopic (absorbs water less rapidly than other nitrates). Because black powder goes dead when it absorbs water, powders made from hygroscopic calcium nitrate [$Ca(NO_3)_2$] and sodium nitrate [$NaNO_3$] have short shelf lives and must be used quickly. As it turns out, one of the main roles of sulphur in black powder (besides being a binding agent) is to improve shelf life by reducing water absorption.

   It is important to know that one can't just mix these chemicals (charcoal, sulfur and potassium nitrate) together and expect to have black powder. The mixing process for black powder is just as important as the formula. black powder MUST be made in a ball mill to work properly.

   A ball mill is a rotating drum with dozens of lead balls inside. The three chemicals are loaded into the ball mill, along with the lead balls, sealed shut and allowed to rotate for anywhere between one hour and 24 hours. As the ball mill rotates, the lead balls will crush the chemicals together, forcing some of the potassium nitrate into the pores of the charcoal and sulfur. At the same time, the entire mass will be reduced to a super fine powder. The longer the ball mill runs, the stronger the black powder will be. A general rule of thumb for all black powder mixtures is "the finer the powder is, the faster it will burn". It is because black powder is "surface burning"; larger the surface area, quicker the burning.

   ONLY lead balls can be used in a ball mill as they are completely non-sparking. Other metal balls could lead to explosions.

   Variant 1: This question has also been asked in PGI, Chandigarh (multiple answers type) as:

Which ingredient is NOT present in black gunpowder?

A. Lead peroxide
B. Arsenic
C. Charcoal
D. Silver nitrate
E. Sulfur

The answer is (A) Lead peroxide, (B) Arsenic and (D) Silver nitrate.

Variant 2: All are components of black gunpowder *except*:

A. Sulphur
B. Charcoal
C. Potassium nitrate
D. Lead peroxide

The answer is (D) lead peroxide.

7. **C.** ***Related facts***: Three chemicals are mostly used as smokeless powders – nitrocellulose, nitroglycerine and nitroguanidine. The are used either singly or in various permutations and combinations. A good mnemonic is to first arrange them in dictionary fashion (i.e. how they would appear in a dictionary).

   1. Nitrocellulose
   2. Nitroglycerine
   3. Nitroguanidine

   Now remember this.

   Single base smokeless powder consists of just no. 1, i.e. nitrocellulose.

   Double base smokeless powder consists of no. 1 and 2, i.e. nitrocellulose and nitroglycerine.

   Triple base smokeless powder consists of all three.

8. **A.** Sometimes the students would see "detonator" as a choice instead of primer, which should be marked as a correct choice.

9. **A.** ***Related facts***: Ballistic co-efficient is a technical term abbreviated as C. Thus $C = \frac{M}{id^2}$. It describes the ability of a bullet to maintain its velocity against air resistance. The better the ballistic co-efficient of a bullet, the less velocity it will suffer over a given distance. The exact derivation of the formula is complicated and beyond the scope of this book, but a brief look at the formula makes it appear very logical and easy to remember. More the weight of the bullet, more must it travel. More the diameter, the more would be air drag and the less it must travel.

   The formula can also be reduced to $C = \frac{M}{d^2} \times \frac{1}{i}$. $\frac{M}{d^2}$ is also known as sectional density, i.e. weight of the bullet in relation to its cross-section.

10. **B.** ***Related facts***: Tracer bullets are special kind of bullets that contain a powder in their base that burns very brightly during their flight. This enables the shooter to follow the bullets' trajectories, and he can adjust his aim accordingly. It is used both in ground as well as aircraft guns. Usually the ratio that is kept is one tracer bullet per four rounds in ground guns, and one tracer bullet per every two or three rounds in aircraft guns. Tracers have been used extensively in machine guns since World War I (1914-1918).

    A tracer bullet is constructed with a hollow base filled with a pyrotechnic flare material. In US and NATO standard ammunition this is usually a mixture of strontium salts and a metal fuel such as magnesium perchlorate. This yields a bright red light. Russian and Chinese tracer ammunition generates green light using barium salts. Due to their pyrotechnic payload all tracers are incendiary in nature. Some bullets called *incendiary tracer bullets* incorporate white phosphorus. These are more effective.

11. **D.** ***Related facts***: Dum Dum bullet was a British military bullet developed for use in India during the late 1890s, so called because it was produced at the Dum-Dum amm-

unition factory near Kolkata. It is a jacketed .303 bullet (meaning its diameter was 0.303 inches) with the jacket nose open to expose its lead core. It immediately balloons out on impact with the target thus increasing the damage. The phrase 'Dum-Dum' is now taken to include any soft-nosed or hollow pointed bullet. It was used by the British on India's North West Frontier and in the Sudan in 1897 and 1898. The Hague Convention of 1899 outlawed the use of dum-dum bullets during warfare. However it is widely alleged that Belgium used Dum dum bullets during the first world war. Germany made such allegations against Belgium. Kaiser Wilhelm II of Germany even wrote a telegram to U.S. President Woodrow Wilson on 7 September 1914 protesting such use. The Belgians however strongly denied these charges.

12. **B.** ***Related info***: Gyrojet cartridges eject small rockets rather than bullets. These rockets contain solid fuel which keeps burning during its flight for much of its course after it comes out of the barrel of the gun. This greatly increases the range. An interesting forensic implication is that the entrance wound caused by such projectiles will show a singeing effect even at very large distances.

13. **B.**

FIREARMS – TYPES

14. **A.** ***Related fact***: Musket is a s**M**ooth bored long-barelled old type **M**ilitary gun, with bayonet at the **M**uzzle end. It fires a single shot at high velocity.

15. **C.** This is a good question and the student would do well to understand the basics behind this question. Many students find it quite odd that this strange formula is used to determine the bore of a gun rather than simple measurement (in cm or inches) of the inside of the barrel of the gun. This has an ancient tradition, when bores of cannons were measured in terms of the weight of the ammunition it would shoot out. Thus a 12 pounder would fire a 12 pound spherical ball (usually of cast iron, but sometimes of lead too). Similarly a 6 pounder would fire a 6 pound (2.7 kg) spherical ball.

Problems arose with smaller cannons and shot guns. One can have one pounder (one which shoots a ball of one pound of lead) or may be half pounder (one which shoots a ball of half pound of lead), but with smaller diameters it is much more comfortable to talk of balls made from one pound of lead. Thus as we go down the diameters, we would come across a gun, which can, say, fire a lead ball, weighing just 1/12 pounds. Instead of calling it, say, "one-by-twelve pounder", it was more comfortable to call it a 12 bore gun; everyone concerned automatically understood that it fired a lead ball weighing 1/12 pounds. In other words, if 12 equal sized balls were made from one pound of lead, each would fit exactly in the barrel of the gun.

This gave us the much touted definition of the bore of a gun as below:

In the smooth-bore gun, the bore is defined as the number of equal sized spherical balls made from one pound of lead, each of which exactly fits the inside of the barrel.

By knowing that the density of lead is 11.352 g/cm^3 and that one pound is equal to 453.5924 g, one can actually calculate the diameter in inches or cms:

Common bores in use vary from 8 bore to 28 bore. It is important to realize that a larger bore indicates a smaller diameter and vice versa. Here is the full conversion (Table 12.1):

The bores marked * are found in punt guns

which are very rarely used now. Punt guns were extremely large shotguns used in the 19th and 20th centuries for shooting large numbers of waterfowls for commercial purposes. They could have bore diameters up to 2 inches. A single shot could kill a whole flock of waterfowl resting on the water's surface. They were too large to hold and the recoil so large that they were mounted directly on the punts used for hunting, hence their name. They have now been banned.

There is one bore which is smaller than even 28. It is commonly referred to as .410 gauge (mainly by convention). In this case the number refers to the internal diameter of the firearm, i.e., 0.41 inches (equal to 10.41mm), and not the number of balls. If we were to convert this into bores, it would be 68 bore, i.e. the internal diameter of this gun is so small that 68 equal sized balls may be made from one pound of lead, each fitting its barrel. This gun is commonly referred to as "four-ten" (from 0.410 inches) or sometimes 10 mm gun (from nearly 10 mm size).

If we were to draw a one inch line and mark all common bores on this, we would find that all would fit within a very narrow spectrum – between 0.5" to 1.0" range (Fig. 12.1). "Four-ten" is the only gun which falls between the 0"-.5" spectrum. Please note that the middle point (0.5") has been referred to as the "break point". This is not a technical terminology. It is just a way to remember that guns lying on right side of it are said to have bores; guns lying on the left side (there is only one though) are known by their actual internal diameters. The break point is technically equal to 32 bore.

16. D. ***Related facts***: Carbine is a light, short-barrelled musket or rifle. The word, the source of which is obscure, seems to have originated in the late or mid-16th century. The carbine, in various versions corresponding to the different full-sized military arms, was chiefly a cavalry weapon until the 18th century. Then some unmounted officers, artillerymen, and other specialists began to carry carbines. By the 1980s the trend toward general use of light assault rifles (e.g., the Soviet AK-47 or the U.S. M16) was making the carbine obsolete as a military weapon. However, its light weight and short length

Table 12.1: Relationship of bore of a gun with the diametre of its barrel. Weight of the shot is also indicated against each bore (bores marked * are found in punt guns which are very rarely used now)

Bore	*Diameter of barrel in inches*	*Weight of the shot in*		
		Ounces	*Grains*	*Grams*
1½ *	–	–	–	–
2 *	–	–	–	–
3 *	–	–	–	–
4	.935 to .955	–	–	–
8	.837	1.925	875	54.4775
10	.777	1.54	700	43.582
12	.729	1.2826	583	36.29758
13	.711	1.1836	538	33.49588
14	.693	1.1	500	31.13
16	.663	0.9636	438	27.26988
20	.617	0.77	350	21.791
24	.578	0.6424	292	18.17992
28	.549	0.55	250	15.565

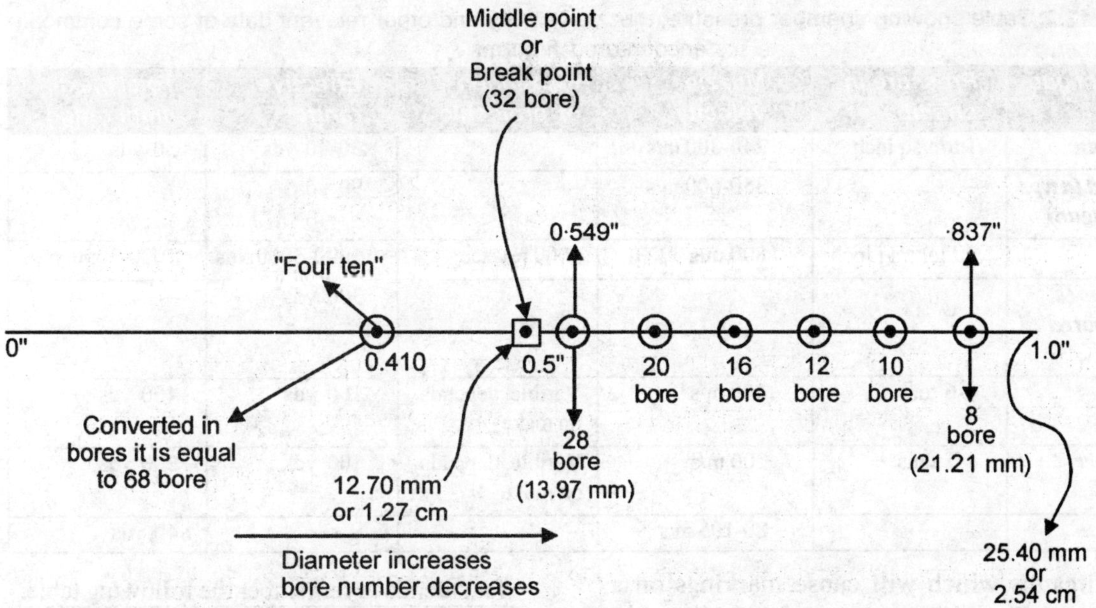

Fig. 12.1: An easy way to understand the concept of bore of a gun (Refer to text for details)

had long made it a popular sporting arm for hunting in heavy brush and also as a scabbard weapon for horseback use.

17. **B.** ***Related fact***: Revolvers never eject cartridge cases. The remaining 3 categories (pistols, shotguns and rifles) all include semiautomatic or automatic versions which eject on firing. But it is useful to remember that all these 3 categories also include versions which are not automatic and thus do not eject on firing.

The standard teaching in this country is that shortguns DO NOT eject cartridge cases, but this is not true. Cartridge ejecting versions of shotguns are well known.

Semi-automatic rifles and shotguns generally eject shells to the right the same way handguns do. Thus a shooter will usually leave cartridges scattered to the right of where he was shooting. The right-hand ejection protects the eyes of right-handed shooters from normal cartridge and powder ejection and especially from the effects of ruptured cases. Left-handed persons sometimes experience some discomfort from powder particle when firing .22 semiautomatics.

Fully automatic shotguns are well known. Shotguns may have tubular, drum or stacked ("clip") type magazines. Not counting drum types, shotguns typically hold between 3 and 8 cartridges.

It is also useful to remember that it is very easy to convert almost any semiautomatic rifle, handgun or shotgun to fully automatic. Sometimes semi autos will fail on their own and turn full automatic.

Fired shotgun shells are referred to as "hulls." You would expect to find hulls at a crime scene if more than one shot was fired quickly from an automatic, semiautomatic, pump or bolt-action shotgun since all of these eject in similar fashion.

18. **C.** ***Related fact***: Markings in a projectile would occur only when it is fired from a rifled firearm. Of all the choices mentioned above, only pistol is the rifled firearm. Other

Table 12.2: Table showing chamber pressure, muzzle velocity and other relevant data of some commonly encountered firearms

Type of gun	*Pressure in chamber*	*Muzzle velocity*	*Revolution of projectile*	*Effective range*	*Total/maximum range*
Shotgun	1 ton/sq inch	240-300 m/s	–	30-40 yds	50 yds
Musket (a type of shotgun)	–	350-600 m/s	–	90 yds	
Rifle	20 tons/sq inch	800 m/s	3000 rev/sec	1000-3000 yds	1000-3000 yds
Carbine (a short barrelled rifle)	–	–	–	300 yds	–
Pistol	4-6 tons	400 m/s	Varible, depends on make	100 yds	400 yds
Revolver	4-5 tons	200 m/s	Varible, depends on make	100 yds	200 yds
Air gun	–	80-105 m/s	–	–	40 yds

firearms which will cause markings on a projectile are (i) revolver and (ii) rifle.

19. B. ***Related facts*****:** When a bullet is fired, important markings known as primary and secondary markings are left on it, which are instrumental in determining the firearm from which it was fired. Handling the bullet with hard objects like toothed forceps, scissors or needle may produce markings of their own, making the job of ballistic expert very difficult. The same precaution must be followed during post-mortem examination. Bullet may also be picked up with a pair of forceps whose tips have been covered with a rubber sheath or cotton.

20. D.

21. C. Effective range (sometimes also referred to as "killing range") is the distance upto which a victim can be hurt or killed. It depends on a number of factors including degree of choking too. 30-40 yards is for a full choke gun. Effective range is often contrasted with total or maximum range, which refers to the total distance upto the missile will travel (without necessarily hurting the target).

This question along with a number of other data are constantly being asked. It is best for stuends to remember the following table.

(Take yards and metres to be practically the same for the purposes of Table 12.2).

22. C. Helixometer was designed by John H. Fisher in 1925 for Bureau of Forensic Ballistics to examine the twist or helix of the rifling in a gun barrel. It found limited application and fell into disuse.

23. D. ***Related facts*****:** The equation guiding the burning of the black powder is:

$$8C + 3S + 10\,KNO_3 \rightarrow 3K_2SO_4 + 2K_2CO_3 + 6CO_2 + 5N_2$$

However this equation represents complete burning. Rarely is burning complete in a cartridge and much unburnt carbon and sulfur is ejected as well.

It is important to realize that the products of burning of black powder in a closed cartridge do not follow any simple equation. Much depends on the exact proportion of chemicals used. A simple, commonly cited, chemical equation for the combustion of black powder is:

$$3C + S + 2\,KNO_3 \rightarrow K_2S + N_2 + 3CO_2$$

It is estimated that one gram of black powder leaves about half gram of residue (composed of unburnt powder and burned products). These residues eject in the form of grayish white smoke, which causes blackening. Some of this residue deposits on the inside of the barrel (known as fouling). Because of this, the barrel of a gun using black powder has to be cleaned again and again (which incidentally is a very arduous and time consuming chore). Immediate cleaning is necessary as this residue is very corrosive in nature, and if allowed to remain for long, may corrode the inside of the barrel.

24. B. FG stands for "fine grain". Since black powder is essentially a surface burning powder, larger the surface area, the quicker it will burn. Larger surface area is produced by griding the black powder very fine.

The four most commonly used granulations are graded as FFFFg, FFFg, FFg, and Fg (also known as 4Fg, 3Fg, 3Fg and Fg respectively). More the F's, finer the grain, with FFFFg being the finest and Fg the coarsest. Thus 4Fg would burn fastest and Fg, slowest.

Elephant Brand black powder (now sold under Schuetzen Powder, LLC) was once made in FFFFFg (5Fg) grain size, the smallest known.

Small (fine) granulations burn faster and are used in small bore guns, where larger (coarser) granulations, are used for larger bore guns and cannons, and for launching Aerial Shells out of mortars. Using a finer granulation for the large bore guns and cannons puts too much strain on the gun (or shell or mortar) because the powder burns much faster and creates a fast pressure increase that could damage whatever one is trying to launch, or the gun/mortar itself.

25. B. ***Related facts***:

- This is also known as paraffin test or diphenylamine test.
- It was introduced in the United States in 1933 by Teodoro Gonzalez of the Criminal Identification laboratory, Mexico City police headquarters.
- This is done to determine whether an individual has fired a firearm or not.
- The principle behind this test is that if an individual has fired a firearm, nitrite and nitrate residues (from burnt gunpowder) would be present in his hands.
- These nitrite and nitrate residues are determined by dermal nitrate test in the following manner:
  - o The hands are coated with a layer of paraffin.
  - o After cooling, the casts are removed and treated with an acid solution of diphenylamine.
  - o A positive test is indicated by the presence of blue flecks in the paraffin.
- False negative results (when the person has not fired a gun, yet the test comes positive) may be obtained in following cases.
  - o If the person has handled fertilizers, urine or cigarettes (all these contain nitrites and nitrates).
- Nowadays dermal nitrate test is rarely performed. Better tests have become available.

Variant: A variant of this question is often asked like this→Paraffin test detects _____on hands (a) Cyanide (b) Gunpowder (c) Blood stains (d) Prints. The answer is (b) Gunpowder.

FIREARM INJURIES

26. A.

27. A. In contact wound, all gases enter the wound. They are under pressure and tend to come back through the same wound, producing the stellate wound.

28. D.

29. B.

30. B.

31. C. When more than one shot have been fired at the cranium, Puppe's rule can often be used to determine the sequence in which the shots were fired. First bullet will cause certain fracture lines to radiate from the hole it causes. The fracture lines emanating from the second bullet hole will stop at the lines caused by the first hole. The fracture lines emanating from the third bullet would stop at the lines caused by first as well as second and so on.

A reference to figure 12.2 would make things clear here. This is the diagram of the skull as seen from the top. This person was hit by three bullets A, B and C. Fracture lines are emanating from all three. The question is to

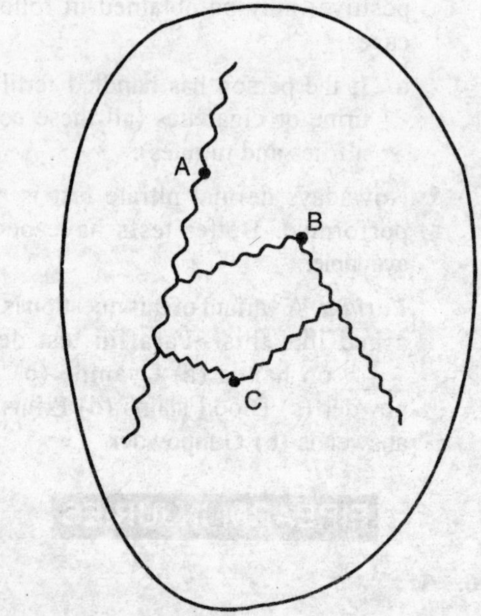

Fig. 12.2: A simple illustration of Puppe's rule – Refer text for details.

determine the sequence of shots. Puppe's rule is useful here. Fracture lines emanating from A are freely expanding both forwards and backwards. One fracture line emanating from B is stopped at the fracture line caused by A, indicating that A was fired first.

Two fracture lines emanate from C; one is stopped by A and the other by B, indicating that both A and B had been fired earlier.

Puppe's rule can also be used to determine the sequence of shots in a glass window or some other similar object. Here cracks in the window instead of fracture lines would be taken into account.

32. C. This is a typical question, which students find hard to answer. The problem is that there are three major classes of guns (pistols and revolves, rifles and shotguns) and three different effects to be remembered (burning and singeing, blackening and tattooing) making a total of nine combinations which need to be remembered.

A few facts to clarify first. Please look at figure 12.3. The figure shows the ejection of flame, smoke and unburnt powder particles from the gun just as it is fired. As can be seen, flame leaps out the shortest distance; smoke goes after that; and unburnt powder particles leap out the farthest.

Now remember the following:

Flame→is responsible for burning, scorching and singeing. These effects can be detected by looking at the hair around, which would be found singed.

Smoke→is produced by *complete* combustion of gun powder. It is responsible for blackening. Smoke simply deposits on the skin, without actually entering inside the dermis. Thus if one takes a wet cotton gauge, sponge or towel and tries cleaning the wound, the blackening would vanish. If one looks at the cotton, one would find it has blackened. Blackening is also known as smudging.

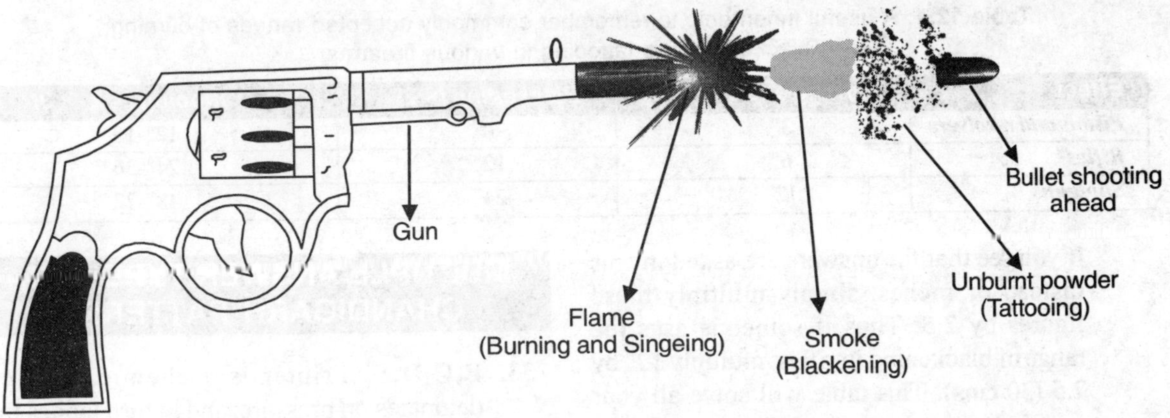

Fig. 12.3: Figure illustrating how burning, singeing, blackening and tattooing are caused

Students often ask, how smokeless powders can produce smoke (and consequently blackening). The term "smokeless powder" is actually a misnomer. They do produce smoke, albeit it is extremely less in amount compared to the black powder. Furthermore the smoke produced by smokeless powders is somewhat greyish white in color, and it produces blackening of a much lighter color.

Unburnt powder particles→are produced by *incomplete* combustion of gun powder. They are of the consistency of very fine sand. They are responsible for tattooing. Unburnt powder particles have so much kinetic energy, that they actually penetrate the dermis and come to lie under it. If one takes a wet towel and tries cleaning the wound, tattooing can not vanish. In decorative tattooing, the artist actually drives the pigment particles inside the dermis, with the help of an electrical gadget. Since the unburnt particles are similarly driven inside the skin, the process has been termed tattooing. It has also been called (i) stippling and (ii) peppering (since it appears as if black pepper has been spread around the wound) (Table 12.3).

Now remember the following table (Table 12.4). You just have to remember one figure– 3", which is the left uppermost numeral. The rule is that as you go to the right or below, you multiply the figure by 2. Tattooing is expressed in range. Thus on reaching the third column, you have to multiply the previous figure first by 2 (to give the lower limit of range) and then by 3 (to give the upper limit of the range).

Table 12.3: Table showing how burning, blackening and tattooing are produced and how best they can be detected

Product of firing a gun	*Responsible for*	*Detected by*
Flame	Burning, scorching and singeing	Looking at singed hair around
Smoke	Blackening	Wiping the wound with a wet sponge Blackeing vanishes. Sponge becomes dirty
Unburnt powder particles	Tattooing	Wiping the wound with a wet sponge Tattooing does not vanish

Table 12.4: A useful mnemonic to remember commonly accepted ranges of burning, blackening and tattooing in various firearms

Effect	Burning and singeing	Blackening (× 2)	Tattooing (× 2 - × 3)
Pistols and revolvers	3"	6"	12"-18"
Rifles	6"	12"	24"-36"
Shotguns	12"	24"	48"-72"

If you see that the answers are asked in cms instead of inches, simply multiply these figures by 2.5. Thus if someone asks the range of blackening in rifles, multiply 12" by 2.5 (30 cms). This table will solve all your questions on ranges.

MULTIPLE ANSWER TYPE (PGI, CHANDIGARH PATTERN)

33. **B,C,D,E.** Primer is a chemical which detonates on pressure, and in turn ignites the gun powder. Calcium carbonate does not belong to this class.

13 Thermal Injuries

1. **Mammalian tissues can survive within a very narrow range of temperatures. This range of temperature is generally taken to be between:**
   A. -12 to 37 degrees Celsius
   B. 5 to 42 degrees Celsius
   C. 20 to 44 degrees Celsius
   D. 30 to 55 degrees Celsius
2. **Burns are classified by which of the following classifications?**
   A. Dupuytren's
   B. Hebra's
   C. Wilson's
   D. All of the above
3. **The lowest temperature that can cause thermal damage to the human body is:**
   A. 40 degrees Celsius
   B. 44 degrees Celsius
   C. 54 degrees Celsius
   D. 80 degrees Celsius
4. **Which of the following burns are most painful? (Classification given by Dupuytren)**
   A. First degree
   B. Second degree
   C. Third degree
   D. Fourth degree
5. **If the burns have caused blisters, it is ....degree burns (Dupytren's classification):**
   A. First degree
   B. Second degree
   C. Third degree
   D. Fourth degree
6. **Dupuytren's classification divides all burns into:**
   A. 3 degrees
   B. 4 degrees
   C. 6 degrees
   D. 8 degrees
7. **Rule of nine is employed to find out:**
   A. The cause of burns
   B. The area of burns
   C. The depth of burns
   D. The prognosis of burns
8. **Heat hematoma is seen inside:**
   A. Cranial cavity
   B. Chest cavity
   C. Abdominal cavity
   D. Uterus
9. **Antemortem burns can be differentiated from postmortem burns by:**
   A. Presence of soot in the finer branches of bronchi

B. Presence of carbon monoxide in the blood
C. Presence of boxer's attitude
D. Both (A) and (B) above

10. **In a completely charred body, in order to determine that the burns were antemortem, the medical officer can best rely on which of the following findings:**
A. Soot in respiratory passages
B. Cyanosis of finger nails
C. Congestion of the kidneys
D. Pale internal organs

11. **If a minimum of ....% of body surface is burnt, the injury may be classified as grievous hurt by the doctor:**
A. 15%
B. 33%
C. 50%
D. 65%

POSTMORTEM FEATURES

External Examination

12. **Heat ruptures show:**
A. Smooth and even margins
B. Irregular margins
C. Ruptured vessels in the floor
D. Clotted blood in the wound

13. **Which of the following is true about "heat ruptures"?**
A. Absence of bleeding
B. Absence of bruising and vital reaction
C. Presence of intact vessels and nerves in the floor
D. All of the above

14. **Antemortem blister can be differentiated from postmortem blisters, by noticing that antemortem blisters:**
A. Have more albumin and chloride
B. Have just gas in them
C. Show a pale base when punctured
D. Do not show any hyperemia around them

Internal Examination

15. **The usual site of Curling's ulcers in burn victims is:**
A. Pharynx and oesophagus
B. Duodenum
C. Caecum
D. Sigmoid colon

MULTIPLE ANSWER TYPE (PGI, CHANDIGARH PATTERN)

16. **Which of the following facts about pugilistic attitude are correct?**
A. It is seen both in severe heat and severe cold
B. It is ten times more common in females than in males
C. It does not occur if burns occur AFTER death
D. Extensors are affected MORE than flexors
E. Stiffening is due to coagulation of muscle proteins

17. **Which of the following facts about *Erythema ab igne* are correct?**
A. It is seen in the form of mottled pigmentation and reddening in front of legs
B. It is seen in people addicted to sitting before an open fire
C. It is typically seen when the skin is subjected alternately to very low and very high temperatures as in certain occupations
D. It is a potentially fatal condition caused by spillage of hot liquids on the body
E. This is the name given to radiation burns caused by X-rays in technicians working in radiology departments

ANSWERS

1. C.
2. D.
3. B. To cause thermal damage at 44°C, the heat would have to be applied for at least 5 hours! This is not just trivia but an important medical fact to keep in mind; of late there have been many medical negligence lawsuits where paramedical personnel have forgotten hot water bottles in the beds of unconscious patients causing burns. As temperature increases, the time required to cause damage drops exponentially; if the temperature is 60°C, only 3 seconds are needed to cause burns.
4. C.
5. B.
6. C.
7. B. ***Related fact:*** According to this rule all areas of the body have areas in multiples of nines (Fig. 13.1).

   Thus head and neck are 9%, front of chest 9%, back of chest 9%, front of abdomen 9%, back of abdomen 9%, right upper limb 9%, left upper limb 9%, front of right lower limb 9%, back of right lower limb 9%, front of left lower limb 9% and back of left lower limb 9%. This makes 99%. The remaining 1% is allotted to genitals.
8. A. ***Related facts:*** Remember the following facts about heat hematoma, which may be helpful in other related MCQs:
   - Heat hematoma is formed in the *Extradural space* (see accompanying figure 13.2 on the next page).
   - The blood in heat haematoma comes either from venous sinuses (it is often found over the superior sagittal sinus) or from the diplöe of the skull. The blood from diplöe, supposedly "boils out" due to great heat and passes through emissary veins, to come to lie just beneath the skull (and outside the dura).
   - Heat hematoma can be differentiated from "normal" traumatic extradural hematoma, by following facts:
     - o Blood in heat hematoma is spongy from gas bubbles.
     - o The color is tawny or chocolate brown.
     - o Heat hematoma would contain carbon monoxide and its levels would match that of peripheral blood.

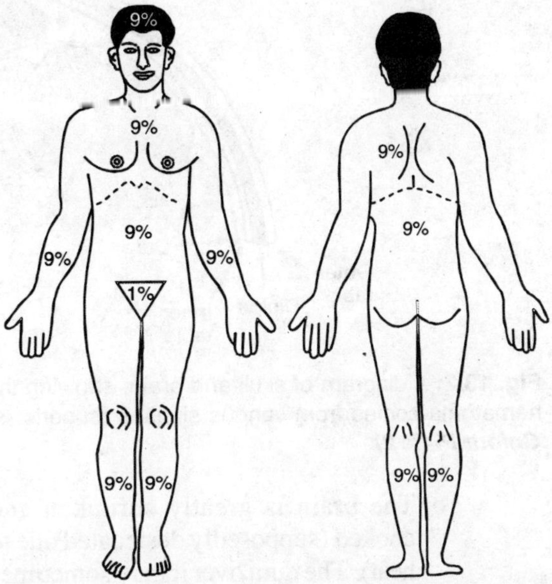

Fig 13.1. Illustration of the "Rule of nine". The body is divided into 12 major areas, 11 of them comprise 9% each, totalling 99%. The remaining 1% is comprised by the 12th region—the genitals

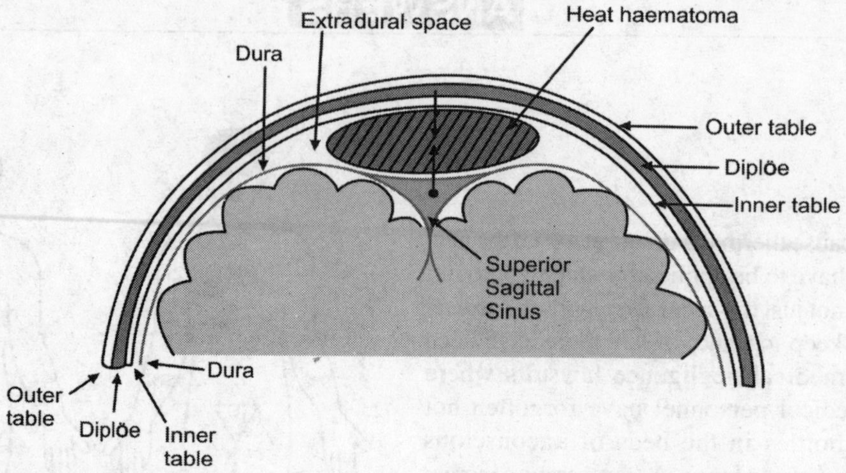

Fig. 13.2: A diagram of skull and brain, showing the position of heat hematoma. Note that the blood in heat hematoma comes from venous sinuses (superior sagittal sinus in the diagram) and from diplöe. ***(See also Colour Plate 2)***

- o The brain is greatly shrunken and cooked (supposedly desiccated due to heat). The dura over it may sometimes be split.

9. **D.** ***Related fact***: Boxer's attitude is seen in both antemortem as well as postmortem burns, so it can not be used to differentiate the two. The other two can genuinely be used to differentiate the two.
10. **A.**
11. **B.** Generally a minimum of 33% of body area (or one-third) must be involved in burns, before burns become dangerous to life. These can then be classified as grievous.

POSTMORTEM FEATURES

External Examination

12. **B.**
13. **D.**
14. **A.**

Internal Examination

15. **B.**

MULTIPLE ANSWER TYPE (PGI, CHANDIGARH PATTERN)

16. **E.** Pugilistic or boxer's attitude is not seen in severe cold. It is not dependent on sex at all. It occurs irrespective of the fact whether burns occur before or after death, so it is NOT a useful criterion to differentiate antemortem from postmortem burns. Flexors are affected more than extensors, that is why there is a boxer like attitude.

Variant 1: A variant of this question is often asked like this→Pugilistic attitude seen in burns resembles the attitude of a (a) Boxer (b) Dancer (c) Athlete (d) Swimmer. The answer is (a) Boxer.

Variant 2: Pugilistic attitude is seen in (a) Drowning (b) Protein coagulation (c)

Electrocoagulation (d) Hanging. The answer is (b) Protein coagulation.

17. **A,B.** *Erythema ab igne* (EAI) is caused by chronic repeated exposure to moderate heat from an external heat source. The exposure, which need not be of long duration, results in cutaneous hyperthermia in the range of 43-47°C, which, in turn, results in histopathologic changes similar to those seen in solar-damaged skin. Pathogenic mechanisms in EAI are poorly understood. However the damage may be due to denaturation of DNA in squamous cells caused by moderate heat acting synergistically with ultraviolet radiation. EAI is most typically seen on the legs of women usually aged between 40-70 years who use indoor fire as a heat source, and on the face and/or palms of cooks who work over an open fire.

14 Explosion Injuries

1. Deaths by which of the following explosion devices are commonly investigated by a forensic pathologist?

A. Letter bombs
B. Car bombs
C. Parcel bombs
D. All of the above

2. In ordinary "civilian" explosions ordinarily encountered by forensic pathologists, the pressures generated may be up to:

A. 150 atm
B. 1,500 atm
C. 15,000 atm
D. 150,000 atm

3. Temperatures of explosive gases in ordinary "civilian" explosions may rise upto:

A. 100°C
B. 300°C
C. 3000°C
D. 10,000°C

4. Death and injury from explosions is caused by:

A. Impact of projectiles derived from the explosive device
B. Impact from surrounding objects and debris impelled by the explosion
C. Blast effects
D. All of the above

5. Which of the following tissue suffers most in a blast caused by an explosion?

A. Lung
B. Liver
C. Skeletal system
D. Nervous system including brain

6. Molotov cocktail is:

A. A special cocktail of strong alcohols which perpetrators take to increase their courage before using explosives
B. A petrol bomb
C. A recently discovered special decoction used for treatment in victims of explosions
D. A special and highly destructive bomb used in Brazil by a gang known as Molotov

7. RDX is one of the most important and useful military explosives. Its full form is:

A. Real death X-ray
B. Red dye xylophone
C. Rightful death explosive
D. Research Department Explosive

8. Typical injury in a bomb explosion is:

A. Abrasion
B. Punctate bruises
C. Puncture lacerations
D. A triad of punctate bruises, abrasions and puncture lacerations

MULTIPLE ANSWER TYPE (PGI, CHANDIGARH PATTERN)

9. Postmortem examination of an explosion victim involves the following objectives?

A. Identification of the victim
B. Conduct a limited postmortem so the mutilated body of the victim is not further disfigured
C. Reconstruction of the events
D. Find the intention of the perpetrator
E. Find how the culprit arranged for the finances to get the explosives

10. Which of the following injuries are typically seen in a victim of explosion?

A. Complete disruption
B. Complete vaporization of bones
C. Flying missile injury
D. Burns
E. Injury from falling masonry

ANSWERS

1. **D.**
2. **D.**
3. **C.**
4. **D.** In addition to these three, death and injury from explosions are also caused by (iv) burns from hot gases and incadescent objects and (v) secondary injuries from falling masonry, beams and furnishings disloged by the explosion.
5. **A.** Blast caused by an explosion is a wave of compression followed by a transient zone of low pressure (below atmospheric pressure). So a rapid double change in pressure is suffered by the body. A blast causes the most damage at an interface between tissues in contact with the atmosphere. This is why lung suffers the most.
6. **B.** ***Related facts:*** A Molotov cocktail (also known as a petrol bomb) consists of a glass bottle partly filled with flammable liquid, usually petrol (gasoline) or alcohol (generally methanol or ethanol). The mouth of the bottle is stoppered with a cork or other type of airtight bung (rubber, glass, or plastic), and a cloth rag is fixed securely around the mouth. The weapon is used by first soaking the rag in a flammable liquid immediately prior to using it, lighting the rag, and throwing the bottle at the target. The bottle shatters on impact, spilling the flammable liquid over the target, which is then ignited by the burning rag.

   It is a common practice to throw several unlit, full, bottles to saturate an area, then finish with a lit one. This avoids some of the risk of throwing several lit devices. If one uses lit bottles each time, the enemy would see the flaming bottles approaching and know which direction to start shooting. There is also the possibility of missing target or dropping the device after being lit.

   Many substances such as white phosphorus, tar, palm oil, acids etc. may be added to the basic Molotov cocktail to enhance its use as a weapon.

   Named after **Vyacheslav Mikhailovich Molotov** (1890–1986) a Soviet politician, who first advocated it.
7. **D.** ***Related facts*:** RDX was discovered as far back as 1899, but not used until World War II. It is also called cyclonite, hexagen, and cyclo-trimethylenetrinitramine.
8. **D.**

MULTIPLE ANSWER TYPE (PGI, CHANDIGARH PATTERN)

9. **A,C.** It is not the duty of the forensic pathologist to find the intention of the perpetrator or to find how the culprit arranged for the finances. These are the duties of the police. The function of the forensic pathologist is to identify the victim (because in most cases his body may be severely disfigured) and the proper reconstruction of events.
10. **A,C,D,E.**

15 Electrocution, Atmospheric Lightning, Radiation Injury

1. **Which of the following tissues is most resistant to electric current?**
   A. Muscle
   B. Skin
   C. Bone
   D. Blood
2. **In India, the voltage of domestic supply is:**
   A. 120 volts, D.C.
   B. 220-240 Volts A.C. at 50 Hz
   C. 220-240 Volts A.C. at 250 Hz
   D. 220-240 Volts A.C. at 500 Hz
3. **In electrocution, death may occur due to:**
   A. Primary shock
   B. Secondary shock
   C. Paralysis of respiratory centre
   D. Coma
4. **In deaths due to electrocution, which of the following factors is the SINGLE MOST IMPORTANT factor in causing fatality?**
   A. Voltage
   B. Amperage
   C. Nature of the current, i.e. AC or DC
   D. Resistance of the body
5. **Which of the following statements regarding electricity is correct?**
   A. A.C. is more dangerous than D.C.
   B. D.C. is more dangerous than A.C.
   C. Both are equally dangerous
   D. Which is more dangerous depends on the fact if one is standing on a wet or a dry surface
6. **Arborescent markings are due to:**
   A. Dry burns
   B. Scalds
   C. Hanging
   D. Lightning
7. **Which of the following is a characteristic postmortem finding of a death due to electrocution?**
   A. Honeycomb liver
   B. Local hemorrhages and/or tears in the muscles
   C. *Taché noir de la sclerotiques*
   D. All of the above
8. **Which of the following facts is correct about judicial electrocution?**
   A. In our country, the condemned prisoner can choose between hanging and judicial electrocution
   B. A current of 2000 volts is passed for 3-5 seconds followed by another impulse of 250-500 volts
   C. A current of 20,000 volts is passed for just one second

D. A current of 120 volts is passed for half an hour, followed by an impulse of 2000 volts for about 10 seconds

9. "Joule burn" is the name given to:

A. Electric entry mark
B. Electric exit mark
C. Flash burns caused by electricity
D. Burns caused by AC rather than by DC

10. "Crocodile-skin" lesions are seen in injuries due to:

A. Low tension currents
B. Currents sustained in bath tubs
C. High tension currents
D. Alternating currents

11. Which one of the following statements is NOT true regarding the joule burn:

A. It indicates exit point of current
B. It is usually round or oval in shape
C. It is usually seen as a shallow crater
D. It has a grayish or pale base

12. Which of the following is the most characteristic feature of a joule burn?

A. It is round in shape
B. It has a depressed base
C. There is an areola of blanched skin at the periphery
D. It is usually green in color

13. Electrocution as a method of judicial execution is followed in:

A. All states of US
B. Only a few states of US
C. United Arab Emirates
D. India

MULTIPLE ANSWER TYPE (PGI, CHANDIGARH PATTERN)

14. Which of the following are genuinely recognized steps to be followed by a forensic pathologist in a case of death due to electrocution?

A. Examine the spleen in great detail
B. Visit the scene of death, especially if there are no burns or electrical injury marks on the dead body
C. Take rectal swabs
D. Call upon an expert electrician and examine all electric equipment at the scene of death immediately
E. Examine the retina in great detail

ANSWERS

1. **B.** The most resistant tissular layer of the body is the skin, followed in order of decreased resistance, by bone, fat, nerve, muscle, blood, and body fluids. Variations in resistance are primarily determined by the water content of the tissues. Dry skin has a higher resistance than skin moist with sweat.

2. **B.** Most students would perhaps correctly remember the voltage. The trick is to remember the correct value of Hz too.

3. **C.**

4. **B.** ***Additional info:*** It is the amperage which is most important, because this is what represents the actual number of electrons passing through the body. Voltage merely represents the "pressure" of electricity, and may not necessarily result in high amperage. Indeed it is said that in high voltage the victim may be thrown clear, while lower voltages (say around 240 volts) cause muscle contraction making the person unable to let go of the conductor. For this reason, in USA the domestic electrical supply is at 120 volts.

5. **A.** ***Additional info***: A.C. is about 4-5 times as dangerous as D.C. It is because of the tetanoid contractions effected by the A.C. An A.C. of 70-80 mA may be lethal, whereas a D.C. with an intensity of 250 mA may be tolerated without damage.

6. **D.** ***Related fact***: These markings are known by several different names, some among them being "arborization", "feathering", "ferning", "filigree burns", "arborescent burns", "Lichtenberg's flowers" [after a pre-eminent German physicist and scientist **Georg Christoph Lichtenberg** (1742-1799) who reproduced similar images with the help of static electricity] or "keraunographic markings". The phenomenon is also known as "keraunographism" from Greek *keraunos*, a thunder bolt (**Keraunomedicine** incidentally deals with medical aspects of lightning injuries and **Keraunopathology** with pathological changes seen in lightning injuries).

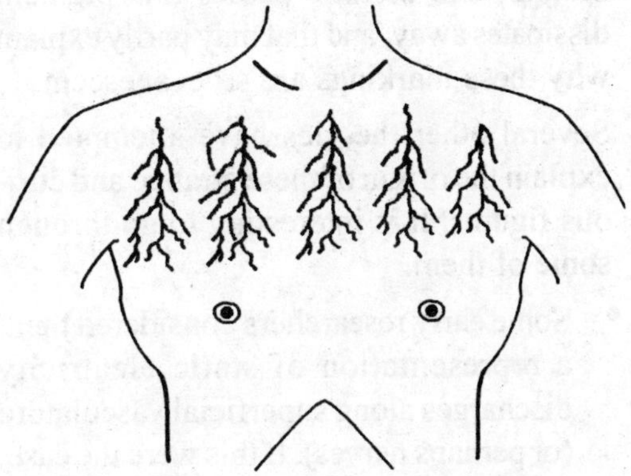

Fig. 15.1: Arborescent markings seen over the chest in a case of death due to lightning

Arborescent markings are one of the most characteristic findings in a lightning death. These are nothing but a fern like pattern on the body. This pattern is usually seen over the shoulders or the flanks. Sometimes it is seen on the front of chest also. In layman's language, this peculiar pattern is usually referred to "lightning marks".

These marks are NOT seen in all cases of lightning. Various studies quote different figures, but most state that these marks are seen in between one-third to one-fifth of all victims (20% to 33%). Curiously, these markings disappear in about 12 hours among survivors of lightning strikes and quite often in the postmortem state too. One might think that these lesions are burns, but they are not.

There are several theories regarding the mechanism of formation of these markings. One of the most popular theories is that these marks arise due to break down of red blood cells within the capillaries of the skin. The red colored pigment **haemoglobin** escapes in the surrounding tissues and stains them, in the pattern of a tree. It is thought that as time passes this pigment dissipates away, and that may partly explain why these markings are so evanescent.

Several other theories have attempted to explain the origin of these strange and curious figures. It is interesting to go through some of them.

- Some early researchers considered them a representation of static electricity discharges along superficial vasculature (or perhaps nerves). If this were the case, they would be seen along the lines of vasculature, but they have been noted to cross body parts, for example, from chest to arm. Vasculature does not cross body parts in this manner, so this theory probably is not true.
- Some persons believe that these dendriform (tree-like) markings may result from electron showers eliciting an inflammatory response in the skin. However if this were really an inflammatory response, the markings would not disappear so soon. Their rapid dissipation without residual scarring thus goes against this theory.
- Some workers have suggested that these markings are the result of current following the lines of skin moisture. However this theory also falls in problems as it is unable to explain their consistent shape under all manner of conditions (whether the person was perspiring or not).
- Some researchers – especially those with a mathematical bend of mind – think that these figures are in fact fractals. Fractals are an interesting mathematical concept, where figures exhibit increasing details with increasing manifestations. Many natural features exhibit fractal like shapes, one notable among them being coastlines (this is especially evident when seen from aircraft at a great height). However how and why these fractals are produced has never been explained satisfactorily.

7. **B.** The hemorrhages/tears are especially abundant in muscles of the extremity. These are due to forcible contraction and spasm induced by the passage of current.

8. **B.** ***Additional info useful for other MCQs*:**

1. The first person to be electrocuted was William Kemmler. The electrocution took place in New York's Auburn Prison on August 6, 1890. In this case an alternating current of 1600 volts at 150 Hz was used. Kemmler was declared dead after 17 seconds. After this electrocution the procedure was changed several times.
2. Of the two electrodes applied to the condemned prisoner, one is shaped like a helmet and is placed on the head. The other is placed on the *right leg* (Watch out for this fact, as this can form a good MCQ).
3. After the application of initial burst of 2000 volts, the victim loses consciousness immediately. It is the second surge (of a lower intensity) which actually kills the victim. It is important to appreciate that there is no uniformity over the amount of current delivered; however two impulses

are indeed given – the first in the range of 2000 volts for a short time (when the victim loses consciousness) and the second in the range of 500 volts for a longer time (when the victim actually dies). Sometimes upto 2,400 volts will be delivered for seven seconds as the first impulse, followed by 600 volts for 17 seconds; the process is repeated. After five minutes, a physician checks the heartbeat. If the heart is still beating, the voltage is delivered again.

4. Beneath the electrodes, the skin temperature may rise as high as 60°C. The temperature of brain in such cases also rises to similar levels. Histologically rupture of neuroaxons and blood vessels can be demonstrated in the brain.
5. Right leg immediately goes into cadaveric spasm.
6. Often sperm ejaculation occurs.

9. A. ***Additional info*:** Remember the following facts which may be helpful in other related MCQs:

1. "Joule burn" is an endogenous thermal burn, i.e. the heat is generated within the body due to the passage of current.
2. It is different from "exogenous burn", where the burn is caused by sparking. Note that in this case, the source of heat is outside the body. The heat is NOT generated within the body, as in case of "joule burn".
3. If the skin touching the conductor is well-moistened, it may not show any electrical burn mark (less resistance would mean less generation of heat). Thick dry skin will show a well-circumscribed electrical burn mark.

Variant: A variant of this question is often asked like this→**Joule burn is seen in** (a) Electrocution (b) Thermal injury (c) Radiation injury (d) Lightning. The answer is (a) Electrocution.

10. C. High tension currents can jump several millimeters across air and cause lesions (it is estimated that in dry air a current of 100 kV can jump upto 35 mm). Such high tension currents can produce extremely high temperatures (upto about 4000°C, just like in the sparking plug of a petrol engine).

These high temperatures can cause the keratin of the skin to melt over multiple small areas. On cooling, molten keratin over these areas fuses into multiple hard brownish nodules, as in the skin of a crocodile—hence the name (Fig. 15.2).

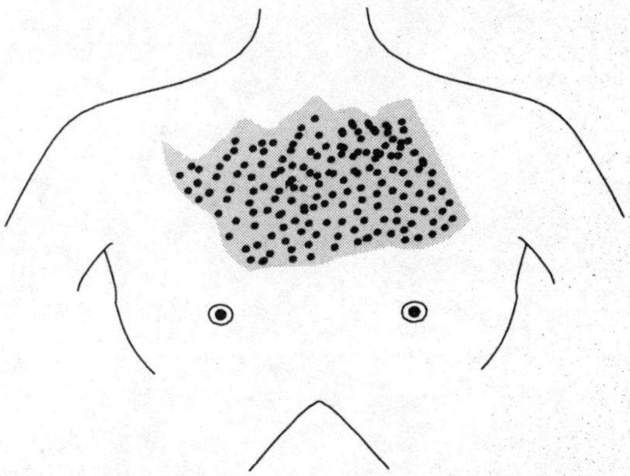

Fig. 15.2: Crocodile skin formed over the chest due to high tension current. Note the characteristic multiple hard brownish nodules

11. A. Exit point of a current is very rarely seen. It is seen in areas where the body was earthed or "grounded". Even when it is seen, it is usually not called Joule burn; it is known simply as "exit point" or "exit mark". Joule burn is usually round or oval in shape, although sometimes it can take a linear shape, reflecting the shape of the conductor (wire).

12. C. An areola of blanched skin at the periphery of the Joule burn is considered the most useful indicator of Joule burn. This is presumably due to arteriolar spasm from the effects of the current. Often there are areas of hyperemia both inside and outside this zone. Thus extending outside from the crater, one can often see a spectrum like this: crater→ reddening→pallor→ reddening.

13. **B.** Only six US states, Alabama, Florida, Georgia, Kentucky, Nebraska and Tennessee, use electrocution for judicial execution.

MULTIPLE ANSWER TYPE (PGI, CHANDIGARH PATTERN)

14. **B,D.** A visit to the scene of crime is essential in deaths due to electrocution. In many cases, the only clues may be the finding of electrical short circuits or defective wiring in electrical home apparatus like hand tools, electrical drills and saws and home laundry machines.

Delay in visiting the scene of death, or impounding the suspicious looking piece of electrical apparatus and keeping it away for subsequent examination may be a big blunder. A good example is the drying away of wet insulation, which may restore the electrical apparatus to its original condition.

Examination of spleen or retina is of no particular value in electrocution.

16 Regional Injuries

GENERAL

1. **"*Plaques jaunes*" is the name given to:**
   - **A.** Old healed cortical contusions
   - **B.** Liver injuries caused by blunt force
   - **C.** Splenic hemorrhages
   - **D.** Testicular injuries
2. **"Retraction balls" are seen after injuries to:**
   - **A.** Liver
   - **B.** Spleen
   - **C.** Lungs
   - **D.** Brain
3. **"Retraction balls" are seen in:**
   - **A.** Cerebral lacerations
   - **B.** Cerebral contusions
   - **C.** Diffuse axonal injury
   - **D.** Injuries to tendons
4. **Kernohan's notch is seen in:**
   - **A.** Lungs
   - **B.** Liver
   - **C.** Spleen
   - **D.** brain
5. **Duret hemorrhages are seen in:**
   - **A.** Endocardium of the heart
   - **B.** Conjunctiva
   - **C.** Middle ear
   - **D.** Brain

HEAD INJURIES

Scalp

6. **Which of the following statements regarding scalp injuries is NOT correct?**
   - **A.** Wounds of scalp may or may not be associated with fractures of the skull
   - **B.** Most scalp wounds take the form of contusions or lacerations
   - **C.** Lacerated wounds over scalp can mimic incised wounds
   - **D.** In the absence of skull fracture, injuries to scalp will not predispose the victim to intracranial infections

Skull

7. **The thickness of outer table of skull is:**
   - **A.** Same as that of the inner table
   - **B.** Twice that of inner table
   - **C.** Half that of inner table
   - **D.** One-third of that of inner table
8. **Average thickness of skull is:**
   - **A.** 1-2 mm
   - **B.** 3-5 mm
   - **C.** 1 cm
   - **D.** 2 cm

FRACTURES

9. Jefferson's fracture is a name given to:

A. A fracture of ribs caused by sudden and inadvertent coughing
B. A fracture of the metatarsals usually seen in soldiers, which entitles them to compensation
C. A fracture of the tibia caused by a speeding car
D. A bilateral bursting fracture of anterior and posterior arches of C1 against the occipital condyles.

10. "*Fractures à la signature*" is a:

A. Depressed fracture
B. Counter coup fracture
C. Fracture dislocation of the 3rd and 4th cervical vertebrae
D. Fracture of the terminal phalangeal bone of the right thumb

11. Pond fracture is:

A. A simple dent of the skull
B. Caused by falling into a deep pond
C. Mostly seen in bones of infants
D. Both (A) and (C) above

12. The percentage of linear fractures of the skull NOT found on X-ray examination is:

A. 0.5%
B. 2%
C. 20%
D. 40%

13. Comminuted fracture is:

A. Breaking of a bone in multiple pieces
B. A cut on a bone extending up to medullary cavity
C. A dent in the skull cap, especially in infants
D. Separation of skull sutures

14. Greenstick fracture is seen mostly in:

A. Females
B. Old people
C. Infants
D. Vertebrae

15. Compound fracture refers to a situation where:

A. A bone gets broken at two places
B. Two or more bones break in a single incident
C. A bone and a cartilage get fractured together
D. A bone breaks and the ends of the broken bone pierce the skin to project out

16. Diastatic fracture refers to:

A. Separation of skull sutures
B. Indenting of skull due to pressure
C. A bone being broken at two or more places
D. Two or more bones fracturing simultaneously

17. Gutter fracture is caused by:

A. A firearm missile glancing along the outer table of the skull
B. Falling into a shallow gutter
C. Falling into a river or any other body of water
D. Both (B) and (C) above

18. A fracture in which a piece of the bone is removed by violence, as by a bullet is known as:

A. Resecting fracture
B. Secondary fracture
C. Segmental fracture
D. Pressure fracture

19. In the skull, fractures caused NOT at the point of impact, but some distance away from it are known as:

A. Diagonal fractures
B. Atypical skull fractures
C. Bursting fractures
D. Depressed fractures

20. Traction fracture is most commonly seen in:

A. Mandible
B. Clavicle

C. Patella
D. Scapula

INJURIES TO BRAIN AND MENINGES

21. Counter-coup injury is seen in:
A. Gunshot wound
B. Head injury
C. Wound in the abdomen
D. Chest wounds

22. The probable diagnosis in a case of head injury where the person loses consciousness transiently; then regains consciousness and then again goes into coma is:
A. Subdural haemorrhage
B. Extradural haemorrhage
C. Subarachnoid haemorrhage
D. Intracerebral haemorrhage

23. In a case of acute subdural haematoma, what is the minimum quantity of blood that must accumulate before the condition becomes life threatening?
A. 1-2 ml
B. 5-10 ml
C. 100-150 ml
D. 500-600 ml

24. Which of the following facts regarding Subarachnoid haemorrhage is NOT TRUE?
A. It is the most common form of intracranial bleeding
B. It can be caused by prolonged hyperextension of the head during bronchoscopy
C. One of its most common causes is rupture of middle meningeal artery in the subarachnoid space
D. It can be caused by asphyxia due to strangulation

25. Which of the following is true of a traumatic porencephalic cyst?
A. It is found in the brain
B. It is filled with CSF
C. It often communicates directly with the ventricular system
D. All of the above

26. The most common type of haemorrhage seen in boxers is:
A. Extradural
B. Subdural
C. Subarachnoid
D. Intracerebral

27. Unconsciousness occurring immediately after a head injury is due to:
A. Cerebral compression
B. Cerebral edema
C. Concussion
D. Cerebral anaemia

VERTEBRAL COLUMN AND SPINAL CORD

28. Which of the following is more dangerous in causing spinal damage?
A. Hyperextension of the neck
B. Hyperflexion of the neck
C. Both hyperflexion and hyperextension of the neck
D. None can cause spinal damage

HEART

29. Rapid accumulation of a minimum of ....c.c. of blood in the pericardium can cause cardiac tamponade?
A. 3 c.c.
B. 30 c.c.
C. 300 c.c.
D. 3000 c.c.

OTHER ORGANS

30. Which of the following facts about "respirator lung" are correct?
A. This condition is seen when a patient dies after several days on a ventilator
B. It is a heavy, stiff, rigid lung
C. Such a pathological entity is unknown
D. Both (A) and (B) above

MULTIPLE ANSWER TYPE (PGI, CHANDIGARH PATTERN)

31. Which of the following is true about "Growing fractures"?
A. They are seen in the skull, especially when the fracture is associated with laceration of the dura
B. They are never seen in children
C. They are sometimes termed cranio-cerebral erosion
D. They are ten times as common in females as in males
E. There is no such term as "growing fracture"

32. Lucid interval is NOT seen in:
A. Extradural haemorrhage
B. Subdural haemorrhage
C. Subarachnoid haemorrhage
D. Subpial haemorrhage
E. Haemorrhage in the lateral ventricles

33. Subdural haemorrhage may come from:
A. Bridging or communicating veins
B. Middle meningeal artery
C. Rupture of dural venous sinuses
D. Injuries to cortical veins
E. Vertebral artery

34. Which of the following statements about "*Dementia pugilistica*" are correct?
A. It is also known as "punch-drunk syndrome"
B. It commonly manifests itself as parkinsonism like symptoms
C. It is commonly seen in car drivers
D. Common findings on autopsy are scars and patches of gliosis throughout the brain tissue
E. It is a peculiar form of rigor mortis seen in boxers

ANSWERS

GENERAL

1. **A.** ***Related facts:*** *"Plaques jaunes"* is a French term meaning "yellow plaques". Also known as *état vermoulu* (worm eaten state), these are old traumatic injuries on the surface of the brain, appearing as depressed, yellowish-brown patches (due to breakdown products of haemoglobin, namely haemosiderin and bilirubin) on the crests of the gyri. Prizefighters often have these injuries, presumably caused during fights. These are considered to be epileptogenic foci, and may cause seizures. Also known as "cerebral cicatrix".
2. **D.** Blunt force that causes sudden angular deceleration or acceleration of the brain can often cause Diffuse Axonal Injury (DAI). The axons are broken; the broken axons retract into a ball like structure, known as "retraction balls" (or "axonal spheroids"). The presence of "Retraction balls" thus indicate axonal damage. They are seen microscopically in the white matter usually after a few days of injury.
3. **C.**
4. **D.** ***Related fact***: Sometimes severe brain swelling or a space occupying lesion such as a large subdural or extradural haematoma may cause increased intracranial pressure above the tentorium. This can cause either unilateral or bilateral compression of the midbrain against the free edge of the tentorium. If unilateral, it causes grooving of a cerebral peduncle known as "Kernohan's notch" (Fig. 16.1). When bilateral, it causes grooving of the uncus on both sides. In extreme cases it can cause infarction of the parahippocampal gyri on both sides.

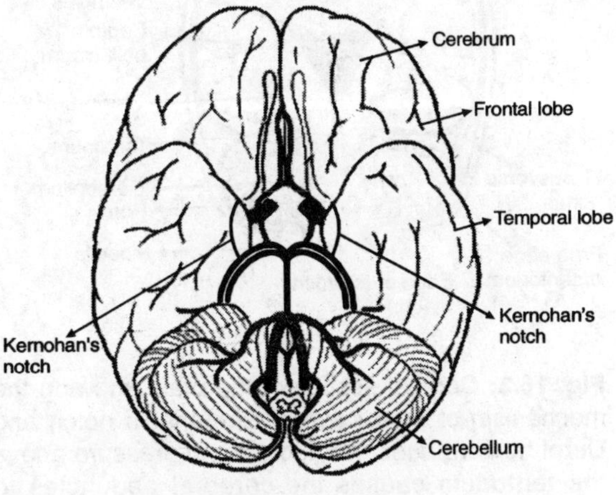

Fig. 16.1: Kernohan's notch, seen on the under surface of brain

5. **D.** Duret hemorrhages are teardrop shape hemorrhages in the brainstem. They are

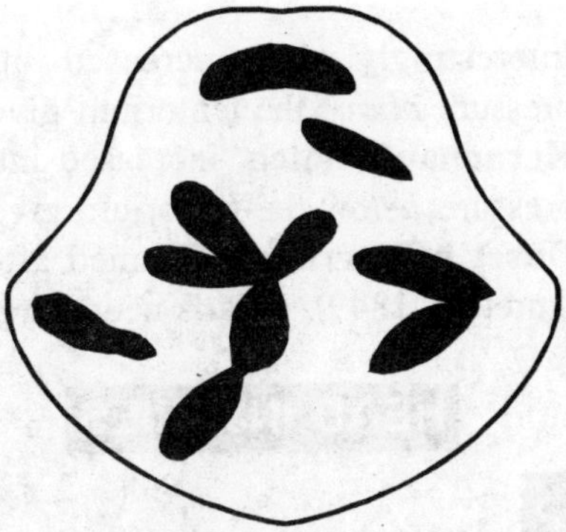

Fig. 16.2: Typical Duret hemorrhages in the brain stem

indicative of raised intracranial pressure, which results in brainstem herniation through foramen magnum. They are thus secondary herniation hemorrhages and range from small streaks to massive confluent Haemorrhage. They commonly occur with asymmetrical herniation of the brain stem.

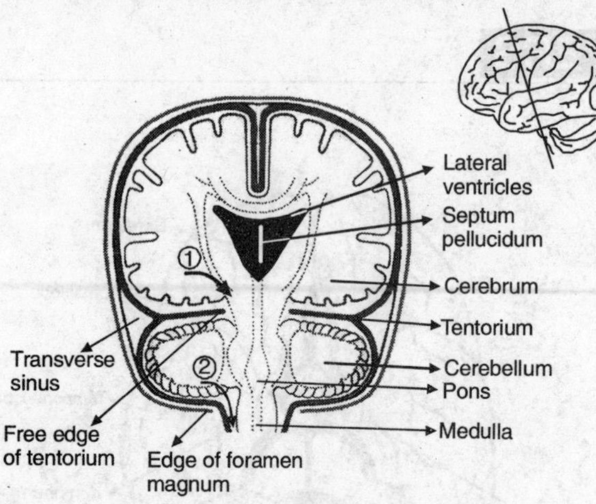

Fig. 16.3: Coronal section of the brain showing the mechanism of production of Kernohan's notch and Duret hemorrhages. An increase in pressure above the tentorium causes the cerebral peduncles to press against the free edge of tentorium causing the notch (arrow shown at 1). An increase in pressure below the tentorium causes the brain stem to herniate through the foramen magnum (arrow shown at 2), in turn causing Duret hemorrhages

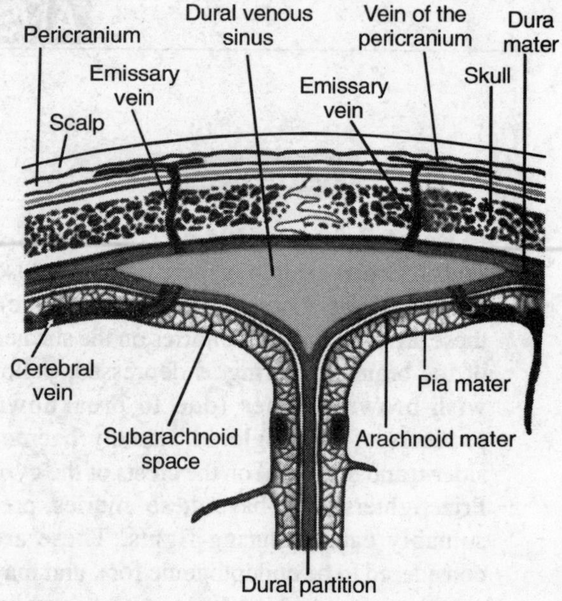

Fig. 16.4: Emissary veins communicate on the outside with veins of the pericranium and the veins of the scalp and face and on the inside with cranial sinuses. Infection from scalp wounds can travel through them to the cranial sinuses causing thrombophlebitis

Interestingly while increased intracranial pressure *above* the tentorium gives rise to **Kernohan's notch**, increased intracranial pressure *below* the tentorium gives rise to **Duret hemorrhages**. Named after Henry Duret (b. 1849), a Paris neurosurgeon.

HEAD INJURIES

Scalp

6. **D.** ***Related fact:*** Diploic veins lying in the spongy tissue between the two tables of the skull are the communication channels between the interior and exterior of skull. On the outside, they communicate with the **veins of the pericranium**, while on the inside they communicate with **meningeal veins and sinuses.**

Another fact to remember is that infected wounds of the scalp and face may cause thrombophlebitis of cranial sinuses. The communication chanel usually attributed here is **emissary veins**, which communicate on the outside with the **veins of the scalp and face** and on the inside with **parasagittal, lateral** and **cavernous sinuses.**

Skull

7. **B.**
8. **B.**

FRACTURES

9. **D.** Jefferson's fracture is caused by an axial loading from the top of the skull.

10. A. ***Related fact:*** These fractures are also known as "signature fractures". They are medicolegally important because their shape resembles that of the striking surface of the weapon. These are mostly seen on the skull. In the case of a hammer, the fracture is circular having the same diameter as the striking surface. Whcn the butt of a firearm strikes the skull full faced, the fracture is rectangular; when the corner of the butt strikes, the fracture is triangular. At the postmortem examination, it is important to preserve the fragments, which can later be reconstructed for demonstration purposes.

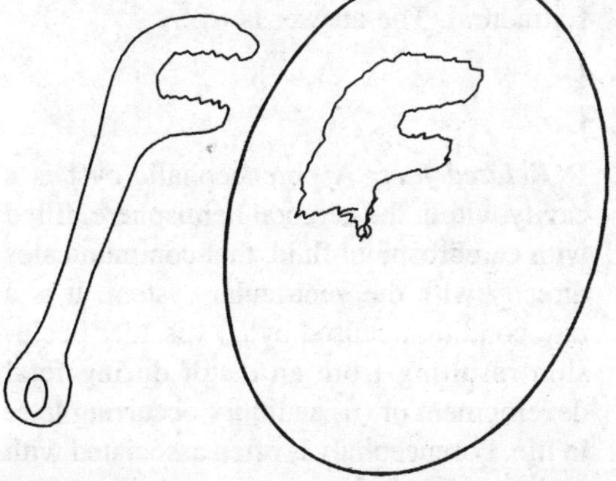

Fig. 16.5: *Fracture à la signature* - A blow on the top of the skull with a spanner would cause a fracture outlining the shape of the spanner itself

11. D. ***Other important facts to remember about pond fracture:*** (i) It is caused often by obstetric forceps (ii) only outer table is fractured (iii) resembles the indentation produced by squeezing a table tennis ball; when elevated it resumes and retains its normal position. Sometimes also known as ping-pong fracture for this reason.

Variant: Pond fracture is common in (a) children (b) adults (c) elderly (d) menopausal women. The answer is (a) children.

12. C.

13. A. ***Related facts:*** Comminute means "to reduce to powder" or "to pulverize". It comes from Latin roots "*com*" and "*minuere*" meaning "to lessen". It is usually seen in the skull, when skull cap is broken into several small pieces.

14. C. ***Additional info:*** In infants bones are not fully calcified. Because of this they behave much like the young green stick of a plant. If one tries breaking it, it would crack, but the two halves would keep adhering to each other, and several twists and turns would be required to separate the two pieces. In young infants too, if a bone breaks, the two halves may keep adhering to each other. This is known as greenstick fracture.

15. D.

16. A.

17. A. ***Related fact:*** These are called so, because the firearm missile glancing along the outer table would create a furrow, which looks like a gutter. This fracture is frequently associated with comminuted depressed fractures of the inner table of the skull.

18. A. ***Related facts:*** Secondary fracture—also known as spontaneous fracture or pathologic fracture—is caused due to weakening of the bone structure by pathologic processes, such as neoplasia, osteomalacia, osteomyelitis, and other diseases. Segmental fracture, also known as double fracture is the fracture of a bone in two places. Pressure fracture is caused by pressure on the bone from an adjoining tumor.

19. C. ***Additional information:*** Bursting fractures of the skull are often seen in falls from heights, when the vertex undergoes sudden flattening. They are also seen in contact firearm wounds of the skull, where the fractures are often seen away from where the bullet enters the skull.

20. C. Traction fractures occur when a bone is pulled apart by traction. The best example is fracture of patella, which may occur when the quadriceps muscle is contracting but the knee joint is straightening (a so-called 'eccentric contraction'; an eccentric contraction occurs when a muscle is contracting, and an external force is trying to lengthen the muscle). When the muscle pulls in this manner, the patella can fracture.

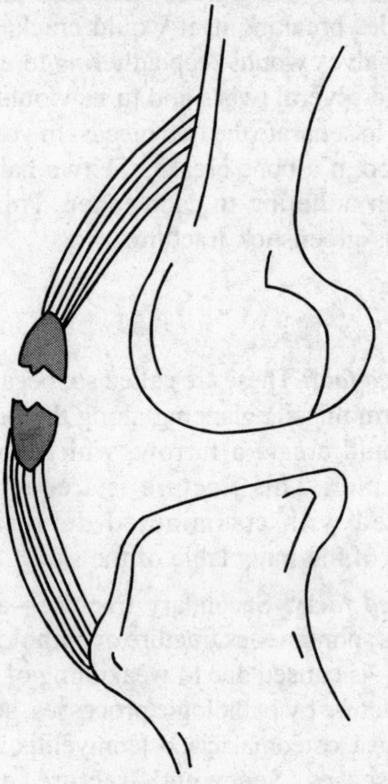

Fig. 16.6: Traction fracture in patella

The above figure illustrates how patella can sustain a traction fracture. Here the muscle is contracting while the knee is bending, trying to "lengthen" the muscle. Since patella is embedded in the tendon of the quadriceps femoris muscle, it experiences opposing forces, causing it to fracture.

INJURIES TO BRAIN AND MENINGES

21. B. A variant of this question is:
Counter-coup injuries are seen in
(a) Brain (b) Heart (c) Liver (d) Pancreas
The answer is (a).

22. B. A variant of this question has been asked like this→Q. A person has been brought in casualty with history of road side accident. He had lost consciousness transiently and then gained consciousness, but again became unconscious. Most likely, he is having haemorrhage of the following type (a) Intracerebral (b) Subarachnoid (c) Subdural (d) Extradural. The answer is (d).

23. C.

24. C.

25. D. ***Related fact:*** A porencephalic cyst is a cavity within the cerebral hemisphere, filled with cerebrospinal fluid, that communicates directly with the ventricular system. It is a rare condition caused by (i) vascular occlusion resulting from an insult during fetal development or (ii) an injury occurring later in life. Porencephaly is often associated with various ophthalmic and neurologic signs (Fig. 16.7).

Pathogenesis is often like this: Patient falls on the head→Haematomas form in frontal or temporal white matter as these are the sites of predilection→Temporal lobe haematomas destroy the optic radiation→If the patient survives, this produces homonymous hemianopsia (loss of one half of vision in each eye on the same side)→Resolution of haematomas form cavities, which often extend medially to communicate with the lateral ventricles→the cavities get filled by

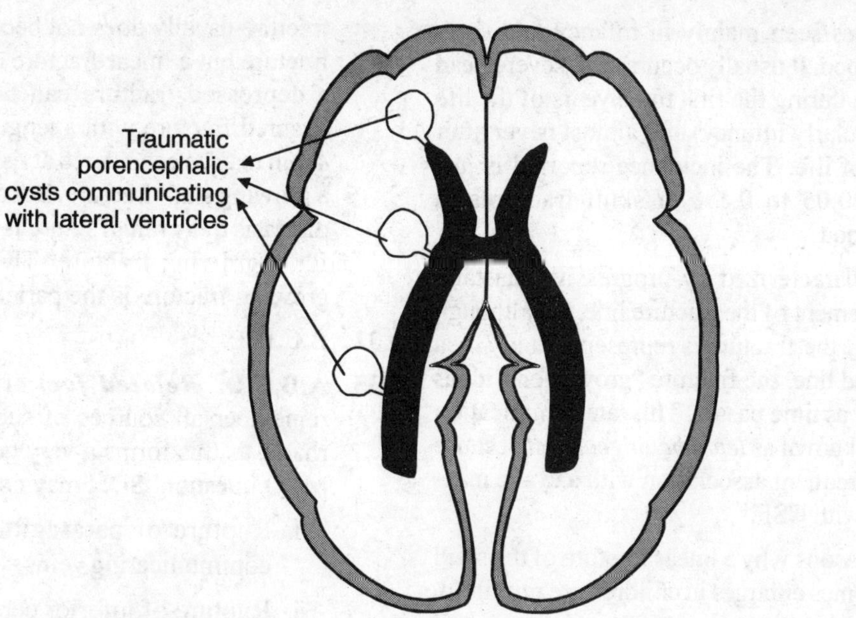

Fig. 16.7: Traumatic porencephalic cysts communicating with the lateral ventricles (Axial section of the brain through inferior corpus callosum)

CSF. These CSF filled cavities are traumatic porencephalic cysts.

26. **B.** ***Additional facts:*** Extradural haemorrhage almost never occurs in boxers, since fractures of skull occur rarely. Subarachnoid haemorrhage may occur rarely if berry aneurysm was present.

27. **C.**

VERTEBRAL COLUMN AND SPINAL CORD

28. **A.** ***Related fact:*** Hyperextension is more dangerous because flexion is protected by the contraction of strong posterior neck muscles. In comparison, the anterior longitudinal ligament (which would protect from injuries during hyperextension) is quite weak.

HEART

29. **C.**

OTHER ORGANS

30. **D.** ***Related fact:*** "Respirator lung" is a well-known entity. The lungs, though heavy do not usually appear edematous. Microscopically the findings are presence of proteinaceous fluid and proliferative cells in the alveoli.

MULTIPLE ANSWER TYPE (PGI, CHANDIGARH PATTERN)

31. **A,C.** ***Additional info:*** Growing skull fracture, sometimes termed as *craniocerebral erosion*, is a rare complication of skull

fractures seen mainly in infancy and early childhood. It usually occurs after severe head trauma during the first three years of the life (particularly infancy) and almost never after 8 yrs of life. The incidence reported is just about 0.05 to 0.1% of skull fractures in childhood.

It is characterized by progressive diastatic enlargement of the fracture line, i.e. although initially the fracture is represented only by a fissured line, the fracture "grows" or widens greatly as time passes. This late complication is also known as *leptomeningeal cyst* because of its frequent association with a cystic mass filled with CSF.

The reasons why a linear fracture of the skull sometimes enlarges in children are multifold. Some major ones are (i) If there is associated epidural haematoma, it may extrude through the fracture line into the subcutaneous tissues. This causes interposition of material (haematoma) between the fractured pieces of skull. This interposition of haematoma prevents osteoblasts from migrating to the fracture site, inhibiting healing (ii) Growing fractures are mostly seen when there is associated laceration of dura mater. It may - in a similar manner - get interposed between the fractured bone pieces, delaying healing (iii) Dura acts as a periosteum of the skull bones, the latter's blood supply coming mainly from dural vessels. Laceration of dura with or without its interposition between the fractured pieces of skull causes nutritional deficiency in the skull bones, causing the skull defect to enlarge. The enlargement starts from the inner table (iv) There is continuous pressure from tissue herniation through the bone gap. This adds to the progression of the fracture line.

These skull fractures, after reaching their maximum extent, cease to grow and remain stable throughout adulthood. A depressed fracture usually does not become a growing fracture but a linear fracture extending from a depressed fracture can become one. A fissured fracture with a length of more than 4 mm may be considered at risk of developing a growing skull fracture. But a post traumatic diastasis of a cranial suture is an unusual site for a growing fracture. The usual site of growing fracture is the parietal region.

32. B,C,D,E.

33. A,B,C,D. ***Related fact:*** It is useful to remember all sources of subdural haemorrhage, as this forms a very good basis of an MCQ question. SDH may come from:

  i. Rupture of parasagittal bridging or communicating veins
  ii. Rupture of inferior cerebral veins (as they enter the dural venous sinuses at the base of the skull)
  iii. Rupture of dural venous sinuses [remember their rupture can also cause EDH. It all depends whether the dural venous sinuses have ruptured on the outside (EDH) or on the inside (SDH) – Refer to **Figure 16.8.**]

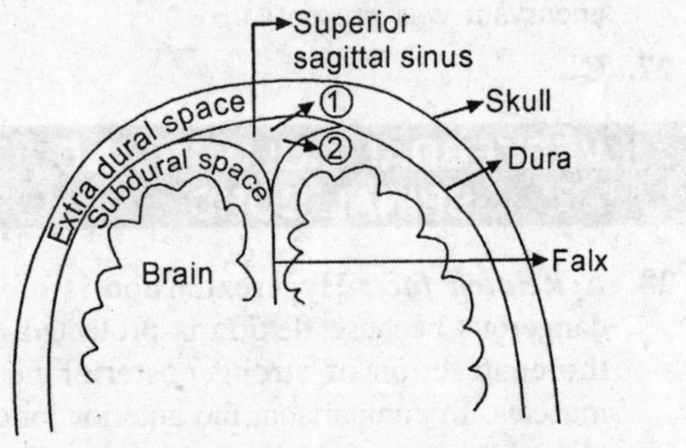

Fig. 16.8: Depending on how the dural venous sinus ruptures, extradural or subdural hemorrhages may form. In the above figure, if the superior sagittal sinus ruptures outside (1), it would give rise to extradural hemorrhage. On the other hand, if it ruptures on the inside (2), it would cause subdural hemorrhage

iv. Laceration of dura and middle meningeal artery. Choice (B) is a surprise choice in this question. Most students think that middle meningeal artery causes extradural haemorrhage only. However the truth is that if there is a laceration of the dura and middle meningeal artery, it may bleed into the subdural instead of the epidural space. It would then cause subdural haemorrhage.

v. Berry aneuryms may rarely bleed directly into the subdural space if arachnoid is torn.

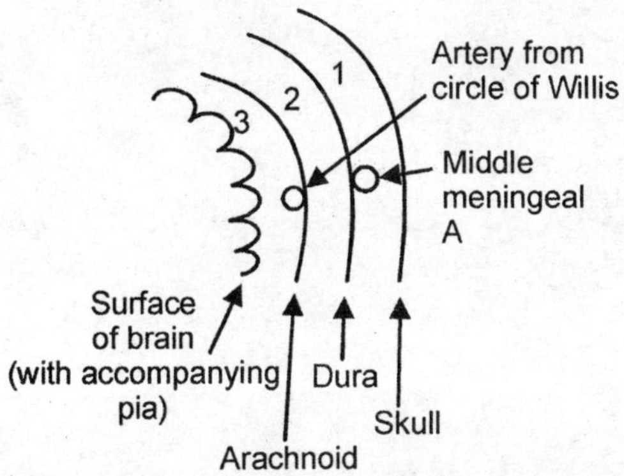

Fig. 16.9: A simplified schematic diagram to understand the causation of various intracranial hemorrhages – refer text for details

Look at the **figure 16.9** to make matters more clear. Space 1 is the extradural space (which is only a potential space, i.e. it does not exist normally, but can be created when bleeding occurs in it). Space 2 is subdural space. Space 3 is subarachnoid space. Normally rupture of middle meningeal artery will cause bleeding in extradural space, but if associated dura is torn, bleeding can come in subdural space. Similarly arteries of the Circle of Willis (where aneurysms are most commonly found) normally cause bleeding in subarachnoid space, but if associated arachnoid is torn, bleeding can come in subdural space.

It must be appreciated that since subdural space is the "middle space" (i.e. between extradural and subarachnoid space), bleedings from both these spaces can come in this space through a tear in the corresponding membrane.

vi. Drugs such as heparin, warfarin or dicoumarol can produce subdural haemorrhage by producing a disturbance in the blood clotting mechanisms.

34. A,B,D. ***Related facts:*** *Dementia pugilistica* is known by several names, among them chronic traumatic encephalopathy, pugilistic Parkinson's syndrome, boxer's syndrome, and punch-drunk syndrome. It is a neurological disorder which affects professional boxers and others who receive multiple serious blows to the head.

The condition develops over a period of years, with the average time of onset being about 15 years after the start of a career in boxing. It appears that the number of years the boxer has been in profession is more important in determining its onset, than the number of serious blows the boxer has suffered in his career. Obviously even minor traumatic events, which may go unnoticed on their own, play their part as they cumulate over the years. Famous boxers who have suffered from this syndrome include Jack Dempsey, Beau Jack, Joe Louis and Muhammad Ali.

The condition is called "punch-drunk" because the victim displays symptoms similar to those shown by a drunk person, and that the state is brought about by repeated punches. The major symptoms are slurred speech, slow thought process, dementia, tremors (much like those seen in Parkinsonism), ataxia and outbursts of violence.

Autopsy shows (i) some cortical atrophy (ii) perforation of septum pellucidum (iii) slight hydrocephalus (iv) thinning out of fornices and adjacent corpus callosum (v) presence of scars and patches of gliosis throughout the brain tissue.

Variant: A variant has been asked like this→"Punch drunkenness" may result from:

(a) Delirium due to acute hashish toxicity (b) Consuming adulterated alcohol (c) A single severe blow to the head (d) Multiple minor cerebral injuries due to boxing. The answer is (d) Multiple minor cerebral injuries due to boxing.

17 Traffic Accidents

GENERAL

1. **Whip lash injury is most often seen:**
   A. When the person is beaten by a whip
   B. In a pedestrian
   C. In an occupant of an automobile
   D. In a cyclist

AUTOMOBILE INJURIES

2. **Which of the following statements regarding "Bumper Fractures" is true?**
   A. Usually the tibia is fractured
   B. Usually the fibula is fractured
   C. Usually calcaneum is fractured
   D. Invariably all three, i.e. tibia, fibula and the calcaneum are fractured

3. **"Bumper fracture" is an example of:**
   A. Primary impact injury
   B. Secondary impact injury
   C. Tertiary impact injury
   D. Quaternary impact injury

4. **If at the time of impact, the vehicle was braking violently, the bumper fractures be:**
   A. At the same height as that of bumper
   B. At a height higher than that of bumper
   C. At a height lower than that of bumper
   D. Seen in the fibula instead of tibia

5. **A proper postmortem examination of a victim of automobile accident must begin with the examination of his clothes because:**
   A. They may show small fragments of paint and glass from the vehicle
   B. There may be grease on the clothes
   C. There may be tire marks on the clothes
   D. All of the above

CYCLISTS AND MOTORCYCLISTS

6. **The so called motorcyclist's fracture is:**
   A. Ring fracture
   B. Division of base of skull into two halves —an anterior and a posterior
   C. Division of base of skull into two halves —a left lateral and a right lateral
   D. Comminuted fracture of the vault

7. **"Under-running" or "tail-gating" is:**
   A. Fracture of lower limb bones in a motorcyclist
   B. Some sharp projecting part of the colliding vehicle entering the chest of the victim, killing him much like a stab
   C. A motorcyclist driving into the back of a large vehicle, usually a truck
   D. Fracture of coccyx occurring in a motorcyclist

8. "Ladder tears" in car occupants are often seen in cases of accident. These tears are seen in:

A. Periosteum of the tibia
B. Pericardium
C. Intima of the descending aorta
D. Liver

9. "Seat belt syndrome" typically seen in drivers of cars involved in collisions involve:

A. Injuries to the abdominal viscera
B. Fractures of the lumbar spine
C. Fracture of multiple tarsal bones
D. Both (A) and (B) above

MULTIPLE ANSWER TYPE (PGI, CHANDIGARH PATTERN)

10. Following types of injuries are seen in pedestrians involved in traffic accidents:

A. Primary impact injuries
B. Secondary impact injuries
C. Quaternary impact injuries
D. Secondary injuries
E. Malingerer's fractures

11. Which of the following injuries may be termed "patterned injuries"?

A. Tyre marks on the legs
B. Graze abrasion on the back
C. Circular abrasion on a driver's chest from impact of steering wheel
D. Lacerations on the thighs
E. Imprint of the headlight on the thigh of a pedestrian

12. Extensive graze abrasions over the body of a deceased pedestrian are seen. Most likely they are:

A. Primary impact injuries
B. Secondary impact injuries
C. Secondary injuries
D. Postmortem abrasions
E. Homicidal injuries

ANSWERS

GENERAL

1. C.

AUTOMOBILE INJURIES

2. A. ***Additional info*:** Usually tibia is fractured, although very rarely fibula may also fracture. The fractured fragment of tibia is triangular in shape. The base of the triangular fragment indicates the site of impact, and the apex points in the direction in which the vehicle was travelling. Occasionally there are no fractures, or even any evidence of external injury, but there may be internal haemorrhage in the calves.

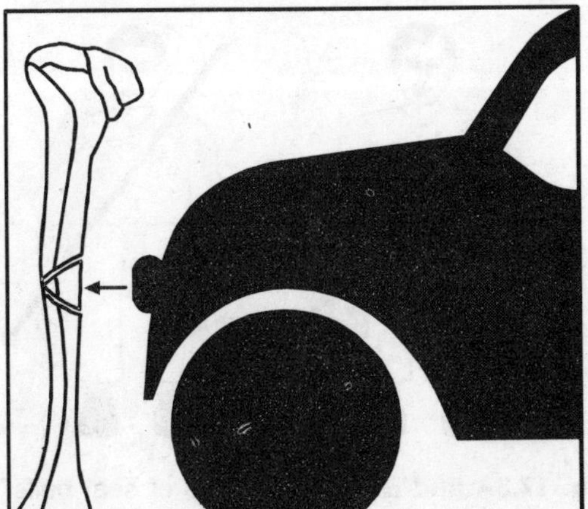

Fig. 17.1: An example of bumper fracture. The tip of the wedge-shaped bone that has fractured is pointing towards the direction in which the offending vehicle was travelling

3. A.
4. C. Usually—if the vehicle was neither accelerating nor decelerating—the fractures of tibia would be *at the same height as that of the bumper*. Indeed the height of the fracture from the heel should be measured by the forensic pathologist, as it can give an idea of the height of the bumper and thus help to identify the car. However if the car was braking violently, the forward portion of the car would dip down, and the bumper fractures would be *at a lower level than that of the bumper*.

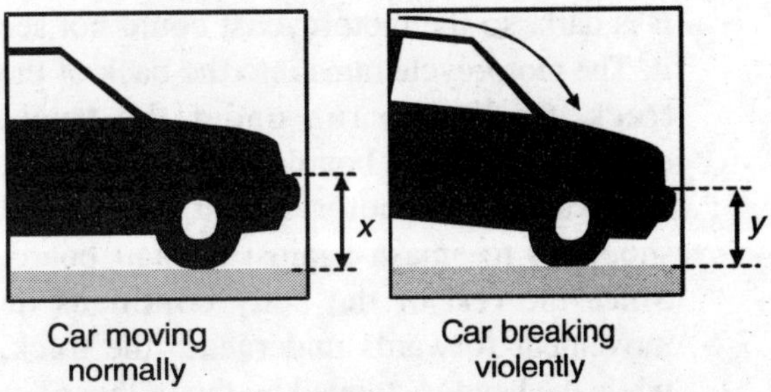

Fig. 17.2: If the car is moving normally, its bumper is at height "x" from the ground, causing fractures of the tibia at that level. If the car were braking violently, the bumper would dip down. The resulting height "y" is less than "x"

5. D. Forensic pathologists usually ignore a proper examination of the clothing of the deceased. Recovery of paint and glass particles from the clothes, or of the grease marks left from the vehicle or tire marks can be very valuable pieces of evidence to link the vehicle to the deceased.

CYCLISTS AND MOTORCYCLISTS

6. **B.** ***Additional info***: Motorcyclists' fracture is seen in motorcyclists as a result of falling on the ground. It is seen as a transverse crack across the middle cranial fossa behind the greater wing of sphenoid bones. It crosses through the pituitary fossa to reach the opposite side. Frequently it continues upwards to the temporal bones as a fissured fracture. It thus divides the skull roughly into two equal halves – an anterior and a posterior. The two halves can be moved independently of each other like a hinge. This fracture is seen both in the driver as well as in the pillion rider.
7. **C.** ***Additional info***: This occurs typically when a motor cyclist is driving fast behind a truck, and it stops suddenly, especially when it is dark, so the motorcyclist could not see it. The motorcycle rams into the back of the truck, tending to run under the truck, especially if its tail board is on a high level. This causes the motor cyclist's head and shoulders to smash against the tail board. Since the rest of the body continues its movement forwards underneath the truck, while the head is stopped by the tailboard, it may result in decapitation.
8. **C.** ***Related facts:*** During accident, the motor vehicle is severely decelerated and the occupants of the car—especially the unrestrained back seat occupants—are forcibly thrown forwards. This causes a severe whiplash effect on thoracic spine and adjacent aorta shows multiple transverse intimal tears in its intima. These appear rather like rungs of a ladder and hence the name "ladder tears".
9. **D.** ***Additional info:*** Seat Belt Syndrome, or SBS, is a phrase that was originally coined by the medical community in the late 1950s and early 1960s to describe injuries that physicians were seeing as a result of occupants wearing lap-belt-only restraints (much like we see in aircrafts today) in frontal collisions. During the collision, the driver was forced forwards violently, causing his body to "jack-knife" over the lap belt, at the waist. This typically caused injury to the abdominal viscera, most typically a tear or perforation of the intestine and its mesentery. It was usually accompanied by fracture or dislocation of the mid-lumbar spine, sometimes leading even to paralysis.

   Because of this defect, modern car seat belts are of lap-strap and shoulder diagonal type. This is the so-called "three point attachment belt" (Fig. 17.3A and B). Seat belt syndrome is seen with much less frequency with these types of belts. A further safety feature is the inertia reel. In this system, a retractor reel lets out the strap or pulls it back as needed, and in the event of an accident the reel locks, preventing any more strap to come out and holding the passenger in the car.

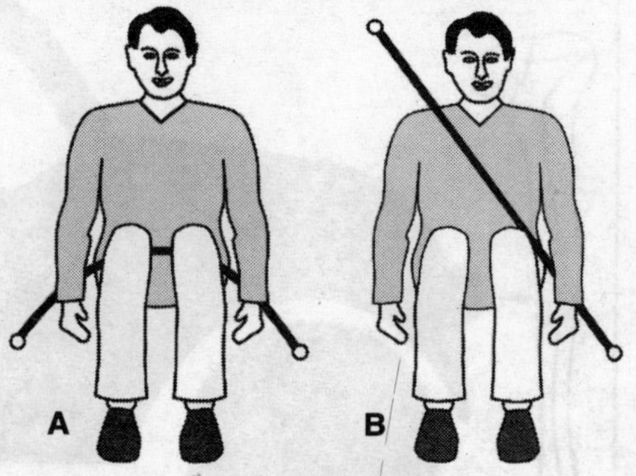

Fig. 17.3A and B: Various types of seat belts: (a) Simple lap strap: Adjustable simple lap strap that goes over the waist. It was used frequently in older cars. Now uncommon except in some rear middle seats. Today it is best seen in modern passenger aircrafts. This can be dangerous to aorta (b) Sash strap: It is the diagonal only kind of strap. This is an adjustable strap that goes over the shoulder. Used mainly in the 1960's, but of limited benefit because it is very easy to slip out of in a collision, leading to strangulation

Contd...

Contd...

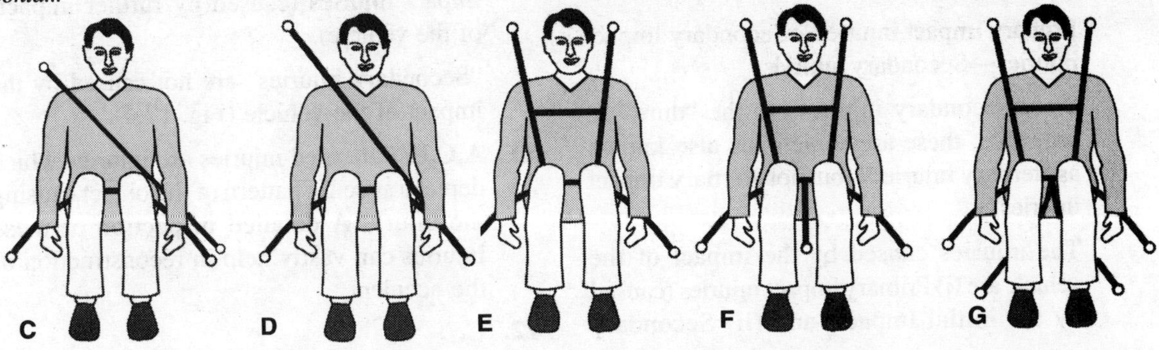

Fig. 17.3C to G: Various types of seat belts: (c) Lap and Sash: Combination of the two above (two separate belts). Mainly used in the 1960s and 1970s, usually in the rear. Generally superseded by three-point design (d) Three-point: Similar to the lap and sash, but one single continuous length of webbing. This is what we use in this country. This appears safest. Both three-point and lap-and-sash belts help spread out the energy of the moving body in a collision over a wide area (chest, pelvis, and shoulders) minimizing the potential for causing injury. Until the 1970's three-point belts were commonly available only in the front seats of cars, the back seats having only lap belts. When it became clear that lap belts could cause "seat belt syndrome", the movement for safer seat belts caught momentum throughout the world, leading to the development of the modern three-point seat belts (e) Shoulder harness: Used in racing cars. It is a belt assembly (one strap for each shoulder) intended to restrain movement of the upper torso and shoulder regions. An optional cross-strap across the chest, called a sternum strap after the bone it bisects, can be used to hold the shoulder harness together. The sternum strap was initially designed to spread belt-tension loads across the chest and include the sternum as a load-dispersing member, but tests have shown it is limited in its effect in a high-deflection (head-on to 30-45 degrees) crash. During side impacts, however, its effectiveness in equalizing shoulder belt loading is increased. There are also questions regarding the mounting of the sternum buckle, including the fact the buckle is close to the driver's chin and could be an obstacle to exiting the car quickly following a crash (f) Five-point harness: It is safer but more restrictive. These are typically found in child safety seats and also in racing cars. The lap portion is connected to a belt between the legs and there are two shoulder belts, making a total of five points of attachment to the seat. The strap between the legs is called the anti-submarine strap. It prevents the pelvis from slipping forward from under the lap belt in the event of an accident (g) Six-point harness: It became popular after the American NASCAR driver Ralph Dale Earnhardt, Sr. (April 29, 1951 – February 18, 2001) died in a racing accident (in turn four of the final lap of the 2001 Daytona 500). Earnhardt was wearing a five-point harness when he crashed and died. Because it was thought at first that his belt had broken, some teams ordered a six-point harness. The additional belt here is an upside-down V, which still attaches to the lap and shoulder belts but mounts to the chassis in two separate, spread locations

MULTIPLE ANSWER TYPE (PGI, CHANDIGARH PATTERN)

10. A,B,D. Primary impact injuries are caused by the initial strike, i.e., the first part of the vehicle that strikes the victim. These are usually the legs. The victim is then thrown back on the vehicle, causing further injuries. These are known as secondary impact injuries. Finally the victim is thrown on the ground. This causes secondary injuries.

The student must be beware of two confusing terms "secondary impact injuries" and "secondary injuries". *Secondary impact injuries* are caused by the vehicle which continues to move as the victim is hit. *Secondary injuries* on the other hand are caused by the victim falling on the ground.

The injuries are caused in this sequence:

Primary impact injuries→Secondary impact injuries→Secondary injuries.

Since secondary injuries are the "third" in sequence, these are sometimes also known as "tertiary injuries" (but not "tertiary impact injuries").

The injuries caused by the impact of the vehicle are (i) Primary impact injuries (caused by the initial impact) and (ii) Secondary impact injuries (caused by further impacts of the vehicle).

"Secondary injuries" are not caused by the impact of the vehicle (Fig. 17.4).

11. A,C,E. Patterned injuries are injuries which depict a specific pattern of the object causing the injury. A detailed inspection of these injuries can vastly help in reconstruction of the accident.

12. C.

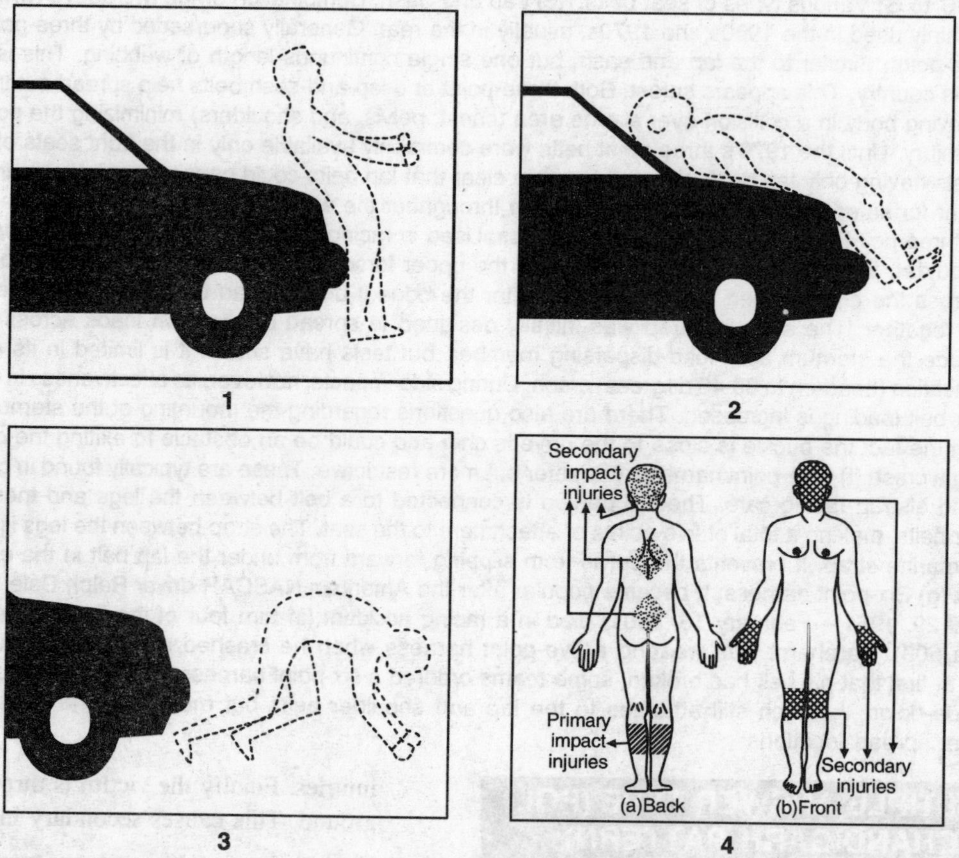

Fig. 17.4: The figure shows the mechanism of production of "primary impact injuries", "secondary impact injuries" and "secondary injuries". The primary impact of the vehicle is upon the back of calves (1). This causes "primary impact injuries" shown on the calves as oblique lines (4). After this impact, the body is thrown backwards causing further injuries to the buttocks, back and even the head if the body slides up the bonnet of the car, the head striking against the pillar of the windshield (2). These injuries are "secondary impact injuries" and are shown as dotted areas (4). Finally the body is thrown forwards on the ground (3). This causes "secondary injuries" to knees, palms and face, shown as cross hatchets(4)

4 DEATHS FROM OTHER CAUSES

18 *Deaths from Asphyxia*

GENERAL

1. **The true etymological meaning of asphyxia is:**
   A. Pulselessness
   B. Breathlessness
   C. Oxygen lack
   D. Difficult breathing
2. **The arterial oxygen tension of 20-40 mm Hg represents**
   A. Hyper oxygenated blood
   B. Normally oxygenated blood
   C. Mild hypoxia
   D. Severe to fatal hypoxia
3. **Diatom test may be useful as an investigational aid in deaths due to:**
   A. Hanging
   B. Strangulation
   C. Drowning
   D. All asphyxial deaths
4. **One of the features in asphyxia is cyanosis. How much should be the concentration of reduced haemoglobin after which it becomes visible?**
   A. 2 grams %
   B. 5 grams %
   C. 6 grams %
   D. 7 grams %
5. ***"le facies sympathique"* was once associated with:**
   A. Hanging
   B. Electrocution
   C. Strangulation
   D. Smothering

A Variant of this question is as below:

6. ***"le facies sympathique"* was once thought to be a sure sign of:**
   A. Antemortem hanging
   B. Postmortem hanging
   C. Both antemortem and postmortem hanging
   D. Masochistic hanging
7. **Horizontal ligature mark is usually seen in:**
   A. Throttling
   B. Ligature strangulation
   C. Complete hanging
   D. Partial hanging

HANGING

8. **Hanging is defined as that form of asphyxia which is caused by:**
   A. Suspension of body by a ligature encircling the neck the constricting force being the weight of the body

B. Suspension of a body by a ligature after death
C. Obliteration of air passages by any means over the level of the chest
D. Any kind of mechanical interference to respiration

9. Most specific and diagnostic feature of antemortem hanging is:
A. Dribbling of saliva
B. Ligature mark
C. Hyoid fracture
D. Thyroid fracture

10. A pressure of .... Kg is required to close jugular veins:
A. 2 kg
B. 5 kg
C. 15 kg
D. 30 kg

11. In a case of hanging where the feet of the victim are touching the ground, which of the following facts is true?
A. It can not be a case of hanging
B. It is a sure case of homicidal hanging
C. It is a case of partial hanging
D. It is a sure case of post-mortem hanging

12. Death in judicial hanging is because of:
A. Vasovagal shock
B. Occlusion of upper airway
C. Fracture dislocation of upper cervical vertebrae
D. Coma

13. Carotid arteries may be torn transversely in:
A. Suicidal hanging
B. Homicidal hanging
C. Judicial hanging
D. All of the above

14. In a case of hanging, ligature marks are most typical examples of:
A. Contusions
B. Pressure abrasions
C. Lacerations
D. Grazes

15. Pin point haemorrhages often seen under the skin, sclera and thoracic serous membranes in some kinds of asphyxial deaths are known as:
A. Gettlers' haemorrhages
B. Tardieu's spots
C. Paltauf's haemorrhages
D. Washer woman's haemorrhages

OTHER FORMS OF ASPHYXIA

16. Which of the following is a combination of homicidal smothering and traumatic asphyxia?
A. Choking
B. Gagging
C. Throttling
D. Burking
Variant 1

17. Burking consists of:
A. Smothering and traumatic asphyxia
B. Choking and drowning
C. Gagging only
D. Traumatic asphyxia only
Variant 2

18. The term "Burking" is derived from the name of:
A. An instrument used for murder
B. A place
C. A person
D. A firearm
Variant 3

19. The method of sitting over the victim's chest and closing his nostrils and mouth to cause asphyxial death is known as:
A. Gagging
B. Overlaying
C. Choking
D. Burking
Variant 4

20. Burking is smothering and:
A. Throttling
B. Gagging

C. Strangulation
D. Traumatic asphyxia

21. Congestion of the face is maximum if the death was due to:
A. Choking
B. Hanging
C. Strangulation
D. Drowning

22. *Café coronary* commonly occurs when a person is:
A. Intoxicated
B. Smoking in an inebriated state
C. Eating fatty food
D. Eating fish

23. In a case of throttling which type of abrasions are seen most often over the victim's neck?
A. Grave
B. Pressure
C. Impact
D. Crescentic

24. When strangulation is effected by compressing the neck of the victim within the bend of the elbow, it is technically termed as:
A. *Bansdola*
B. Mugging
C. Garrotting
D. Throttling

DROWNING

25. The average specific gravity of human body is about:
A. 0.89
B. 1.08
C. 1.23
D. 1.65

26. All are seen in drowning *except*:
A. Miosis
B. Wet heavy lungs
C. Water and weeds in stomach and lungs
D. Froth from nose and mouth

27. Most common consistent feature in a child who has died from drowning in a pond is:
A. Water in the alveoli of lungs
B. Petechial hemorrhages in the lungs
C. Washer woman's hands
D. Cyanosis

28. Most common type of drowning is:
A. Suicidal
B. Accidental
C. Homicidal
D. Immersion syndrome

29. Which of the following signs would indicate that the death was antemortem?
A. Cutis anserina
B. Washer woman's hands
C. Weed and grass in the hands
D. Cyanosis

30. Which one of the following is a definite sign of death due to drowning?
A. Sand and mud in the mouth and nostrils
B. Fine lathery froth in the mouth and nostrils
C. Washerwoman's hands and feet
D. Diatoms in the bone marrow

31. Gettler's test is done in:
A. Hanging
B. Strangulation
C. Drowning
D. Throttling

32. The term "near drowning" refers to:
A. A person who was about to drown but just saved himself from drowning
B. A person who drowned but was brought out and he survived for at least 24 hours
C. A person, who survived drowning for 1 week
D. Dry drowning

33. Dry drowning is defined as:
A. Drowning in sea water

B. Falling in a deep well which has dried
C. Drowning in very cold water with death occurring due to cardiac arrest
D. Drowning where death is due to laryngospasm

34. Dry drowning is said to occur in ....% of all drownings:
A. 1-2%
B. 10-15%
C. 25%
D. 30-35%

35. Paltauf's hemorrhages are seen in:
A. Drowning
B. Firearm injury
C. Hanging
D. Strangulation

36. Bleaching of the cuticle becomes quite evident after ....hours of immersion:
A. 2
B. 12
C. 24
D. 48

37. Floatation of the body in our country in summers occurs in:
A. 12 hours
B. 24 hours
C. 3 days
D. 6 days

38. Besides drowning, froth at the mouth may be seen in a few other conditions. Identify that condition below:
A. Opium poisoning
B. Sulphuric acid poisoning
C. Head injury
D. Tetanus

39. How many species of diatoms are there?
A. About 100
B. Between 500-1000
C. Between 2000-5000
D. About 15,000

40. Oligohalophilic diatoms live in:
A. Fresh water
B. Brackish water
C. Sea water
D. Sewer water

41. Diatom test may be negative in a case of:
A. Freshwater drowning
B. Seawater drowning
C. Drowned body but decomposed
D. Dry drowning

42. For diatom test, the best site for taking samples is:
A. Lungs
B. Bone marrow in ulna
C. Bone marrow in femur
D. A large and fleshy muscle

43. Emphysema aquosum is seen in:
A. Wet drowning
B. Dry drowning
C. Secondary drowning
D. Immersion syndrome

44. Hyperventilation before underwater swimming:
A. Causes dry drowning
B. Causes immersion syndrome
C. Can result in unintentional drowning
D. Is a surefire method to prevent drowning

45. The term "Kotzwarraism" or "Kocz-warism" refers to:
A. Manual strangulation
B. Choking
C. Autoerotic asphyxia
D. Traumatic asphyxia

MULTIPLE ANSWER TYPE (PGI, CHANDIGARH PATTERN)

46. Which of the following facts are true about lynching?
A. It was the public hanging of females who were found to be infidel
B. It is a form of homicidal hanging
C. It is another name for masochistic hanging

D. It was mostly practised in North America
E. It was mostly practised by Negroes on White people

47. Which of the following facts are correct regarding autoerotic asphyxia?
A. It is suicidal in nature
B. It is also known as masochistic hanging
C. Pornographic material is often found around the scene
D. There is usually a layer of padding between the ligature and the neck
E. It is exclusively seen in females

48. Which of the following are generally considered to be the "classic" signs of asphyxia?
A. Congestion of internal organs
B. Bleeding inside splenic capsule
C. Increased fluidity of blood
D. Engorgement of right side of heart
E. Abnormal stretching and tearing of muscles of the diaphragm

49. In deaths due to which of the following causes are petechiae *seldom* demonstrable?
A. Fall from height
B. Drowning
C. Traumatic asphyxia
D. Plastic bag suffocation
E. Entering an atmosphere full of carbon dioxide

50. What are the major differences in gross appearances of lungs in sea water and fresh water drowning?
A. The lungs are ballooned and heavy in salt water drowning while in fresh water drowning they are ballooned and light
B. Color of lungs in fresh water drowning is pale pink while it is purplish or bluish in salt water drowning
C. The consistency of lungs is emphysematous in salt water drowning while it is soft and jelly like in sea water drowning
D. After removal from the body the lungs in fresh water drowning tend to flatten out while in sea water drowning the tend to retain shape and do not collapse
E. There are no appreciable differences in the gross appearances of lungs in fresh water and salt water drowning

ANSWERS

GENERAL

1. **A.** Although this term signifies lack of oxygen, its true etymological meaning is pulselessness. The term derives from Greek words "*a*" (not), plus "*sphyzein*" (pulse). [*sphyzein* also gives rise to the word sphygmanometer, or an instrument which measures pulse pressure]. Because it was seen that cases in which there was lack of oxygen, were associated with a feeble or depressed pulse, this term came to be applied to these conditions.
2. **D.** Normal saturation of arterial blood is around 90-100 mm of mercury (or 12-13.5 kPa). Persons over 60 years of age may have a somewhat lower saturation – around 60-85 mm Hg (8-10 kPa). Mild hypoxia is said to occur when the oxygen levels fall to around 60 mm Hg (8 kPa). Severe to fatal hypoxia results when the oxygen tension falls to between 20-40 mm Hg (3-5 kPa). Thus in a way, fatal hypoxia results when the oxygen levels fall to about 1/5 of normal.
3. **C.**
4. **B.**
5. **A.** ***Related fact***: "*Le facies sympathiques*" is more or less a mythical phenomena, and no serious forensic pathologist believes in this phenomenon anymore. It was once believed to be a hallmark of antemortem hanging.

   In this phenomenon, the right eye was believed to remain open and the left closed with the left pupil small and right dilated. It was believed to result as a result of unequal tension on the neck structures.

   The only justification of inclusion of this question is that this question is still being asked in various examinations.
6. **A.**
7. **B.**

HANGING

8. **A.**
9. **A.** ***Related fact***: This is supposed to be due to pressure and irritation of the parotid gland caused by the knot.
10. **A.** ***Related fact:*** The pressures required to close various structures in the neck were determined by experiments conducted in 1897 by Professor Brouardel (1837-1906), a professor of legal medicine at the University of Paris. The usually accepted figures are:

    Jugular veins→2 kg
    Carotid arteries→5 kg
    Trachea→15 kg
    Vertebral arteries→30 kg.
11. **C.** ***Related fact:*** It is wrong to think that if the feet are touching the ground, it can not be case of hanging. Several cases of genuine suicidal hanging are seen where the feet are touching the ground. These cases are known as partial hanging. If no part of the body is touching the ground, it is known as "complete hanging".
12. **C.** ***Additional info:*** For "judicial hanging" remember the following additional points, which may be helpful in other MCQs:
    1. The body of the victim is made to drop from a height. The drop is usually *5-7 metres*, depending on the build of the person. Heavier the person, lesser the drop.
    2. Fracture dislocation occurs usually at the level of "2-3rd" or "3-4th" Cervical vertebrae. Less commonly it is at "atlanto-

occipital" (or skull-1st) or "1-2nd" vertebrae (in which case, the odontoid process of the axis vertebrae fractures and causes pulping of the spinal cord).

3. Death is instantaneous, but heart continues to beat for about 10-15 minutes afterwards. Respiratory movements and spasmodic muscular jerking may continue for the same period.

13. C. ***Related fact:*** Damage to the carotid arteries is seen mainly in judicial hanging. This damage is because of the big drop.

14. B.

15. B. ***Related info:*** In 1866, French Professor Ambroise Auguste Tardieu (1818-1879) demonstrated petechial haemorrhages in the visceral pleura of the bodies of infants who were claimed to have died due to overlaying. These spots later came to be known as Tardieu's spots, and were thought to be present in all asphyxia deaths. Remember the following facts about Tardieu's spots:

- Tardieu's spots vary in size between 0.1 to 2 mm. If they are larger than this, they are technically known as *ecchymoses*.
- They are caused by an acute rise in venous pressure, which is most often brought about by compression of the neck (as in strangulation) or chest (as in traumatic asphyxia). It is *rare* to see these petechial haemorrhages in asphyxial deaths *unaccompanied by such compression* (e.g. drowning, plastic bag suffocation and deaths due to entering inert atmospheres).
- It is hypothesized that hypoxia of the vein wall is another mechanism causing these haemorrhages – hypoxic vein walls allowing easier leaking of blood. But this claim has not been verified experimentally and is at best conjectural. The rapidity with which petechial haemorrhages appear in asphyxial deaths makes this mechanism quite unlikely.
- Petechiae are rarely seen in **p**arietal **p**leura and **p**eritoneum except in deaths due to haemorrhagic diatheses. In the thorax, they are most commonly seen on the visceral pleura especially around the hilum and in the interlobar fissures.
- Petechiae – both cutaneous and visceral - can not only enlarge after postmortem, they can appear *ab initio* as a postmortem phenomenon. It has been shown by some workers that the number of petechiae seen on the body are directly proportional to the number of hours the person has been dead, although no attempts have been made to mathematically link the two.

OTHER FORMS OF ASPHYXIA

16. D. ***Related facts:*** The term Burking derives from the name of **William Burke** (1792-1829), who along with his friend **William Hare** killed almost 16 poor beggars and supplied their dead bodies for dissection to an anatomist **Dr. Robert Knox**, who would pay them handsomely for this favor. Burke and Hare would invite poor beggars to their home and intoxicate them with liquor. When the victim was drunk enough, Hare would wrestle him to the floor and close his mouth and nostrils with his hands (smothering), while Burke would sit on the victim's chest (traumatic asphyxia). Thus the death was due to an effective combination of smothering and traumatic asphyxia. Burke was hanged for his crimes on 28 January 1829. Hare turned approver so he was forgiven.

17. A.

18. C.

19. D.

20. D.

21. C.

22. A. ***Related fact:*** *Café coronary* is the term given to death occurring due to impaction of food in trachea, when an intoxicated person is eating. Death is not typically due to asphyxia; it is due to vagal inhibition of the heart.

23. **D.** ***Related facts:*** These are semilunar type abrasions produced due to the nails of the assailant.

24. **B.** An assailant can strangulate his victim in a number of ways. Different terms are used depending on how the strangulation was brought about. If the neck was compressed within two bamboo rods, or wooden poles, it is known as *bansdola* (literally "doing away with bamboos"). It is quite common in India. If the strangulation is achieved by compressing the neck in the bend of the elbow, it is known as mugging. Many blacks in USA

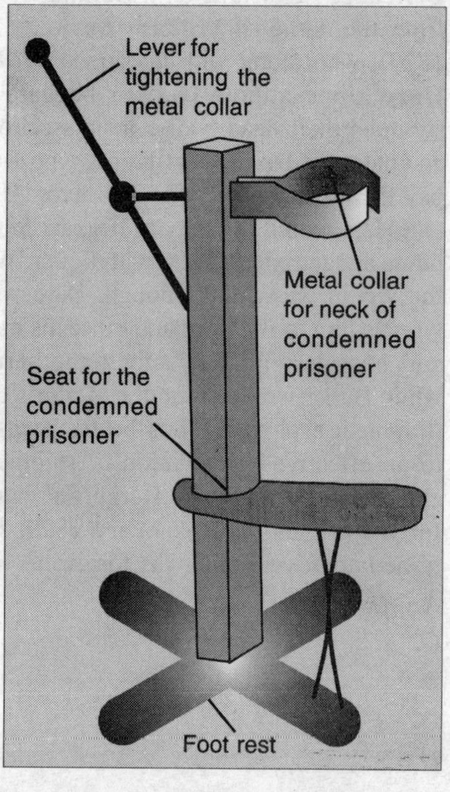

18.1: The official Garrotte once used in Spain

are known to extort money from their victims in this way; they are known as "muggers". Garrotting was once used as a method of execution in Spain (it is no more used now, the last garrotting occurring in 1974).

Interesting fact: Garrotting developed from the early Chinese form of execution known as the bow-string, in which the criminal was tied to an upright post with two holes bored in it. Ends of a cord from a long bow were passed through these holes. These were pulled tight round the neck by the executioner until the condemned strangled.

The Spanish equivalent had several versions. In one version the prisoner was made to sit on a shorter post with his back to the main post and a rope loop was placed round his neck and around the post. The executioner twisted a stick inserted in the loop to tighten the rope and slowly strangle the prisoner.

Another form comprised a wooden stool on which the prisoner sat with his back to the post (see Fig. 18.1). In yet another form, a strong wooden chair was used and the condemned was strapped at the wrists, arms, waist and legs. In both types, behind the seat, was a substantial post to which was affixed a heavy screw operated by a handle or a weighted lever in both cases connected to a spike or a small star shaped blade which ran through the post. When the screw/lever mechanism was operated the blade entered the criminal's neck and severed the spinal column. This was done in order to achieve a quick death; in earlier forms the victim strangled slowly.

Throttling is another name for manual strangulation. In this form the compression of the neck is effected by hands. Multiple crescentic nail marks on the neck of the victim are the hallmark of this form of strangulation.

DROWNING

25. B. *Related facts:* Each tissue in the human body has a different specific gravity. The specific gravity of bone is about 2.01, of muscle 1.08 and of fat 0.92. Thus the average specific gravity of human body would depend on the relative ratio of fat and muscle in the body too, more fatty people having lower specific gravity. However the value of 1.08 is generally accepted as an average value. Seawater has an average specific gravity of 1.028 with 3.5 g of dissolved salts for every 100 g of pure water.

The specific gravity of water in the saltiest ocean—the Dead Sea—is 1.166. Thus the human body will not sink in it. Bathing, however, in the Dead Sea can hardly be styled a pleasure, as the water is very irritating to the skin and eyes.

26. A.

27. A.

28. B.

29. C. *Related fact:* Cutis anserina and washer woman's hands are not signs of antemortem drowning. Cutis anserina may be seen in any death due to rigor mortis of erector pilae muscles. Washer woman's hands are merely signs of submersion.

Variants of the choices in this question:

Other correct choices can be (i.e. changes which indicate antemortem drowning).

- Copious froth at mouth and nostrils.

Other incorrect choices can be (i.e. changes which DO NOT indicate antemortem drowning).

- Postmortem lividity over the face, neck, and front of chest. (Postmortem lividity over the face etc. indeed develops in drowning deaths, but it is **NOT** a sign of antemortem drowning. It is simply because the centre of gravity of the dead human body is so placed, that the body comes to lie face downwards when suspended in water, and hence the development of postmortem lividity in face in cases of drowning. This phenomenon would occur in postmortem drowning as well).

30. B. *Related facts:* This is a tricky question, many students believing (with some justification perphaps) that the correct choice should be (d). Diatoms in the bone marrow indeed is a good sign of antemortem drowning, but when compared with "fine lathery froth in the mouth and nostrils", it pales in significance. In fact there are several objections to the so-called "diatom test", many skeptics saying that since diatoms are ubiquitous (they are present in all bodies of water, even in the water that we drink and the air that we breathe), they may gain access to our bone marrows already during life. To confirm that the deceased indeed died of drowning, one therefore needs to carefully compare the species found in the bone marrow with those found in the body of water where the dead body was found. In the absence of this comparison, it would be far fetched to say the person died of drowning, just by observing diatoms in the bone marrow.

If you do not see the choice "fine lathery froth in the mouth and nostrils", then of course "diatoms in the bone marrow" becomes the right choice. Remember this is a tricky question.

31. C. *Related fact:* Also known as "Gettler chloride test". The test was suggested by Alexander O. Gettler in 1921. The presumption is that normally the chloride content is equal in all chambers of the heart (about 600 mg per 100 ml). Fresh river water contains almost no chloride while sea water contains chloride far above this level.

If antemortem drowning occurs in fresh water, the water will enter the lungs (along with respirations). From there it will enter the capillaries and ultimately find its way to the *left heart*. Thus the chloride concentration of the left heart will decrease (upto 50% lower).

By the same reasoning left heart chloride is *more* if the drowning occurs in sea water.

Checklist for other related questions on Gettler's test:

- It can be used to differentiate antemortem from postmortem drowning.
- If it is a known case of antemortem drowning, it can be used to differentiate between fresh water and sea water drowning.
- A 25% difference in chloride content in the two sides of the heart is considered significant. If the difference is less than this, or there is no difference, no definite conclusions could be drawn.
- The test is useless in the following circumstances:
  - o If either of the heart septa is patent (e.g. patent foramen ovale).
  - o If the water is brackish (i.e. its salt content is somewhat between that of freshwater and seawater). Brackish water has almost the same chloride content as the blood.
  - o If putrefaction has occurred.
  - o This fact has been asked in MCQ as→ Gettler test is not of help (i) if the deceased had patent foramen ovale (ii) if death was due to drowning in brackish water (iii) in advanced stages of putrefaction (iv) all of the above. The intended answer is (iv) all of the above.
- The test is controversial, and not many forensic pathologists believe in this test today.

32. B. This definition does not take into account whether the individual subsequent survives or, if he survives, whether he has any neurological impairment. "Near drowning" victims are important to resolve the issue whether electrolyte disturbance occurs in the blood in drowning victims or not. In "near drowning" victims physicians found that electrolyte disturbances were mild and rarely had any clinical significance.

33. D.

34. B.

35. A. Paltauf's hemorrhages are seen in lungs. These were first described by Arnold Paltauf (1860-1893), professor of forensic medicine at the German university in Prague.

36. B. ***Related fact:*** This bleaching (and other immersion related changes) are attributed to the imbibtion of water into the outer layers of the skin. Also remember that these changes are **NOT** diagnostic of antemortem drowning. They merely indicate submersion, which could be antemortem as well as postmortem.

Watch out for other related MCQs. Important pointers are:

- **2 hours**→Wrinkling of skin starts.
- **12 hours**→Bleaching of cuticle.
- **24 hours**→Bleaching, corrugation and soddening of cuticle becomes very much pronounced.
- **48 hours**→Cuticle begins to separate from palm of hand and sole of foot.
- **3-4 days**→Cuticle can be peeled off like a glove.

37. B. ***Related fact:*** Floatation occurs in 2-3 days in winters. It might be confusing to some students that the cuticle is peeled off in 3-4 days, while floatation occurs in 2-3 days maximum. This can happen if the body was tied with a weight, or it gets entangled in weeds etc. In these conditions, it might remain underwater for longer periods, explaining peeling off of the skin like a glove.

38. A. ***Related fact:*** Conditions where froth may be produced are:

- Opium poisoning.
- Organo-phosphorus poisoning.
- Strangulation.
- Epileptic attacks.
- Electric shock.
- Acute pulmonary edema.
- Putrefaction.
- Snake bite.

39. D.

40. A. ***Related facts:*** Oligohalophilic diatoms live in fresh water with a salinity of less than 0.05%. Polyhalophilic diatoms live in sea water. Mesohalophilic diatoms live in water midway in salinity between freshwater and seawater, i.e. brackish water.

Additional info on diatoms: Diatoms belong to phylum Bacillariophyta. They are found floating in all the waters of the Earth. Diatoms may be either unicellular or colonial. The silicified cell wall forms a pillbox-like shell (frustule) composed of overlapping halves (known as epitheca and hypotheca) that contain intricate and delicate markings. These markings are useful in testing the resolving power of microscope lenses. Because of their beautiful symmetry and design, they are sometimes called "jewels of the sea".

Diatoms are divided into two orders on the basis of symmetry and shape: the round, nonmotile *Centrales* ("centric" diatoms) have radial markings; the elongated *Pennales* ("pennate" diatoms), which move with a gliding motion, have pinnate (featherlike) markings. Food is stored as oil droplets, and the golden-brown pigment fucoxanthin masks the chlorophyll and carotenoid pigments that are also present. Diatoms, among the most important and prolific sea organisms, serve directly or indirectly as food for many animals. Diatomaceous earth, a substance composed of fossilized diatoms, is used in filters, insulation, abrasives, paints, and varnishes.

For forensic pathologists diatoms are important as they may be found in peripheral organs (bone, brain, liver, spleen etc.) in cases of antemortem drowning.

41. D.

42. C. ***Variant:*** Sometimes the question is asked in this form→Antemortem drowning can best be confirmed by demonstrating diatoms in (a) Brain and bone marrow (b)Liver and anal canal (c) Pancreas and lungs (d)Lungs and stomach. The answer is (a) Brain and bone marrow.

43. A. ***Related fact:*** The terms *"Emphysema aquosum"* (also known as *emphysème hydroaérique*) and *"Oedema aquosum"* are rarely used, if at all, by serious forensic pathologists today. The only justification of this question being included here is that this question is still being asked in various examinations.

It is important to appreciate the mechanism supposed to be working behind the production of "*Emphysema aquosum*" and "*Oedema aquosum*".

A live person can either jump himself in water (often with suicidal intention), or someone may throw him in water after first striking him unconscious (homicidal drowning). In the first instance the victim is "conscious" and thus makes violent efforts to breathe. This causes lot of foam to be created, as the water gets churned up with mucus of the air passages. This appears to give a rather emphysematous appearance to the lungs (*Emphysema aquosum*).

If on the other hand, the victim was unconscious at the time of entry into water, no such conscious violent efforts to breathe are made. Water simply enters the passages with each breathing movement. There is no violent churning of the water with mucus, and thus almost no froth. The latter appearance is traditionally known as "Odema aquosum".

To summarize:

Person alive at the time of entry into water:

Conscious→Emphysema aquosum.

Unconscious→Oedema aquosum.

Person dead at the time of entry into water→*Post mortem drowning.*

44. C. Some swimmers hyperventilate before underwater swimming, so they can remain longer under water. This does raise their blood O_2 levels, but simultaneously lowers their CO_2 levels in the blood quite significantly. CO_2 is required to stimulate the respiratory centre. After some time of underwater swimming, the blood oxygen is used up, but carbon dioxide levels do not rise enough to cause air hunger. The swimmer does not feel the need to come up. Lowered oxygen levels cause him to loose consciousness and the swimmer drowns inadvertently.

45. C. ***Related facts:*** It is an archaic term but may still be asked as an interesting MCQ. The term comes from the name of an 18th Century Czech composer Franz Kotzwara, who was fond of this practice. On September 2, 1791 he paid a visit to a prostitute Susannah Hill in a London brothel and asked her to asphyxiate him partially, so he could get sexual pleasure. She did accordingly but in the process Kotzwara died accidentally. Susannah Hill was arrested and charged with murder (on September 16, 1791) at the Old Bailey. But she was acquitted after testimony proved her innocence. The court records were destroyed to prevent the scandalous case from going public. A secret copy was however made which was intended to be sold and published at a later time. It never was, but the manuscript is preserved and kept in the Francis Countway Library of Medicine in Boston. The term Kotzwarraism comes from his name. Koczwarism is just a corruption of that name.

MULTIPLE ANSWER TYPE (PGI, CHANDIGARH PATTERN)

46. B,D. Lynching is a name given to execution of criminals by hanging in 18th Century America. The person responsible for this practice was Charles Lynch (1736-96). With three other respected members from Lynchburg, he formed an ad hoc court to hear crimes and grievances. Lynch's court however had no legal authority. Major crimes such as rape (especially rape of a white woman by a black), horse stealing, and cattle rustling, were punished by public hanging on a tree (known as lynching). Since the mob hanged the accused without the benefit of a fair trial, the hanging was clearly homicidal in nature. Lynch clearly exceeded his authority, but he was later exonerated by the state legislature.

Some authorities believe that the name comes from another Virginia resident William L. Lynch (1724-1820), whose actions were similar to those of Charles Lynch.

47. B,C,D. Autoerotic asphyxia, autoerotic hanging, sexual hanging, Sexual asphyxiophilia, hypoxyphilia or masochistic hanging are synonymous terms. The following features are typical of autoerotic asphyxia:

- The person does it for getting heightened sexual pleasure.
- It is well-known that masturbation during a state of partial cerebral anoxia can lead to heightened and more intense sexual orgasm. The person achieves this by passing a noose round his neck, placing a padding (usually a towel) between the noose and the neck. This is done to avoid pain due to rope biting in the neck, as well

as to avoid getting tell-tale marks on the neck. The other end of the rope is fixed to some point in the ceiling/overhead fan etc. The length of the rope is such that the legs of the victim can easily touch the ground, but he can tighten the noose voluntarily by slumping against the noose. This produces partial cerebral anoxia by blocking carotid arteries. He masturbates simultaneously to get heighted sexual pleasure.

- There is evidence of masturbation combined with partial or complete nudity.
- Pornographic material is usually kept around to stimulate him sexually.
- There is often a mirror in front of him, so he can observe himself masturbating.
- Usually he is a transvestite. He wears female clothings, padded bra, panties etc.
- Some element of bondage is usually present, e.g. binding of the body and/or the extremities and/or genitals with ropes, chains etc.
- It is most commonly seen in males. Although females are also known to engage in this activity the incidence is much less.
- There is no obvious or apparent wish to die. Suicide note is never found, because suicide is never intended in the first place. Death is always accidental. The victim slumps on the noose to achieve partial cerebral anoxia, but he may lose consciousness sometimes and this may be his undoing. His whole weight begins to act on the noose producing complete asphyxia. Since he is unconscious he can not retrieve himself and dies of asphyxia. Thus this is always a case of accidental hanging.
- Opinion by forensic pathologist whether the hanging was suicidal or accidental is important, as some life insurance policies don't pay if the death was suicidal in nature.

48. A,C,D. The classic signs are asphyxia are generally considered to be (i) Cyanosis (ii) Congestion of internal organs (iii) Petechial haemorrhages (iv) Oedema (v) Engorgement of the right side of the heart (vi) Increased fluidity of the blood (see square boxes in figure 18.2 on next page).

The mechanism of these classic signs of asphyxia is complex but can be grasped by referring to figure here. Application of ligature, pressure of chest or restriction of respiration by other means generally results in compromise of the movements of the chest, which normally facilitates venous return. This causes (i) Obstruction of venous return (ii) Acute rise in venous pressure and (iii) Back pressure in the venous system. Since lungs cannot expand fully it also results in (iv) Collapse of pulmonary vasculature. Refer to the figure to understand how these in turn produce classic signs of asphyxia.

Hypoxia that results from lack of oxygenation is supposed to release fibrinolysins which are supposed in turn to increase the fluidity of blood.

It must be stressed however that these "classic signs" of asphyxia are *no more considered pathognomonic of asphyxia.* These are supposed to be very general signs seen in almost any autopsy. The explanations given above are however generally advanced for these signs as seen in asphyxia.

49. A,B,D,E. It is usually believed that petechiae are seen in *all* asphyxial deaths, but this is not true (see answer to a question above). Asphyxial deaths unaccompanied by compression of either the neck or thorax rarely show pethechiae. Furthermore the rapidity with which people die in plastic bag suffocation and in atmospheres devoid of

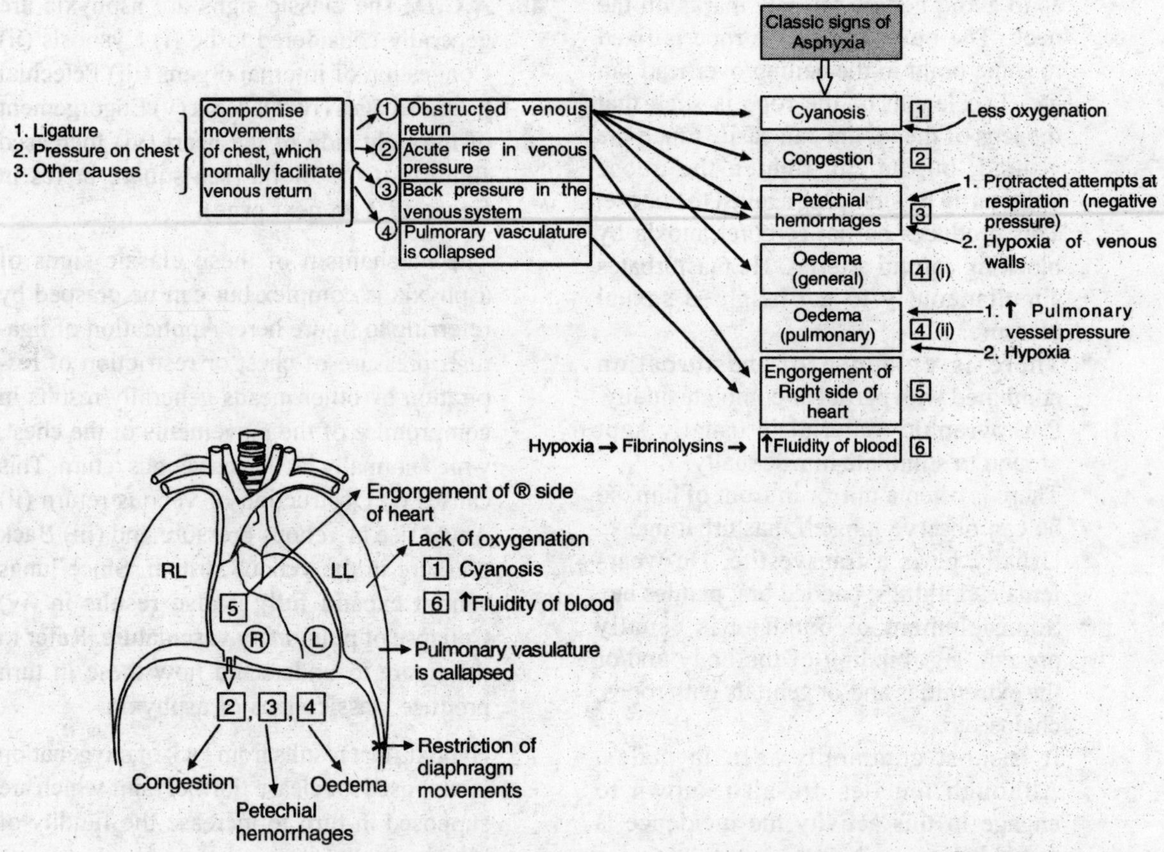

Fig. 18.2: Mechanism of all six "classic" signs of asphyxia

oxygen, makes one think they do not die of asphyxia in the first place; instead some rapid vasovagal cardio-inhibitory mechanism might be at work.

50. E. Most textbooks taught in this country would have us believe that fresh water and sea water drowning could be easily differentiated by looking at the lungs and the usual differences cited are the ones mentioned in rest of the choices (from A till D). The fact is that there are little or no differences in appearances of lungs in the two forms of drowning. Some workers have sought to differentiate between the two by looking for unique diatoms (found in fresh or sea water) or even by looking at fresh water plankton (with varying rates of success). But this is obviously not to do with the gross appearances of lungs. The fact remains that there are *no appreciable differences in the gross appearances of lungs in fresh water and sea water drowning.*

19 Deaths from Starvation

1. **During starvation, how much of the body weight should be lost when life is threatened?**
   A. 20%
   B. 40%
   C. 60%
   D. 70%

2. **Total lack of food, when water is available, is likely to cause death in about:**
   A. 10-12 days
   B. 30-35 days
   C. 50-60 days
   D. 90-100 days

3. **How many calories are needed to maintain body weight in active adults?**
   A. 800-1000 calories
   B. 1500-1900 calories
   C. 2000-2500 calories
   D. 2500-3000 calories

4. **In acute starvation, the feeling for intense hunger lasts for how many days?**
   A. Just for about first two days
   B. For first 7 days
   C. For first 15 days
   D. It lasts till starvation continues

5. **In how many days would a normally nourished person die, if both water and food are withdrawn?**
   A. 5-7 days
   B. 10 days
   C. 20 days
   D. 30 days

6. **In death due to starvation, what is the major finding in the gall bladder?**
   A. Its walls show numerous ulcerations
   B. It is empty
   C. It shows several small stones
   D. It is full

7. **Biochemical manifestations of starvation include:**
   A. A low blood sugar
   B. A low non-protein nitrogen
   C. High level of chlorides
   D. High levels of cholesterol

8. **A political prisoner has gone on a hunger strike and the jailor requests the jail doctor to force-feed the prisoner in order to save his life. The current legal situation in this country is:**
   A. That the doctor should force feed the prisoner

B. That the doctor should not force feed the prisoner
C. That the doctor should inform the prisoner's family and then go according to the family's wishes
D. Ambiguous

MULTIPLE ANSWER TYPE (PGI, CHANDIGARH PATTERN)

9. Chronic starvation may result in following situations:
A. Famine
B. Being trapped in pits
C. Oedema of legs
D. Myocardial infarction
E. Neglect on the part of parents or guardians

10. Following facts about starvation are CORRECT?
A. The very young and the very old suffer the worst
B. Females withstand starvation for a longer period
C. Obese people can not withstand starvation
D. Exposure to warmer conditions is more deleterious than exposure to colder conditions
E. Active physical exertion hastens death

11. Postmortem findings of starvation include:
A. Weight of brain is reduced to 800 g
B. Muscles are darker in color
C. Fat is completely absent in the subcutaneous tissues, but retained in the omentum, mesentery and around the internal organs such as kidney
D. Subepicardial fat is replaced by a watery gelatinous material
E. Trophic changes in the skin

12. In starvation, which organs retain fat till the very last?
A. Female breast
B. Hips
C. Orbits
D. Abdomen
E. Folds of neck

ANSWERS

1. B.
2. C.
3. B.
4. A.
5. B.
6. D. An interesting related fact: Parenteral nutrition leads to the formation of gall stones.
7. A.
8. D. ***Related facts***: The legal situation in this country currently is quite ambiguous. There are arguments that if the doctor does not force feed the prisoner, he may be sued for abetment of suicide (under section 306 of IPC). On the contrary if the doctor force feeds the prisoner against his wish, he may be sued for using criminal force under section 350 and 352 of Indian Penal Code. A good lawyer could argue the case from either side. World Medical Association has however given guidelines to doctors in its **Declaration of Tokyo** (adopted in 1975 and amended in 2005) and **Declaration of Malta** (adopted in 1991 and amended in 1992).

Declaration of Tokyo basically gives guidelines to physicians concerning torture and other cruel, inhuman or degrading treatment or punishment in relation to detention and imprisonment. Among other things it says that "Where a prisoner refuses nourishment and is considered by the physician as capable of forming an unimpaired and rational judgment concerning the consequences of such a voluntary refusal of nourishment, he or she shall not be fed artificially. The decision as to the capacity of the prisoner to form such a judgment should be confirmed by at least one other independent physician. The consequences of the refusal of nourishment shall be explained by the physician to the prisoner."

Declaration of Malta is specifically on the role of doctor in case of Hunger strikers. It realizes that the doctor indeed is under a serious conflict. On one hand, "there is a moral obligation on every human being to respect the sanctity of life. This is especially evident in the case of a doctor, who exercises his skills to save life and also acts in the best interests of his patients" and on the other hand "it is the duty of the doctor to respect the autonomy which the patient has over his person. A doctor requires informed consent from his patients before applying any of his skills to assist them, unless emergency circumstances have arisen in which case the doctor has to act in what is perceived to be the patient's best interests." Following guidelines are given to resolve this conflict:

- The doctor should ascertain on a daily basis whether or not the patient wishes to continue with his hunger strike.
- The ultimate decision on intervention or non-intervention should be left with the individual doctor without the intervention of third parties (such as jailor etc) whose primary interest is not the patient's welfare. However, the doctor should clearly state to the patient whether or not he is able to accept the patient's decision to refuse treatment or, in case of coma, artificial feeding, thereby risking death. If the doctor cannot accept the patient's decision to refuse such aid, the patient would then be entitled to be attended by

another physician (article 4 of the preamble of this Declaration).

- The hunger striker must be professionally informed by the doctor of the clinical consequences of a hunger strike, and of any specific danger to his own particular case. An informed decision can only be made on the basis of clear communication. An interpreter should be used if indicated.
- The doctor has a responsibility to inform the family of the patient that the patient has embarked on a hunger strike, unless this is specifically prohibited by the patient.
- When the hunger striker has become confused and is therefore unable to make an unimpaired decision or has lapsed into a coma, the doctor shall be free to make the decision for his patient as to further treatment which he considers to be in the best interest of that patient, always taking into account the decision he has arrived at during his preceding care of the patient during his hunger strike, and reaffirming article 4 of the preamble of this Declaration.

Basically both these Declarations respect the autonomy of the patient, and very much weighed towards the opinion that the doctor should **NOT** force feed such cases.

MULTIPLE ANSWER TYPE (PGI, CHANDIGARH PATTERN)

9. A,B,E.

10. A,B,E. ***Related facts***: Obese people can withstand starvation better because they have a better reservoir of fat. Exposure to colder climate hastens death because of increased metabolic demands (to keep the body warm).

11. B,D,E. Size and weight of all organs is reduced except that of brain. Muscles are atrophied and darker due to lipochrome. Fat is completely absent in the subcutaneous tissues, and is ALSO ABSENT IN the omentum, mesentery and around the internal organs such as kidney. This situation is generally not seen in wasting diseases such as tuberculosis and cancers.

12. A,C.

20 Anaesthetics and Operative Deaths

1. The first successful public demonstration of general anaesthesia was done in the year ....by ....using ....?

A. 1812, Joseph Priestley, chloroform
B. 1831, Humphry Davy, pancuronium bromide
C. 1845, Horace Wells, nitrous oxide
D. 1846, William T.G. Morton, diethyl ether

2. If death has occurred during anaesthesia, which of the following is the most appropriate step?

A. The body must be sent for post-mortem
B. Death certificate should be signed by the Head of the Department of Surgery
C. Death certificate must be signed by Head of the Department of Anaesthesia
D. Death Certificate should be jointly signed by anaesthetist, surgeon and the medical superintendent of the hospital

3. The term "etheromania" refers to:

A. Delirium due to ether overdose
B. Idiosyncrasies due to ether anaesthesia
C. Addiction to use of ether
D. Psychosis induced in a patient after administration of ether

4. All of the following are true about malignant hyperthermia *except*:

A. It can follow administration of anaesthesia
B. It is inherited as an autosomal dominant trait
C. There is dark brown coloration to urine
D. Blood chemistry shows decreased blood levels of creatine phosphokinase (CPK)

5. In a medicolegal investigation of alleged death due to Anaesthesia, all of the following are correct statements *except:*

A. Blood samples of the cadaver must be taken
B. Devices introduced into the patient, such as endotracheal tubes, catheters etc. must be removed before starting autopsy
C. Injuries due to resuscitative measures may mimic strangulation
D. Radiographs of the dead body must be taken before autopsy

6. Barbiturates used for clinical anaesthesia are:

A. Sodium thiopental
B. Thiamylal
C. Methohexital
D. All of the above

7. The incidence of halothane producing fulminant hepatic necrosis is:

A. 1 in 500 patients
B. 1 in 5,000 patients
C. 1 in 10,000 patients
D. 1 in 100,000 patients

8. Halothane hepatitis has a fatality rate of:
A. 10%
B. 25%
C. 50%
D. >80%

MULTIPLE ANSWER TYPE (PGI, CHANDIGARH PATTERN)

9. Which of the following are genuine complications arising from anaesthetic procedures?
A. Pulmonary oedema
B. Smothering
C. Malignant hyperthermia
D. Transection of trachea
E. Aspiration of gastric contents

10. Among the following anaesthetic agents which ones are the parenteral anaesthetics?
A. Propofol
B. Halothane
C. Etomidate
D. Isoflurane
E. Ketamine

ANSWERS

1. **D.** ***Additional info*:** Combinations in choice (A) and (B) are completely fictitious. In 1845, Horace Wells, a dentist, did try to publicly demonstrate general anaesthesia by nitrous oxide at the Massachusetts General Hospital in Boston, but the patient cried out in pain, and the demonstration was deemed a failure. In 1846, William T.G. Morton–surprisingly still a second year medical student–successfully demonstrated anaesthesia with diethyl ether (again at the Massachusetts General Hospital). Although in the beginning the crowd which had gathered as well as the surgeon who had to conduct the operation (Dr. Warren) were sneering at Morton, they were all appreciative at the end, as the patient did not feel any pain whatsoever. At the end of the operation, Dr. Warren turned to the audience and made this famous statement, "Gentlemen, this is no humbug". Another famous surgeon Dr. Henry J. Bigelow, who had come to attend the demonstration, said, "I have seen something today that will go around the world".
2. **A.**
3. **C.** ***Additional info:*** Recreational ether-drinking (ether-sniffing or inhalation is an equally popular form of intake) began on a serious scale only after its anaesthetic properties were discovered in 1846 by Thomas Morton, who marketed it as 'letheon'.
4. **D.** Blood CPK is increased in malignant hyperthermia. Also increased are blood potassium, uric acid and phosphate. Hyperkalemia, raised CPK and myoglobinuria, can be explained by damaged cell membranes.

   Additional info: Malignant hyperthermia—often noted for the first time during administration of anesthesia—is a group of inherited muscle problems characterized by muscle breakdown following certain stimuli—such as anesthesia, extremes of exercise (particularly in hot conditions), fever, or use of stimulant drugs. The problems associated with this condition result from over-excitable muscles that contract uncontrollably, severe fever, abnormal heart rhythms, and kidney failure.

   The anesthetized patient rapidly develops a high fever and muscle rigidity. During these episodes, muscle tissue is destroyed and break-down products of muscle may damage the kidneys and cause acute renal failure. The urine may turn dark due to released muscle pigments (rhabdomyolysis).

   The best course of action for this condition is prevention. If a general anesthetic is to be given, pretreatment with dantrolene sodium is recommended.
5. **B.** Devices introduced in the patient must not be removed, as it is very important to know their position within the body. Blood samples are necessary for analytical tests. Radiographs of the body are necessary in order to know the correct position of various devices such as endotracheal tubes.
6. **D.** ***Additional info:*** Although all these three barbiturates are used for anaesthesia, sodium thiopental is most commonly used.
7. **C.** ***Additional info:*** This is known as "halothane hepatitis".
8. **C.**

MULTIPLE ANSWER TYPE (PGI, CHANDIGARH PATTERN)

9. **A,C,E.**
10. **A,C,E.** Halothane and Isoflurane are inhalational anaesthetics.

21 Hypothermia

1. **Cold is endured longer by:**
   A. Men
   B. Women
   C. New born infants
   D. Old people
2. **"Systemic hypothermia" is a condition when the core body temperature drops below:**
   A. 37°C
   B. 35°C
   C. 30°C
   D. 0°C
3. **In hypothermia, which is the "cut off" rectal temperature in degrees Celsius below which death will usually ensue?**
   A. 35
   B. 31
   C. 26
   D. 15
4. **In hypothermia, the surface of the body becomes:**
   A. Hyperemic
   B. Pale
   C. Blackish brown
   D. Light greenish in color due to production of haematoidin
5. **The mechanism of death in hypothermia is:**
   A. Cessation of circulation usually preceded by ventricular fibrillation
   B. Hypothermic coagulation of proteins
   C. Asphyxia brought about by inability to breath cold air
   D. Paralysis of the diaphragm
6. **How many times faster is body heat lost in water than in dry, cold air at the same temperature?**
   A. It looses equally fast in both cases
   B. 3 times
   C. 12 times
   D. 20 times

MULTIPLE ANSWER TYPE (PGI, CHANDIGARH PATTERN)

7. **Which of the following facts are true about Trenchfoot?**
   A. It is due to exposure to temperatures below 0°C
   B. It is named after the condition suffered by many soldiers in the trenches during World War I
   C. Dampness is an important factor in producing this condition

D. Usually affected body parts are the extremities
E. If this condition develops, amputation of the affected limb is the only remedy

8. Which of the following is the correct treatment of frostbite?
A. Rub snow on the affected part
B. Rapidly rewarm in clean water at 40°–42°C for about 10-30 minutes or until the extremity becomes pliable again
C. Rapidly rewarm with a heater or fire directly in front of the limb
D. Thaw the frozen part and let it freeze again
E. Allow the person to smoke as it will provide warmth to the lungs

ANSWERS

1. **B.** This is because of higher fat content in women. The aged and the infants are most vulnerable to cold.
2. **B.** 35°C is equivalent to 95°F, so keep this choice in mind too.
3. **C.**
4. **B.**
5. **A.**
6. **B.** ***Related fact:*** Body heat is lost faster in water, because it conducts heat away from the body faster. Because of this reason, immersion hypothermia is extremely dangerous.

MULTIPLE ANSWER TYPE (PGI, CHANDIGARH PATTERN)

7. **B,C,D.** Cold injuries are divided into two general groups: those that occur without any freezing of the body tissues and those that result from the freezing of the skin or a body part (generally the fingers, toes, ears, nose and cheeks). Examples of cold injuries *without tissue freezing* include chilblains and "trench foot" (also known as immersion foot). Examples of cold injuries *with tissue freezing* include frostnip and frostbite.

   Frostbite is a cold injury that is associated *with tissue freezing*. It occurs at temperatures below 0°C. In this injury, ice crystals form in the skin and deeper tissue. Ice crystals exert osmotic force, causing water to move from intracellular space. This causes swelling of tissues (filling up of intercellular spaces with fluid). At the same time there is cellular dehydration and hyperosmolarity. There is also denaturation of proteins and destruction of enzymes. The skin is numb and discolored; it is purple in most severe cases. On touching the skin, it does not feel like normal "bouncy" skin; instead it feels just like a rock, block of ice or perhaps like a piece of chicken from the freezer. Blisters appear, which may become hemorrhagic. **Frostnip** is an early – and least serious—stage of frostbite. The symptoms are numbness and tingling, but no actual tissue injury occurs. The symptoms occur when the blood vessels supplying the affected tissues constrict. The skin appears white and waxy or gray and mottled but feels normal to touch.

   Trench foot is less severe than frostbite, and there is no permanent injury in trench foot. Trench foot occurs generally at 5-8°C (no tissue freezing occurs at this temperature), while frostbite appears at temperatures less than 0°C (tissue freezing occurs here). Dampness is an important factor in production of trench foot.

8. **A.** Rubbing snow on the affected part is a folk remedy. It is not only useless, but dangerous. Dry heat (to thaw the affected part) must be avoided, as it can desiccate the damaged tissue. Heating in clean water is the desirable course. Avoid smoking (nicotine contracts blood vessels), but alcohol may be helpful (it dilates blood vessels). Frostbite is a tetanus prone wound. Tissue injury is greatest when tissue is partially thawed and allowed to refreeze. Blisters must not be punctured.

22 Deaths due to Heatstroke and Related Causes

1. **The body's basal metabolic rate (BMR) is:**
   A. 10-20 kcal/h/m^2
   B. 25-35 kcal/h/m^2
   C. 50-60 kcal/h/m^2
   D. 500-600 kcal/h/m^2

2. ***Insensible perspiration*** **is the name given to:**
   A. Perspiration through nostrils and mouth
   B. Loss of moisture from the nonsweating body
   C. Loss of moisture large enough to cause a dulling of senses
   D. Perspiration through the hairy portions of the body such as scalp, axilla etc.

3. **Evaporation of 1 mL of sweat results in the loss of .... kcal of heat:**
   A. 0.18
   B. 0.58
   C. 58
   D. 580

4. **In response to thermal stress which of the following types of sweat glands respond maximum?**
   A. Eccrine glands
   B. Apocrine glands
   C. Hypothermal glands
   D. Hyperthermal glands

5. **At the upper limits of temperature tolerance, sweat can amount up to:**
   A. 0.5 liters per hour
   B. 1.5 liters per hour
   C. 2.5 liters per hour
   D. 3.5 liters per hour

6. **Generalized or Jacksonian (focal) convulsions are most typically seen in:**
   A. Heat cramps
   B. Heat exhaustion
   C. Heat syncope
   D. Heatstroke

7. **The external temperature within which the haemostatic mechanism of thermo-regulation in humans is not stressed is:**
   A. 18°C
   B. 21° C
   C. 29° C with a 2° C variation on either side
   D. 35° C with a 2° C variation on either side

8. **Biological adaptation that reduces physiologic strain, improve physical work capabilities, improve comfort and protects vital organs from heat injury is known as:**
   A. Heat safety mechanisms
   B. Heat syncope
   C. Heatstroke
   D. Heat acclimatization

9. Degeneration of neurons in brain – mostly in the Purkinje cell layer of cerebellum—are seen in:
A. Heatstroke
B. Heat cramps
C. Heat exhaustion
D. Heat syncope

10. Which of the following factors can aggravate the causation of heatstroke?
A. Alcoholism
B. Humid atmosphere
C. Dysentery
D. All of the above

11. Which of the following conditions, if not treated immediately, can lead to heatstroke?
A. Heat syncope
B. Heat exhaustion
C. Heat cramps
D. Miner's cramps

12. The classical triad of increased temperature, dry skin and neurological deficit are typically seen in:
A. Heatstroke
B. Miner's cramps
C. Heat prostration
D. All of the above

13. Which of the following may be confused with heatstroke?
A. Falciparum malaria
B. Morphine poisoning
C. Dhatura poisoning
D. Both (A) and (C) above

14. Neurological deficit is most characteristically seen in:
A. Heat exhaustion
B. Heatstroke
C. Heat syncope
D. Miner's cramps

15. Sweating ceases completely from the trunk and limbs, but continues in face and neck in:
A. Thermogenic anhidrosis
B. Heat hyperpyrexia
C. Heat cramps
D. Heat syncope

16. This condition is caused by exposure to the sun. Its most typical symptom is erythema which occurs in about 2-6 hours. Name the condition:
A. Prickly heat
B. Heat oedema
C. Sunburn
D. Miliaria rubra

17. Sweating ceases completely in:
A. Heat cramps
B. Heatstroke
C. Heat exhaustion
B. All of the above

18. This condition is caused by prolonged wetting of the skin with sweat and without evaporation. Its probable pathogenesis is sweat duct obstruction due to sodium chloride from the evaporated sweat continuing to lie on the skin. Name the condition:
A. Heat cramps
B. Heat oedema
C. Sunburn
B. Miliaria rubra

19. Which of the following is most serious heat related disorder in which thermoregulation is maintained?
A. Heat syncope
B. Heat cramps
C. Heat exhaustion
D. Heatstroke

20. In a heat acclimatized individual, sweating is:
A. Delayed and greater
B. Earlier and greater
C. Earlier and lesser
D. Delayed and lesser

21. Most serious heat related disorder is:
A. Heat cramps
B. Heat syncope
C. Heatstroke
D. Heat exhaustion

22. Heat acclimatization generally occurs in:
A. 2 hours
B. 2 days
C. 2 weeks
D. 2 months

23. In a heat acclimatized individual:
A. Core Temperature is reduced
B. Body heat production is lower
C. Thirst is improved
D. All of the above

24. The maximal temperature tolerance limits for human cells range from:
A. 0°C to 37°C
B. 0°C to 45°C
C. 10°C to 40°C
D. 10°C to 50°C

25. Miner's cramps result from:
A. Low altitude
B. Mountaineering
C. Exposure to excessive heat
D. Scuba diving

26. Which of the following is the simplest and least obnoxious of the following heat related disorders?
A. Heatstroke
B. Heat exhaustion
C. Heat prostration
D. Heat cramps

27. Which of the following factors predispose an individual to heatstroke and other heat related disorders?
A. Obesity
B. Alcohol
C. Intake of anticholinergics
D. All of the above

28. Which of the following statements about heatstroke are correct?
A. Nonexertional heatstroke is classically seen among the elderly
B. Exertional heatstroke is classically seen among young persons who perform strenuous tasks in hot and humid climate
C. The two forms of heatstroke are clinically indistinguishable
D. All of the above

29. In which of the following conditions, there is no water or salt depletion?
A. Heat syncope
B. Heat exhaustion
C. Heat cramps
D. Heatstroke

30. Which of the following disorders is divided in three types: pure salt depletion type, anhidrotic and pure water deficiency types?
A. Heat exhaustion
B. Heat cramps
C. Heatstroke
D. Heat syncope

31. Which of the following conditions has the worst prognosis?
A. Heat syncope
B. Heat exhaustion
C. Heatstroke
D. Heat cramps

32. Decerebrate rigidity may be seen in:
A. Heatstroke
B. Heat cramps
C. Heat exhaustion
D. Heat syncope

ANSWERS

1. **C.** The body's basal metabolic rate (BMR) is 50-60 kcal/h/m^2 (approximately 100 kcal/h for a person weighing 70 kg). In the absence of adequate thermoregulatory mechanisms, the BMR may lead to an increase in body temperature of approximately 1.1°C/h. The rate of increase may be significantly higher during periods of heavy exercise or in the setting of high environmental heat loads.

2. **B.**

3. **B.**

4. **A.** ***Related facts:*** There are two types of sweat glands: eccrine and apocrine. Eccrine glands are "true" sweat glands, which respond to thermal stress. Found in large numbers only in man and some primates, they are distributed over the entire skin surface. The duct from eccrine glands opens directly onto the skin surface. These glands are innervated by sympathetic cholinergic fiber. Thermal sweating occurs over most of the body integument. Emotional stress can induce eccrine sweating, in selected areas like the palms, soles, axillae and forehead by a mechanism that is not well understood.

   Apocrine glands on the other hand produce an oily fluid (not sweat) which acquires a scent only after it interacts with skin surface bacteria. These glands are found in many mammals. In man they are localized mainly to the **a**xillary, **a**reolar, **a**nus and genital regions; (modified apocrine glands are found in the breast and the external auditory canal). The ducts from these glands open into the hair follicle above the entrance of the sebaceous duct. Myoepithelial cells, surrounding the gland, help to force the secretions outward. Apocrine glands continuously produce their secretions. Their function is presumed to be the production of sexual olfactory messages.

   Apocrine glands are better developed in women than in men, are best developed in the Negro race and their secretion does not appear before puberty.

> **Memory aid**→Remember **A** for Apocrine and **A** for **A**xilla. This should remind us that apocrine glands are located only at a few places and thus have specialized functions. However they can better be remembered by their actualy etymology, which is like this:
>
> **Apocrine**→Greek prefix "*apo*" means "from". Latin "*crinis*" means "hair". Thus the term literally means "coming from hair". Recall that apocrine glands appear mainly in hairy areas and their ducts open in hair follicles. The Greek root "*apo*" is seen also in apomorphine (from morphine) and apothecary (from a box or chest).
>
> **Eccrine**→Greek prefix "*ec*" means "away from". Thus eccrine means "away from hair". Eccrine glands are true sweat glands, which appear all over the body – not just on hairy regions. The root "*ec*" is also seen in "eccentric" (away from the circle) or "ecbolic" (a drug which throws something away from the uterus. "*bole*" means "throw").

5. **D.**

6. **D.**

7. **C.** The external temperature within which the haemostatic mechanism of thermoregulation is not stressed and the basal heat production rate is at its minimum is called the *zone of thermoneutrality*. In the resting person, this is 2°C on either side of 29°C depending on whether the person is clad or not. Deviation from this zone sets the homeostatic thermo-

regulatory mechanism in action. On the hotter side; the heat loss is increased while on the cooler side the heat conservation is stimulated. Body loses and gains heat by conduction, convention and radiation. In addition heat loss occurs by evaporation as well.

8. D.

9. A.

10. D.

11. B.

12. A.

13. D. Both Falciparum malaria and Dhatura poisoning cause the classical triad of dry skin, rise in body temperature and neurological deficit as is seen in heatstroke. Morphine does not present this classical picture. Skin is cold and clammy in morphine poisoning.

14. B.

15. A.

16. C.

17. B.

18. D. *Miliaria rubra* is another name for Prickly heat. Other synonyms are lichen tropics and heat rash.

19. C. Heatstroke is a still more serious condition, but in this condition, thermoregulation breaks down.

20. B.

21. C.

22. C.

23. D. The following things occur in a heat acclimatized individual.
- Thermal Comfort—Improved.
- Exercise Performance—Improved.
- Core Temperature—Reduced.
- Sweating—Earlier and Greater.
- Skin Blood Flow—Earlier.
- Body Heat Production—Lower.
- Heart Rate—Lowered.
- Thirst—Improved.
- Salt Losses (sweat and urine)— Reduced.
- Organ Protection—Improved.

24. B. At 0°C there is ice crystal formation. At about 45°C there is thermal coagulation of intracellular proteins.

25. C. Also known as heat cramps.

26. D.

27. D.

28. D.

29. A. This condition is caused by an intense peripheral vasodilatation which leads to peripheral pooling and hypotension. Blood is diverted away from brain which is responsible for syncopal attack. There is no water or salt depletion in this condition.

30. A.

31. C.

32. A.

STUDY MATERIAL

GENERAL

Humans are warm-blooded animals. They maintain their body temperature within a narrow range (within 1 or 2 degrees of 98.6° F) despite large fluctuations in external temperatures. This internal temperature range must be maintained for the body to function normally. Body temperature that gets too high or too low can result in serious injury to organs or death.

The body regulates its temperature by balancing heat production and heat loss. Heat disorders are caused by too much heat production or by too little heat loss.

Too much external heat encourages excessive sweating. It depletes the body of fluids and salts (electrolytes), which can lead to *low blood pressure* and painful muscle contractions. Which heat disorder develops depends on the severity of body fluid and salt depletion. **Heat cramps** – the mildest of heat disorders–results from mild or moderate depletion; **heat exhaustion**, from moderate or severe depletion; and **heatstroke**, the most serious of the heat disorders, often from severe depletion.

During high ambient temperature even under resting conditions shunting of blood to skin occurs (to promote heat loss). It produces a fall in BP and rise in heart rate. This phenomenon is further aggravated by dehydration. During exercise, blood is shunted to working muscles in addition to the skin. In unacclimatized persons, this can lead to cardiovascular instability characterized by rising heart rate and fall in stroke volume.

PREDISPOSING FACTORS

Factors which contribute to ineffective heat loss (predisposing factors) are:

i. Hot and humid conditions (sweat unable to evaporate).
ii. Heavy, tight, waterproof clothing (prevents sweat from evaporating from the skin surface).
iii. Drugs (antipsychotics, anticholinergics)—Sweating is impaired.
iv. Diseases (cystic fibrosis, scleroderma, psoriasis, eczema, severe sunburns)—Sweating is impaired.
v. Obesity—Impairs sweating because (i) it requires the heart to work harder, thereby depleting the reserve needed to increase pumping for sweating (ii) thick layer of fat in obese people slows heat loss from internal organs (iii) Since metabolic heat is produced in proportion to the bulk of tissue and is lost in proportion to surface area, the larger volume-to-area ratio creates an added risk.
vi. Alcohol—Interferes with sensible responses that could prevent heat disorders. For example, an inebriated person may not move to a cool environment, remove heavy clothing, or turn on an air conditioner.

ACCLIMATIZATION

When a person is exposed to longer periods of heat and humidity, the body gradually adjusts and is better able to maintain normal body temperature. This process is called acclimatization. An acclimatized individual has a greater ability to sweat under similar conditions. The salt content of the sweat is also less in an acclimatized individual (thus conserving body salt).

CLASSIFICATION OF HEAT DISORDERS

There is no universally accepted classification of heat disorders. Various authors, books and institutions have classified these disorders in their own ways, with lot of overlap and consequent confusion. However the International classification of diseases divides Heat disorders into several categories of which the following are medicolegally most important:

1. Heat Cramps
2. Heat Syncope.
3. Heat Exhaustion.
   a. Type 1: Pure salt deficiency.
   b. Type 2: Anhidrotic.
   c. Type 3: pure water deficiency.
4. Heat Hyperpyrexia.
5. Heatstroke.

Other heat disorders, which are medicolegally less important are:

1. Sunburn.
2. Prickly heat.
3. Heat oedema.
4. Hidromeiosis.

Heat Cramps

Also known as **Stoker's cramps, Miner's cramps, Fireman's cramps, Cane cutter's cramps.**

Heat cramps—the simplest of all heat disorders—are severe muscle spasms resulting from a combination of prolonged exercise, heavy sweating, and *excessive water replacement* in extreme heat. During sweating, salts (electrolytes) and fluids are lost, but drinking large quantities of water lowers the effective salt concentration, causing cramps.

Heat cramps are rhythmic, painful contractions in muscles of the hands, calves, feet, thighs, arms or abdomen. They usually last from 1 to 3 minutes but may recur for several hours.

Heat cramps are common among manual laborers, such as engine-room personnel, steel workers, roofers, and miners. Heat cramps may also develop in athletes, especially mountain climbers or skiers, whose many layers of clothing may keep them from noticing their heavy sweating. Cramps are common in tennis players and runners who do not take time to replace salts lost in sweat.

Mild heat cramps can be treated by drinking beverages that contain salt or eating salty food. Severe heat cramps are treated with fluids and salts given intravenously.

Heat Syncope

Also known as **Heat Collapse.**

It is another relatively mild disorder. There is no water or salt depletion. There is intense peripheral vasodilatation which leads to peripheral pooling and hypotension. The one factor which is usually present is *sudden change* (change from cool to hot environment; from hot to very hot environment; from dry heat to humid heat, or when there is sudden increase in physical work). Prolonged standing is another precipitating factor. Usually seen in unacclimatized individuals.

The main symptoms are giddiness and fainting (that's why it is called heat syncope or heat collapse). The main reason for this is the diversion of blood from the brain to the skin (peripheral pooling). Other symptoms are nausea, epigastric distress, urgency to defecate and blurring to vision. Main signs are pallor, tachycardia and hypotension.

Shifting the patient to a cool or shaded area in a head low position will usually restore consciousness.

Heat Exhaustion

Also known as **Heat Prostration.**

Heat exhaustion is the most serious heat disorder in which thermoregulation is maintained (heatstroke is a still more serious disorder, but in this, the power of thermoregulation is lost). It is also the most common heat disorder encountered clinically. It results from severe dehydration after a huge amount of sweat has been lost. It occurs typically in otherwise healthy young individuals who undertake prolonged physical exertion (exertion-induced heat exhaustion), such as marathon runners, outdoor sports players, military recruits, coal miners and construction workers. The basic feature of this disorder is circulatory deficiency due to water and/or salt depletion. Most characteristic symptom is *extreme fatigue* characterized by muscle aches, nausea, and fever.

The condition may be considered an incipient stage of heatstroke, and if left untreated, it may eventually progress to heatstroke.

It is divided into three types – Type 1, Type 2 and Type 3 heat exhaustion.

Type 1 (Pure salt deficiency or depletion)

It typically occurs in *unacclimatized* individuals (e.g. troops from a cold country landing suddenly in hot climate). Since these individuals are unacclimatized, the salt content in their sweat is relatively higher (their body does not conserve salt, since they are unacclimatized). When sweating occurs, the individual drinks water to quench thirst. Thus although water is replaced, salts get depleted gradually. Vomiting and diarrhoea contribute to this condition for similar reasons (salts are lost through vomiting and diarrhea).

- Symptoms
  - Lassitude, anorexia, headache, giddiness and vomiting. Muscle cramps in about 50% of cases.
  - Thirst is *not* a feature.
  - This condition usually *does not* predispose to heatstroke.
- Signs→skin remains moist. Fall of blood pressure. Tachycardia.
- Laboratory investigations show raised blood urea and low sodium and chloride levels.
- Treatment→IV isotonic saline since oral salt would cause vomiting.
- Prevention→Take 15-25 g salt daily.

Type 2 (Anhidrotic)

Also known as Thermogenic anhidrosis, Desert syndrome, Tropical anhydrotic asthenia.

- First described late in 2nd World war (1944) by Australian, American and British authorities almost simultaneously in their troops in the tropics.
- Usually does not occur until 4-7 months in a hot climate.
- Almost always preceded by skin eruptions of small gray papules like rice grains, often with fluid vesicles on the trunk and limbs. It is different from prickly heat (there is no surrounding erythema and no itching in eruptions seen in thermogenic anhidrosis, while this is so in prickly heat).
- Temperature is usually 99-100°F, but may go upto 102°F (39°C).
- A very important feature is that while sweating ceases on trunks and limbs, it continues on face and neck.

Type 3 (Pure water deficiency or depletion)

It occurs in acclimatized (or trained) individuals because of their increased ability to sweat. Water is inadequately replaced, as when water supply is inadequate. At times it is due to increased loss of water due to vomiting/diarrhea.

As salt is not lost proportionately (because of acclimatization), there is rise in serum sodium and chloride with rise in osmolarity.

- Most important symptom is thirst, which may become an obsession.
- Mild headache and giddiness, but far less than that seen in salt deficiency type.
- No muscle cramps.

- Moderate increase in temperature 100°F -104°F (38°C - 40°C).
- Sweating decreased. Urine output decreased.
- The process of "water depletion heat exhaustion" is far more rapid than "salt depletion heat exhaustion".
- Delirium, which may proceed to coma and death.

Treatment→Rehydration by mouth as vomiting is rare. Upto 6-8 Litres of fluid with normal salt intake in 24 hours. In unconscious individuals replace fluids IV.

Mixed Type
International classification of diseases does not mention this type. This is a mixed type where there is both water and salt depletion. This may be the most common type of heat exhaustion.

Heat Hyperpyrexia

Most authorities consider heat hyperpyrexia as synonymous to heatstroke, but international classification of diseases considers them differently. Heat hyperpyrexia is a milder version of heatstroke. There may be some sweating in this condition, while in heatstroke sweating ceases completely. Secondly the mind remains clear in heat hyperpyrexia while in heatstroke there is complete clouding of senses.

Heatstroke

Also known as **sunstroke** or **thermic fever**

- This is the *most* serious disorder caused by heat.
- There is a complete breakdown of thermoregulatory mechanism.
- Pathophysiology: Initially, the body attempts to lower the core temperature via renal and splanchnic vasoconstriction with concomitant peripheral vasodilatation, thereby shunting blood to the periphery. Eventually, the vasoconstriction needed to keep the blood in the periphery fails; cutaneous (i.e., peripheral) blood flow decreases, less heat is carried away from the core, and hyperthermia results. This hyperthermia causes cerebral edema and cerebrovascular congestion, which culminate in increased intracranial pressure (ICP). This increased ICP combined with a decreased mean arterial pressure (from the failure of renal and splanchnic vasoconstriction and decreased peripheral resistance) causes cerebral blood flow to decrease. This is manifested clinically as CNS dysfunction.
- Temperature rises to above 41°C (>106°F). Temperatures of 108°F are common and 113°F has been recorded. This extreme rise in temperature is instrumental in organ damage, especially the CNS. Neurological deficit is most characteristically seen in heatstroke.
- Two forms are mainly seen:
  - o Classical or nonexertional heatstroke—Seen among elderly, debilitated persons often in epidemic fashion during heat waves of hot season. Persons taking anticholinergics, antiparkonians or diuretics are most susceptible (causing either inhibition of sweating or increased water loss through urination).
  - o Exertional heatstroke→unacclimatized young persons who perform strenuous tasks in hot and humid climate (athletes, soldiers, laborers).
  - o The two forms are defined by the underlying etiology but are clinically indistinguishable.
- Factors aggravating heatstroke are (i) wrong clothing (ii) alcoholism (reason mentioned above) (iii) recent – if not

present–toxic pyrexia (iv) dysentery with resulting dehydration (v) humid atmosphere (vi) no breeze and (vii) absence of a full acclimatization for a foreigner.

- Symptoms
  - o Headache, giddiness, nausea, vomiting, general weakness, lack of energy.
  - o Cessation of all sweating.
  - o Tachycardia.
  - o Signs showing neurological deficit - Clouding of senses, speech difficulties, bizarre behavior, delirium, muscular twitching, generalized or Jacksonian convulsions, opisthotonus, hallucinations, decerebrate rigidity, cerebellar dysfunction, oculogyric crisis, fixed and dilated pupils, coma.
  - o Subarachnoid hemorrhages in some cases.
- Prognosis is bad, as mortality is very high.
- Diagnosis→Based on classical triad of (i) increased temperature (ii) dry skin (iii) neurological deficit.
- Differential diagnosis→(i) Falciparum malaria (ii) dhatura poisoning.
- Treatment
  - o Cool the body by sponging or immersing the patient in cool bath. The body should be cooled to just about 39°C (102°F) and not below this. When the temperature has been brought to this level, further cooling continues despite the cessation of active treatment. If it does not occur then active cooling should be recommenced, but it is a bad prognostic sign.
  - o Temperature should be recorded every 10-15 minutes so that excess cooling does not occur.
- If hyperpyrexia continues for more than 4 hours, prognosis is bad. Even if the condition is not fatal, the patient may have permanent neurological deficit.
- Postmortem features:
  - o Findings lack specificity.
  - o There may be presence of visceral hemorrhages. This may be due to (i) hepatic damage due to increased temperature and consequent prothrombin depletion (ii) thrombocytopenia and decrease in plasma fibrinogen seen in heatstroke (iii) increased capillary fragility coincidental to anoxia and circulatory collapse seen in heatstroke.
  - o CNS findings:
    - Brain and leptomeninges are congested.
    - Convolutions are flattened.
    - Scattered petechiae all over the brain, especially in the walls of third ventricle and floor of fourth ventricle.
    - Degeneration of neurons in brain – mostly in the Purkinje cell layer of cerebellum. Degeneration also seen in cortical neurons. Degeneration of neurons is least in globus pallidus.
    - The heat dissipation center (preoptic and supraoptic regions) and the heat conservation and heat-production centers (caudolateral portions of the hypothalamus) have been subjected to extensive investigation, but there is no general agreement on the changes seen.
  - o If patient survived for more than 24 hours, following changes may be seen:
    - Degeneration of megakaryocytes.
    - Lobular pneumonia.
    - Acute tubular necrosis.
    - Adrenal hemorrhages.
    - Frank adrenal cortical necrosis.
    - Centrilobular necrosis of the liver.

Differences between heatstroke and heat exhaustion may become clear from the figure 22.1:

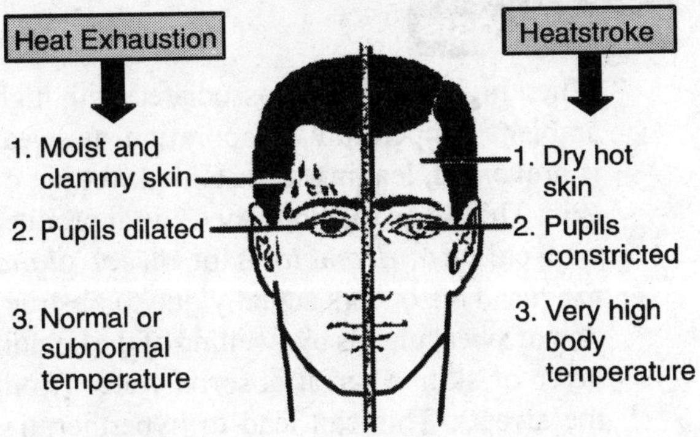

Fig. 22.1: Comparison between heat exhaustion and heatstroke

MEDICOLEGAL IMPORTANCE

Heat related disorders become medicolegally important when there is sudden death in factories or, say, in an overheated engine room with an extremely hot environment with poor facilities for ventilation. They also become important in situations where people are overcrowded in hot and humid, confined, ill ventilated spaces such as railway carriages, trucks and prison cells. Many deaths in prison cells occurring due to heatstroke may be ascribed wrongly by an overenthusiastic press to police excesses. On the contrary, police may claim that a prison death has occurred due to heatstroke, while it may actually be due to police beating. Forensic pathologist has to be very careful in conducting autopsy in all these cases.

OTHER HEAT DISORDERS

These are less significant medicolegally. These are:

1. Sunburn.
2. Prickly heat.
3. Heat oedema.
4. Hidromeiosis.

Sunburn

Caused by exposure to the sun. Erythema occurs in about 2-6 hours. Without further exposure, comes back to normal. Skin is oedematous. Edge of erythema, which is usually the edge of exposure, is raised. Capillaries and small arterioles become prominent and blisters may form.

Prickly Heat

Synonyms→**Miliaria rubra, lichen tropics, heat**

- Rash on anterior surface of elbows, posterior surface of knees, sternum, clavicle, waist, axillae. Palms and soles are not affected.
- Caused by prolonged wetting of the skin with sweat and without evaporation. Hence worse with humid climate.
- Probable pathogenesis→Sweat duct obstruction and the periductal oedema due to sodium chloride from the evaporated sweat continuing to lie on the skin→ inflammation of sweat glands occurs.
- Infants and obese are especially affected.
- Males suffer more frequently than females.
- Non absorbent drip dry man made fibers aggravate the condition.
- D/d→Anhidrotic heat exhaustion. In prickly heat, sweating is present while in anhidrotic heat exhaustion it completely ceases from trunk and limbs.

Heat Oedema

Synonyms→**Deck ankles, Colombo flop**

[Persons travelling in ship may roam on decks to pass time. They may develop heat oedema; hence known as *deck ankles*.]

- Swelling of the hands and feet.
- People often notice this first when their

shoes feel too tight or one their rings won't fit the finger that they used to wear it on.
- Unacclimatized people arriving in the tropics may notice mild pedal edema, which usually resolves in a few days.
- The exact cause is not known, but it is postulated to be due to the adaptive mechanisms (cutaneous vasodilatation, aldosterone and antidiuretic hormone hyperactivity) resulting in venous stasis and / or expansion of extra cellular fluid volume.
- Women more commonly affected than men.

Hidromeiosis

When high humidity is associated with high ambient temperature, evaporation of sweat is prevented, leading to sustained wetting of skin. This leads to diminished sweat production called *hidromeiosis* or *sweat gland fatigue*. This occurs actually due to obstruction of sweat glands by swelling of the keratin layer of skin when it absorbs water (from the sweat). This can lead to hyperthermia. Shifting the patient to dry environment reverses this process.

5 MEDICOLEGAL ASPECTS RELATING TO SEX AND MARRIAGE

23 Impotence and Sterility

DEFINITIONS

1. Which of the following females would ordinarily be called a sterile woman?
- **A.** A woman who is incapablé of having a normal sexual intercourse
- **B.** A woman who can not be sexually aroused
- **C.** A woman who can not conceive
- **D.** All of the above

2. Which of the following males would ordinarily be called a sterile male?
- **A.** A person who is unable to beget children
- **B.** A person who is unable to have normal sexual intercourse
- **C.** A person who has a premature ejaculation
- **D.** All of the above

3. Inability to perform or take part in sexual intercourse by a male is known as:
- **A.** Sterility
- **B.** Impotence
- **C.** Frigidity
- **D.** Fertility

4. A person who is *impotent quoad hoc* is:
- **A.** Medically impotent but legally potent
- **B.** Medically potent but legally impotent
- **C.** Impotent both medically and legally
- **D.** Impotent towards one particular woman only

5. *Fecundatio ab extra* refers to:
- **A.** Conception occurring in a woman, when she is already pregnant
- **B.** Conception occurring in a woman when the semen was deposited on her thighs or on the vulva
- **C.** Superfecundation
- **D.** Pregnancy advancing beyond the legal limit of 280 days

6. Artificial introduction of semen into the vagina, cervix or uterus to produce pregnancy is known as:
- **A.** Extramarital conception
- **B.** Premarital conception
- **C.** Illegal insemination
- **D.** Artificial insemination

7. When only the semen of husband is used for artificial insemination, the procedure is known as:
- **A.** AIH
- **B.** AID
- **C.** AIHD
- **D.** Fecundatio ab extra

8. When the semen of donor is mixed with that of the infertile husband, the procedure is known as:
- **A.** AIH
- **B.** AID
- **C.** AIHD
- **D.** None of the above

9. Sterilization done in order to prevent danger to the life of the woman due to a future pregnancy is known as:
   A. Compulsory sterilization
   B. Therapeutic sterilization
   C. Eugenic sterilization
   D. Contraceptive sterilization

MULTIPLE ANSWER TYPE (PGI, CHANDIGARH PATTERN)

10. Following methods are employed for artificial insemination:
   A. AIHD
   B. Insemination through laparoscopy
   C. AIT
   D. AIH
   E. AID

ANSWERS

DEFINITIONS

1. C.
2. A.
3. **B.** ***Related fact:*** Frigidity is a term reserved mainly for females. It means inability to respond warmly to sex arousal stimuli. This fact is often asked – though rather incorrectly – as follows→The feminine of impotence is (a) Rigidity (b) Frigidity (c) Sterility (d) Nymphomania. The intended answer is (b).
4. **D.** ***Related fact:*** "*Quoad hoc*" is a Latin phrase meaning "As to this" or "with respect to this". Thus "*impotent quoad hoc*" would literally mean "impotence with respect to". Because of psychological factors it is perfectly possible for a person to be impotent towards one particular woman, but not towards the rest.
5. **B.** ***Related fact:*** If a person is impotent, he may not be able to penetrate the vagina. Instead the semen may be deposited on the woman's thighs or on the vulva. Rarely spermatozoa in such cases can travel up the genital passage and give rise to pregnancy. This is known as "*Fecundatio ab extra*".

   It is important to note that impotence at the time of marriage is a ground for annullment of marriage if marriage has not been consummated (i.e. there has been no sexual intercourse after marriage) because of this. If a baby is born to a couple after marriage, and sometime after this, the wife files a suit for annullment of marriage on the ground that the marriage has not been consummated, it is possible for her to get the marriage annulled if she can prove that the pregnancy was as a result of "*fecundatio ab extra*". This can perhaps be proved if it could be shown that her hymen was intact.

   To be sure, the husband on his part, may try proving, she was a case of "false virgin", i.e. a proper intercourse did take place but the hymen remained intact because of its abnormally high elasticity. Much would depend on the doctor's testimony here.

   "*Fecundatio ab extra*" does not constitute consummation of a marriage.
6. **D.**
7. **A.**
8. **C.** AIHD stands for Artificial Insemination by Husband and Donor. It is sometimes also known as Artificial Insemination Mixed (AIM). This method offers no special advantage over AID, except that the husband may believe that he could be the father of the child. In fact AIHD has been criticized since semen from the infertile husband may contain antibodies which could interfere with normal sperm function. However studies have not confirmed this. In some foreign jurisdictions AIHD is outlawed. Indian law is silent on this.
9. **B.** ***Explanation of other terms:*** Compulsory sterilization is referred to when sterilization is done against the wishes of a person. Reports of compulsory sterilization trickled in during the Emergency period in India. It may also be done on mentally defective people, or as a punishment for sexual crimes. It is not legal in India. Sterilization performed to prevent the conception of children who are likely to be physically or mentally defective is known as eugenic sterilization. Contraceptive sterilization is used for family planning.

MULTIPLE ANSWER TYPE (PGI, CHANDIGARH PATTERN)

10. A,D,E. AIH stands for Artificial Insemination Husband or Homologous. AID stands for Artificial Insemination Donor. AIHD stands for Artificial Insemination Husband and Donor. This is also known as Artificial Insemination Mixed or AIM. All these are genuinely recognized methods of artificial insemination. AIT is a fictitious term. Insemination through laparoscopy is never done.

24 Virginity, Pregnancy and Delivery

VIRGINITY

1. **Which of the following facts about human hymen is correct?**
   A. The broadest part of the hymen lies anteriorly
   B. It is a fold of mucus membrane about 5 mm thick
   C. An average hymen consists of folds of membrane having annular or crescentic shape
   D. Both (B) and (C) above
2. **A *virgo intacta* is:**
   A. Another name for an intersex
   B. A woman who has never had any sexual intercourse
   C. A woman who does not have any hymen
   D. A woman who has a congenitally torn hymen
3. **An 18-year-old unmarried female has been brought to a doctor. On examination the hymen is found to be intact, labia majora are separated and flabby, the labia minora are cutaneous in appearance and separated, the fourchette is torn and the vagina is roomy and enlarged. Most probably the woman is:**
   A. A true virgin
   B. A false virgin
   C. Sterile
   D. In premenstrual stage
4. **All of the following could be seen in a false virgin *except*:**
   A. Flabby breasts
   B. Tight and narrow vagina
   C. Labia separated
   D. Thick and elastic hymen
5. **The most important finding/sign of defloration is:**
   A. Enlarged nipple
   B. Dilation of vaginal canal
   C. Enlarged breasts
   D. Ruptured hymen
6. **When a virgin has her first intercourse, the hymen is most often torn at:**
   A. 12 O' clock position
   B. 3 O' clock position
   C. 6 O' clock position
   D. 9 O' clock position
7. ***Carunculae myrtiformes* are:**
   A. A type of bacteria found in bacterial secretions
   B. Healed tags of hymeneal tissue remaining attached to the margin after the hymen is torn

C. Prominent tubercles found on the areola of the breast
D. Fresh tears of the hymen

8. In cases of sexual assault on a female child, the hymen often escapes injury because it is:
A. Deeply seated
B. Very tough
C. Absent in children, developing only at puberty
D. Very elastic

9. *Sola pith* is sometimes used by prostitutes to:
A. Dilate the vagina of very young girls
B. Repair their own torn hymen so they can pass off as virgins
C. Enlarge their breasts
D. Strengthen the vaginal muscles

10. All of the following are likely to cause rupture of hymen *except*:
A. Insertion of sanitary tampons
B. Ulceration from diphtheria
C. Riding, jumping and dancing
D. Masturbation

11. Hymen can be ruptured by:
A. *Sola pith*
B. Masturbation
C. Sanitary tampons
D. Any of the above

12. Which one of the following types of hymen can resemble a torn hymen?
A. Crescentic
B. Semilunar
C. Fimbriated
D. Cribriform

13. Of the following types of hymen mentioned, which one is never found?
A. Annular
B. Septate
C. Vertical
D. Cruciate

14. Which of the following is the most common type of hymen?
A. Semilunar
B. Annular
C. Cribriform
D. Septate

15. When the hymenal membrane is pierced by many small perforations it is known as .... hymen:
A. Semilunar
B. Septate
C. Annular
D. Cribriform

16. When the hymen has two openings with a broad vertical septum dividing them, it is known as:
A. Vertical
B. Semilunar
C. Septate
D. Annular

PREGNANCY

17. During pregnancy, abdomen gradually enlarges in size after the:
A. 8th week
B. 12th week
C. 16th week
D. 20th week

18. If a woman sentenced to death is found pregnant, which of the following courses of action HAS TO BE TAKEN by law?
A. The sentence of death has to be commuted to that of life imprisonment
B. The sentence of death has to be postponed
C. The woman will be given amnesty

D. The woman will be sent to a women's welfare board, where she will work till death

19. Weight of a virgin uterus is:

A. 30-40 g
B. 100-120 g
C. 200-250 g
D. 400-500 g

20. The earliest Aschheim-Zondek test is able to detect pregnancy is after .... days of conception:

A. 2-4 days
B. 6-10 days
C. 10-14 days
D. 28-30 days

21. Male frogs or male toads were once used in the diagnosis of pregnancy in the following test:

A. Hogben test
B. Friedman test
C. Galli-Mainini test
D. Aschheim-Zondek Test

LEGITIMACY AND PATERNITY

22. For a child to be termed *LEGITIMATE*, he must be born within .... days of the dissolution of the marriage of his mother:

A. 266 days
B. 270 days
C. 280 days
D. 296 days

23. Which of the following is a "suppositious child"?

A. A child fictitiously claimed by a woman to be hers
B. The second child born in a twin pregnancy
C. A child born out of wedlock
D. A child who was conceived by AIH

DELIVERY

24. On pressure, colostrum can be squeezed out of breasts for about .... after delivery:

A. 24 hours
B. Ten days
C. 3 weeks
D. 6 weeks

25. The intermittent contractions of the uterus, known as after-pains are usually present for .... after delivery:

A. 4-5 hours
B. 4-5 days
C. 3 weeks
D. 6 weeks

ANSWERS

VIRGINITY

1. **C.** ***Related fact:*** (i) The thickness of hymen is about 1 mm. (ii) The broadest part lies posteriorly (iii) Hymen may even be cartilagenous sometimes (iv) At 10 years of age, the tip of small finger can be passed through it; at puberty, one finger can be passed.

2. **B.**

3. **B.** ***Related facts:*** Traditionally it has been believed that if the hymen of a female is intact, she is a virgin, i.e. she has not experienced sexual intercourse. However this has proved to be false on a number of occasions. There are several cases on record where a female has had sexual intercourse and yet her hymen was intact. Hymen has been found intact in women coming for delivery, and even in prostitutes. The following definitions are important:

   True virgin: A woman who has never experienced sexual intercourse. Her hymen may or may not be intact.

   False virgin: A woman who has experienced sexual intercourse, but her hymen is intact.

   To differentiate between a true and a false virgin, accessory signs of virginity are to be seen to ascertain if the woman was a true or a false virgin. In the given question, all accessory signs are in favour of sexual intercourse having taken place, so the girl is a false virgin.

4. **B.**

5. **D.**

6. **C.** ***Related fact:*** 6 O' clock is same as posteriorly. Watch out for this, as the examiner may ask the question in this form.

7. **B.** ***Related info:*** Another name for Carunculae myrtiformes is Carunculae hymenales. Watch out for both names.

8. **A.**

9. **A.** ***Additional info:*** *Sola* is an Indian plant with stems containing woody pith. This pith - the "Sola Pith" - is sponge wood with great absorptive powers. (It is often carved into delicate flowers, toys and deities. Sola topee is sun helmet, made from *sola pith*).

   To initiate very young girls into the business of prostitution, their mentors have to dilate their vagina. This is done by inserting a piece of *sola pith* into their vagina (the piece is as large as the vagina can contain), and then asking the girl to sit in a tub of water. The absorbent sponge wood absorbs water and swells up, enlarging the vagina. The process is repeated with bigger pieces of *sola pith*, till the vagina is roomy enough for sexual intercourse.

   The hymen is torn in this process. So this is one of the causes of torn hymen too.

10. **C.** ***Related facts:*** Situation of the hymen is such that riding, jumping and dancing are not likely to cause rupture of hymen. Forcible separation of thighs will not usually cause rupture until and unless perineal tears are produced.

11. **D.** ***Related fact:*** *Sola* is an Indian plant with stems containing pith. It can absorb water like a sponge and swell. A piece of *sola* pith – as large as the vagina can accommodate –

is inserted into the vagina of the young girl, who is then made to sit in a tub of water. The pith absorbs water, swells, grows bigger, and dilates the vagina. The size of the pith is gradually increased for further dilatation. This tears the hymen. This practice is followed by prostitutes to initiate young girls into prostitution.

12. C. Various types of hymen can best be appreciated by having a look at them. Here are the diagrammatic representation of some common types of hymen (Fig. 24.1A,B).

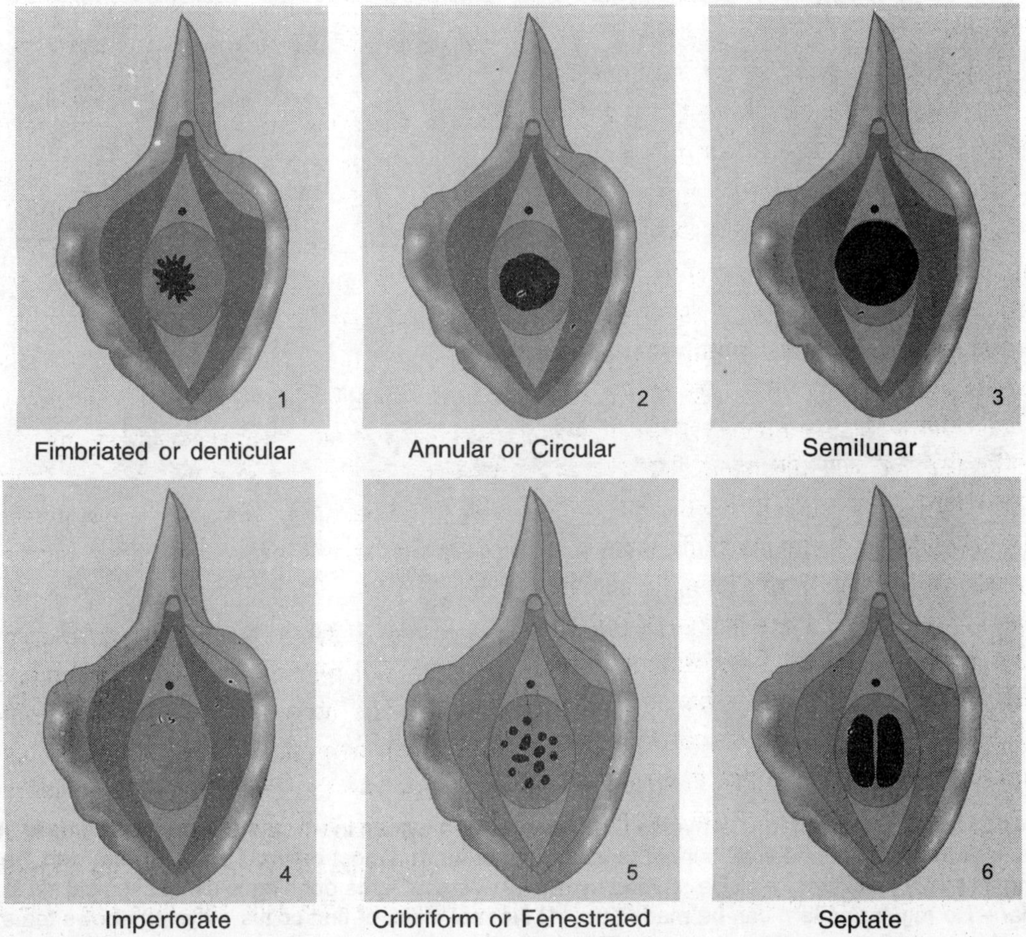

Fig. 24.1A: Some common types of hymen.(1) Fimbriated or denticular – the free edges of hymen show indentations, but the indentations do not reach the peripheral margin. Compare it with a torn hymen (11), where tears are reaching up to the periphery. This is the usual criteria to distinguish between these two types of hymen (2) Annular or Circular – the hymen has an almost circular central opening (3) Semilunar – The hymen looks like a crescent (4) Imperforate – The hymen has no opening at all. In such cases, at the onset of menstrual cycle, the doctor needs to make a surgical opening to let menstrual blood out. If this is not done, it may lead to collection of blood within the distensible vagina (hematocolpos) or uterus (hematometra) (5) Cribriform or Fenestrated - a hymen pierced by many small perforations. This type of hymen lets menstrual and other fluids out with no problem, but sexual activity and the insertion of tampons can be problematic (6) Septate - a hymen in which the opening is divided by a narrow septum. If the septum is somewhat broader, it has been called hymen bifenestratus or hymen biforis. ***(See also Colour Plate 3)***

Contd...

Contd...

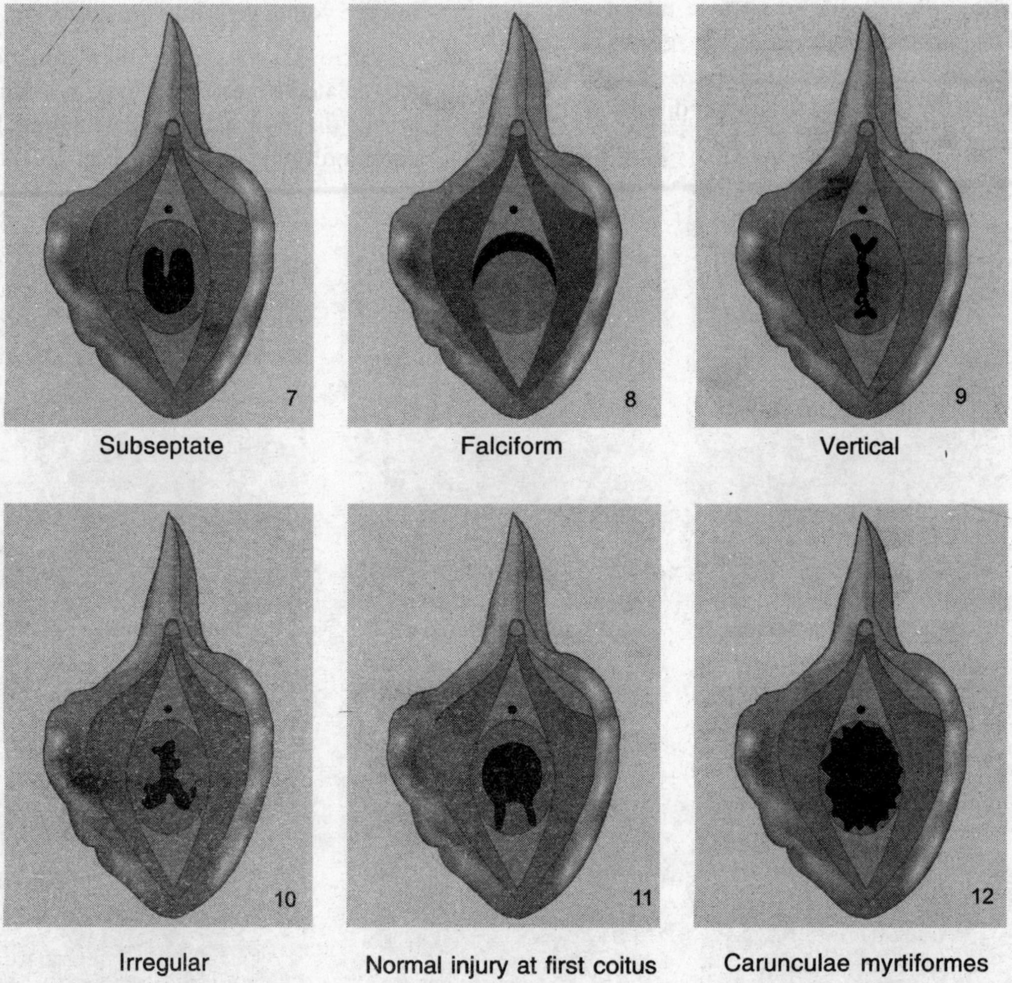

Fig. 24.1B: Some common types of hymen (7) Subseptate - a hymen in which the opening is partially filled by a septum growing out of one wall, but not reaching the other. It almost reminds one of throat with the uvula hanging down (8) Falciform - a sickle-shaped hymen (9) Vertical – the opening is almost vertical slit like (10) Irregular – No regular pattern can be made out (11) Normal injury at first coitus – hymen shows tears. Note that the tears reach the peripheral margin. This is an important feature to note. Please look at fimbriated hymen (1) and see that the indentations in that case do not reach up to the peripheral margin (12) Caruncular myrtiformes – In a woman having experienced multiple acts of intercourse, the hymen almost disappears giving rise to just small minuscule tags of tissue at the periphery. ***(See also Colour Plate 4)***

13. D.

14. B.

15. D.

16. C. ***Related fact:*** Other name for septate hymen is biforis hymen.

PREGNANCY

17. B.

18. B. Section 416 of *Criminal Procedure Code* states, "If a woman sentenced to death is found to be pregnant, the High Court shall order the execution of the sentence to be postponed, and may, it thinks fit, commute the sentence to imprisonment of life".

This section makes it mandatory for the High Court to stay the order of execution. Till what time the order of execution will be stayed is not clearly defined in this section. Many students wrongly believe that the period upto which the order of execution will be stayed is legally fixed as 6 months (or one or two years) after birth of the child. This is not so. Generally it would be upto the delivery of the baby and perhaps for some period after that.

The sentence may even be commuted to that of life imprisonment, but it is not mandatory. It depends on the judgment of the High Court.

19. A ***Related facts:*** Remember these additional facts, which may be asked as MCQ questions:

- Adult uterus measures 7.5 cm x 5 cm x 2.5 cm.
- It is divided into two parts – Body or corpus (5.0 cm) and cervix uteri (2.5 cm).
- In fetal life, cervix is considerably larger than the body.
- After parturition, the uterus nearly regains its usual size, weighing on an average the same as the virgin uterus, but its cavity is larger than in the nulliparous state.

Note: The size and weight of ovaries has rarely been asked in examination, yet it is useful to know the figures. The size of each adult ovary is 3 cm x 1.5 cm × 1 cm. Interestingly the same figures in inches would give you the size of the uterus! Alternatively remember that uterus is about 2.5 times bigger (in every dimension) than each ovary. The weight of each ovary in a non pregnant state is between 2 to 3.5 gm.

20. **D.** ***Related facts:*** Aschheim-Zondek test is one of the several biological tests of pregnancy that were in vogue before 1960s. They are no more used now, and do not find a place in modern text books of obstetrics or forensic medicine. Yet sometimes the student may face an odd question related to these tests. The facts to remember about these tests are:

- All biological tests for pregnancy become positive about 2 weeks after the first missed period, i.e. about 4 weeks after conception.
- There are four main biological tests namely (i) Aschheim-Zondek test (ii) Friedman test (iii) Hogben test (iv) Galli-Mainini test.
- All biological tests aim to detect Human Chorionic Gonadotropin (hCG) in the woman's urine.
- In all tests, woman's urine is injected in the animal. In some tests the animal has to be killed.
- The details of test (See Table 24.1).

21. **C.**

LEGITIMACY AND PATERNITY

22. **C.** ***Related fact:*** This is prescribed in Section 112 of *Indian Evidence Act*. The usual interpretation is that the marriage dissolved either by divorce or death of the husband. [*For discussion on all related IEA sections, please see, chapter 25 (sexual offences and sexual perversions), where s114A is discussed.*]

23. **A.** ***Related facts:*** A woman may produce a suppositious child in order to extort money from some rich male with whom she has had sexual relations and now claims that the

Table 24.1: Biological tests of pregnancy

S.No	Test	Scientists who discovered	First came into use in	Animal used	Area where urine injected	Animal killed or not	What is seen as a positive reaction	Time taken for completion of test	Comments
1	Aschheim-Zondek or A-Z test	German researchers Selmar Aschheim (1878-1965) and Bernhard Zondek (1891-1966)	1928	Immature female mice 3-4 weeks old (weighing between five and eight grams)	Subcutaneously twice daily for three days	Yes. Killed after 100 hours	Presence of corpora lutea and hemorrhages in enlarged ovaries	5 days	Very first scientific pregnancy test. Developed in Germany
2	Friedman test	Maurice H. Friedman (1903-1991)	1931	Virgin female rabbit	10 cc of morning urine once in the marginal ear vein	Yes. Killed 24-30 hours after injection	As above	2 days	Its advantages were the availability of the animals, a reduced error rate, and the reduced time required for completion of the test.
3	Hogben test	British biologist Lancelot Hogben (1895-1975)	1939	Female African clawed toad (*Xenopus laevis*)	1 cc of urine into the dorsal lymph sac	No	Toad ovulates and extrudes visible eggs within four to twelve hours.	12 hours	—
4	Galli-Mainini test	—	—	Male frogs (*Rana pipiens*) or male toads (*Bufo marinus*)	Few ccs of urine into the dorsal lymph sac	No	1-4 hours later Frog /toad releases spermatozoa through cloaca, which are observed under low power of microscope	2-5 hours	—

child was his. Sometimes she may indeed have become pregnant as a result of such relationship, but may have given birth to a dead child. In such cases, she may try to switch the dead child with a live child (stolen from somewhere). This is also a suppositious child. A widow may in certain situations (as in order to inherit family property) produce a suppositious child supposedly fathered by her own husband who is now deceased.

In all such cases, the medical officer can tell that the child is suppositious by the following:

- Comparing the age of the child with the period when she was pregnant. A gross dissimilarity would prove that the child is suppositious. This is helpful in cases, when the woman was indeed pregnant and gave birth to a baby, albeit dead.
- If the woman was never pregnant and simply feigned pregnancy, it would be useful to look for signs of pregnancy and recent delivery, such as (i) enlarged, tense and knotty breasts, lax abdomen, striae gravidarum and linea nigra etc.
- If facilities for DNA profiling are available, comparing the DNA profiles of mother with that of the child.

DELIVERY

24. B.

25. B.

25 Sexual Offences and Sex Perversions

GENERAL

1. **Under which section of the Indian law is rape defined?**
   A. 320 I.P.C.
   B. 375 I.P.C.
   C. 375 Cr.P.C.
   D. 376 I.P.C.
2. **A valid consent for sexual intercourse cannot be given by a girl below:**
   A. 15 years
   B. 16 years
   C. 18 years
   D. 21 years
3. **In India a boy below .... years cannot be charged with rape?**
   A. 7 years
   B. 12 years
   C. 14 years
   D. There is no such age limit
4. **According to Indian law, all of the following would be instances of rape *except:***
   A. The sexual intercourse is done via anal route without consent
   B. The sexual intercourse is done vaginally without consent
   C. Sexual intercourse is done with a 20-year-old prostitute without her consent and against her will
   D. Sexual intercourse is done with a 14-year-old girl with her consent
5. **If a man has married a girl below 15 years of age, which of the following statements is true?**
   A. He can have sexual intercourse with her but only with her consent
   B. He can have sexual intercourse with her even without her consent, as she is deemed to have given unconditional consent for sexual intercourse at the time of marriage
   C. He can have vaginal intercourse with her, but not anal intercourse, which is permissible only after 16 years of age
   D. It is illegal for him to have sexual intercourse with her
6. **Under which section of the Indian law is rape punishable?**
   A. 320 I.P.C.
   B. 375 I.P.C.
   C. 375 Cr.P.C.
   D. 376 I.P.C.

7. Under the Indian law, the punishment for rape is:

A. Capital punishment
B. Not less than 7 years, but which may extend to life
C. Maximum 7 years
D The judge may give any sentence without mentioning any justifications in the judgment

8. In which of the following circumstances, a man can legally rape his own wife?

A. When she has not consented for sexual intercourse
B. When the wife is menstruating
C. When the wife is below 15 years of age
D. Both (A) and (C) above

9. Statutory rape is:

A. Rape on a girl below 16 years
B. Rape of another person's wife
C. Intercourse with one's own wife without her consent
D. Intercourse through anus

10. Gang rape has been defined in Indian law as:

A. Rape committed on a woman by a member of a criminal gang
B. Rape committed by a member in order to induce the woman to join their gang
C. A rape by one or more in a group of persons acting in furtherance of their common intention
D. Rape followed by killing of the woman

11. A rape by a woman on a man is:

A. Possible in Indian law
B. Not possible in Indian law
C. Possible only in very special circumstances, which are not explicitly defined in Indian law
D. Possible only if the woman is a hirsute and the man a *zenana*

12. If a man has sexual intercourse with his own wife without her consent, who is living separately from him under a decree of separation or under any custom or usage, he shall be punished with:

A. Maximum imprisonment of 7 years but no fine
B. Maximum imprisonment of 7 years but with fine
C. Minimum imprisonment of 2 years but no fine
D. Maximum imprisonment of 2 years and fine

13. If the superintendent or manager of a jail, remand home or a women's or children's institution takes advantage of his official position and induces or seduces any female inmate of such jail, remand home or institution to have sexual intercourse with him, and such sexual intercourse *does not* amount to the offence of rape (i.e. committed with her valid consent), which of the following statements is true?

A. Such a person cannot be charged under any section of Indian Penal Code
B. Such a person would not be punishable under Indian Penal Code but under Police Act
C. He can be charged under section 376C of Indian Penal Code, for which the punishment is up to a maximum of five years and fine
D. He will still be charged under rape, as he has used his official position to obtain consent.

14. Which of the following is NOT rape?

A. Sexual intercourse with wife below 15 years of age with her consent
B. Sexual intercourse with wife above 20 years without her consent

C. Sexual intercourse with a girl below 16 years with her consent
D. Sexual intercourse with a woman above 20 years without her consent

15. The court shall presume the absence of consent in certain prosecutions for rape. This provision is provided in which of the following sections?
A. Section 375 I.P.C.
B. Section 376 I.P.C.
C. Section 114A Indian Evidence Act
D. Section 327(2) Cr.P.C.

16. Whoever discloses the identity of a victim of rape by printing or publishing shall be punished with imprisonment of either description for a term extending to two years and shall also be liable to fine. This punishment is provided in which of the following sections?
A. Section 228A of I.P.C.
B. Section 375 of I.P.C.
C. Section 376 of I.P.C.
D. Section 327(2) of Cr.P.C.

17. The enquiry into and trial of rape shall be conducted *in camera*. This provision is provided by which of the following sections?
A. Section 375 I.P.C.
B. Section 376 I.P.C.
C. Section 113 of Indian Evidence Act
D. Section 327(2) of the Cr.P.C.

18. Which of the following can be called incest?
A. Anal intercourse
B. Intercourse with one's daughter
C. Oral intercourse
D. Intercourse with an animal

19. Under which section of the Indian law is incest punishable?
A. 498 I.P.C.
B. 375 I.P.C.
C. 377 I.P.C.
D. It is not punishable

UNNATURAL OFFENCES

20. Bestiality is:
A. Having intercourse with an animal
B. Cruelty to animals
C. Cruelty to fellow humans
D. Beast like behavior of an insane

21. Under which section of the Indian law is homosexuality punishable?
A. 375 I.P.C.
B. 376 I.P.C.
C. 377 I.P.C.
D. 375 Cr.P.C.

22. Under Indian law, the maximum punishment for homosexuality is:
A. 3 years
B. 5 years
C. 7 years
D. 10 years

23. Sin of Gommorrah is another name for:
A. Anal intercourse
B. Lesbianism
C. Buccal coitus
D. Tribadism

24. Pedophilia is having anal intercourse with:
A. Older women
B. Children
C. Homosexual adult
D. Hijra

25. *Zenanas* are:
A. Male prostitutes whose genitalia are intact, but they wear female clothings to give an impression that they are females
B. Male prostitutes who have been castrated and in whom artificial vaginas have been constructed
C. Another name for female prostitutes
D. Female pseudohermaphrodite

MULTIPLE ANSWER TYPE (PGI, CHANDIGARH PATTERN)

26. **Sexual perversions as understood by Indian law include:**
    A. Zoophilia
    B. Fetishism
    C. Incest
    D. Homosexuality
    E. Urophilia
27. **In which of the following cases of rape, the culprit would be punished with a minimum sentence of ten years rigorous imprisonment?**
    A. A police officer committing rape on a woman in his custody
    B. A person who commits rape on a woman knowing her to be pregnant
    C. Rape on a girl below 12 years of age
    D. Gang rape
    E. Anal intercourse with a woman
28. **Sexual intercourse by a man with a woman is rape if:**
    A. Sexual intercourse is done with her consent but against her will
    B. Sexual intercourse is done with her will but without her consent
    C. Sexual intercourse is done with one's own wife above 21 years of age during her menstruation and without her consent
    D. Sexual intercourse is done without the consent of one's own wife above 21 years of age, when she is visiting her parents
    E. Sexual intercourse is done both against her will and without her consent

ANSWERS

GENERAL

1. **B.**
2. **B.**
3. **A.** According to Section 82 of I.P.C., a child below 7 years can not be charged for any offence whatsoever.
4. **A.** If the intercourse is done via anal route, the offence is classified NOT as rape, but as unnatural sexual intercourse, which is punished under section 377 of IPC.

   Additional info: According to Indian law, if one has legally married a woman above 15 years, he can have intercourse with her even against her will and without her consent, as his wife is deemed to have given an unconditional consent for intercourse at the time of marriage.
5. **D.** Sexual intercourse with or without consent of wife below 15 years is illegal and it would be termed as rape. However the sentence given to the husband for raping his own wife (between 12 and 15 years of age) is much less – a maximum of two years of imprisonment (simple or rigorous) and/or fine.
6. **D.**
7. **B.** Punishment for rape is defined u/s 376 (1). The punishment is for a minimum of 7 years (simple or rigorous). However if the court wants to give a lesser sentence for some adequate and special reasons, these reasons have to be mentioned in the judgment.
8. **C.** ***Related facts:*** In Indian law, a denial of consent by wife is not a ground for constituting the offence of rape, as she is deemed to have given unconditional consent for sexual intercourse at the time of marriage.

   The correct answer here is (c). This choice is often confusing to students, because the legal age of marriage for girls in India is 18 [section 5 (iii) *Hindu Marriage Act 1955*]. But the fact is that younger girls are getting married in our society. According to section 18 (a) of the *Hindu Marriage Act 1955* (Note that the section is 18 which may act as a good mnemonic), if a boy below 21 years, or a girl below 18 years do marry, the punishment is simple imprisonment of a maximum of 15 days or fine upto 1000 Rupees or both. The marriage is NOT dissolved, because it is considered a very sacred institution in India.
9. **A.** ***Related facts:*** Section 375 of I.P.C. lays down that sexual intercourse with a girl under 16 years shall be regarded as rape, whether or not the intercourse was done with her consent. This is known as "statutory rape".

   Explanation: In English law—from which Indian law mostly derives—two varieties of law are recognized: **common law** and **statutory law**. Common law is the unwritten law and it is based mostly on usage and custom. Statutory law on the other hand is duly passed by legislature and is properly written and codified. Any act proclaimed as an offence by statutory law is known as **statutory offense** or **statutory crime.** Since it is written in our law that sexual intercourse with a girl under 16 years of age – with or without her consent - is to be regarded as rape, it is known as **statutory rape**.
10. **C.** ***Related facts:*** An example would make the concept clear. If there is a group of five people, four of whom merely restrain the limbs of the woman (say one limb restrained by each person) and actual rape is committed

by just the fifth person, each person will be deemed to have committed gang rape. Interestingly according to this definition, even a woman can legally rape a woman, if she happens to be one of the group!

11. B.

12. D. This maximum imprisonment of 2 years can either be simple or rigorous in nature. This is prescribed under section 376A of Indian Penal Code.

13. C.

14. B. ***Related fact:*** It might appear that sexual intercourse with a non-consenting wife is rape. But this is not true. Sexual intercourse with wife below 15 years—even with her consent—is rape.

15. C. ***Related fact:*** Section 114 of IEA deals with the presumption by the Court of certain facts. An example is that if a man is in possession of stolen goods soon after the theft, and can not account for his possession, he may be presumed by the court to be either the thief, or has received the goods knowing them to be stolen.

In 1983, by the Criminal Law (Amendment) Act, 1983, Section 114 A was added to this section, because it deals with the presumption by the court regarding the consent. In essence, the section says that if the sexual intercourse by the accused is proved and the question is whether it was without the consent of the woman alleged to have been raped and **she states in her evidence before the court that she did not consent**, the **Court shall presume that she did not consent.**

Additional Notes: Chapter VII of Indian Evidence Act (s.101-114) deals with "burden of proof", and several sections are of interest to us as medical professionals.

- S.105→A man wants to take defence u/s 84 IPC. The burden of proving that he was insane at the time of committing that offence is on him. If he enjoys lucid interval, the presumption will be that he committed the offence during the lucid interval.
- S.107→***Presumption of life***: Court will presume a person to be alive if he is shown to be alive within last 30 years. The burden on proving that he is dead lies on the person who asserts this.
- S.108→***Presumption of death***: Court will presume a person dead, if he is not heard of within last 7 years, by the persons who should normally have heard from him. The burden of proving that he is alive is on the person who asserts this.
- S.112→***Period of Legitimacy***: A child is legitimate, if he is born within **280 days** after the dissolution of marriage.
- S.113A→***Presumption as to abetment of suicide by a married woman***: Woman within 7 years of marriage subjected to cruelty. It is shown she was subjected to cruelty (meaning of cruelty explained in s498A of IPC) by husband→Court will presume abetment of suicide by the husband.
- S.113B→***Presumption as to dowry death***: Question is of dowry death of a woman. It is shown that a person subjected her to cruelty in connection with dowry. The presumption is that, that person caused dowry death.

Note: Difference between 113A and 113B is that in the former there is NO mention of dowry, while in the latter there is a mention of dowry.

- S.114A→***Presumption of absence of consent***: Prosecution for rape. Female asserts she did not consent. The court will presume she indeed did not consent.

16. A. ***Related fact:*** Section 228 of IPC deals with intentional insult to public servant sitting in judicial proceeding. In 1983, by the Criminal Law (Amendment) Act, 1983, section 228A was added. According to this section, neither the name of the accused, nor the name of the victim can be published or printed (say, in a newspaper). However there are a few riders to this. The following things are **not** covered by this section.

   i. When the investigating officer is publishing such information for investigation purposes.
   ii. When the victim gives authorization in writing.
   iii. When the victim is dead, or minor, or of unsound mind, then next of kin can give consent. Such consent by the next of kin can only be given to any recognized welfare institution or organisation. This rider is not applicable if the victim herself is giving authorization.
   iv. Printing or publication of the judgment of any High Court or the Supreme Court does not attract the provisions of this section.

17. D. ***Related fact:*** Section 327 of the Cr.P.C. prescribes that Criminal courts will be open for general public (so far as the same can conveniently contain them). This was causing embarrassment to the victims of rape, who were not coming forward with their allegations.

   So in 1983, by the Criminal Law (Amendment) Act, 1983, this section was added to Section 327, and original section was renumbered as 327(1). The section says that notwithstanding anything contained in section 327(1), the trial for rape shall be conducted *in camera.*

18. B.

19. D. Strangely incest is not punishable in Indian law. We can only guess the reasons why this is so. When the English formulated the Indian Penal Code in 1860, they must have observed that marriages between cousins (and other close relatives) was common in many tribes and cultures. Eager to maintain social norms, they did not make it a criminal offence, although in their own law, incest is punishable. Interestingly Indian Government too – after coming to power in 1947 – has preferred not to disturb this law.

   Variant: This question is asked in several variants. One variant is like this→Which of the following is not an offence in India? (i) Bestiality (ii) Sodomy (iii) Incest (iv) Paedophilia. The correct answer is (iii) Incest.

   Interesting fact: Incest is not a crime in India, but a crime in Britain. Homosexuality even between two consenting adults is a crime in India (under section 377 of IPC) but not in Britain!

UNNATURAL OFFENCES

20. A.

21. C.

22. D. ***Related fact:*** The imprisonment can be of any description. No minimum punishment has been prescribed, as in Sect 376. In addition, he is also liable to fine.

23. C. ***Related fact:*** According to the Bible, buccal coitus was prevalent in a town called Gomorrah. Hence the name.

   Note all the other major sexual perversions, which can be asked as MCQs. These are also known as paraphilias:

   - **Algolagnia**→Same as sadism. See below.
   - **Anilingus**→Oral stimulation of the anus
   - **Bestiality**→Sex with animals.
   - **Buccal coitus**→Intercourse through mouth. Sin of Gomorrah.
   - **Buggery**→Same as sodomy.
   - **Coitus per os**→Same as buccal coitus.

- **Coprolalia**→Sexual stimulation by making obscene telephone calls, or by conversing with a member of the opposite sex in an obscene language.
- **Coprophilia**→Sexual arousal by faeces.
- **Cunnilingus**→Oral stimulation of the female genitalia.
- **Dippoldism**→Sexual gratification from beating children. Supposedly named after Dippold, a German schoolmaster.
- **Ecouteurism**→Sexual gratification by listening to stories of sexual encounters of others or to sounds of others produced during intercourse, either live or recorded.
- **Electra complex**→These are intended sex between father and daughter.
- **Eonism**→These are same as transvestism. The term is derived from the name of a Frenchman **Chevalier d'Eon de Beaumont** (1728-1810), who suffered from this.
- **Exhibitionism**→These are obtaining sexual arousal by exposing genitals to an unsuspecting stranger.
- **Fellatio**→Oral manipulation or stimulation of the penis.
- **Fetishism**→Obtaining sexual arousal using or thinking about an inanimate object or part of the body. The inanimate object is generally a piece of cloth such as a handkerchief or undergarments of the opposite sex.
- **Frotteurism**→Obtaining sexual arousal and gratification by rubbing one's genitals against others in public places.
- **Gerontophilia**→Sex with old people.
- **Klismaphilia**→Sexual arousal by giving or receiving of enemas.
- **Lesbianism**→Sex between two women. The term comes from the name of an island, the Isle of Lesbos, mentioned in Greek mythology, where women used to practice homosexuality. Also known as tribadism.
- **Masochism**→Reverse of sadism. Sexual arousal through getting pain inflicted on oneself through another person, usually a partner of the opposite sex. Named after an Austrian novelist **Leopold Sacher Masoch** (1836-1895), who suffered from this perversion. Also known as passive algolagnia.
- **Masochism**→Sexual arousal by having pain and/or humiliation inflicted upon oneself.
- ***Ménage a trois***→Same as Troilism.
- **Mixoscopia**→Observing the sex performance of other couples.
- **Mixoscopic bestialis**→Sexual delight in watching an intercourse between a person and an animal.
- **Mixoscopic zoophilia**→Sexual delight in watching animals copulate.
- **Mysophilia**→Sexual arousal by filth such as by sweaty underwears or used menstrual pads.
- **Narrotophilia**→Sexual stimulation from reading erotic materials.
- **Necrophagia**→Sexual gratification through eating the flesh of dead people (psychiatric disorder).
- **Necrophilia**→Intercourse with dead people.
- **Nymphomania**→Excessive sexual desire in females (cf. Satyriasis).
- **Oedipus complex**→Intended sex between mother and son.
- **Olfactory eroticism**→Getting sexual stimulation by the odour of vaginal secretions.
- **Paederasty**→Same as Pedophilia.
- **Passive algolagnia**→Same as masochism.
- **Passive scopophilia**→The desire to be looked at by others. A form of exhibitionism.
- **Pedophilia**→Sex or sexual activity with children who have not reached puberty. Also known as Paederasty.

- **Peeping Tom**→Observing nude individuals without their knowledge. Also known as voyeurism.
- **Playing the bagpipes**→Having intercourse under the armpits.
- **Pyromania**→Getting sexual stimulation by seeing flames and destruction of a building. It is a psychosexual disorder.
- **Sadism**→Sexual arousal through inflicting pain on another person. From the name of a French person **Marquis de Sade** (1740-1814), who wrote books in which the characters suffered from this condition. Also known as Algolagnia.
- **Satyriasis**→Excessive sexual desire in male (cf. Nymphomania).
- **Scopophilia**→Getting pleasure by seeing a nude woman in her privacy. Also known as scoptophilia. Another name for this is voyeurism.
- **Scoptophilia**→Same as scopophilia. Don't confuse with Scotophilia, which is love of darkness (from Gk *skotos*, dark).
- **Sin of Gomorrah**→Buccal coitus.
- **Sodomy**→Anal intercourse between two men or a man and a woman. Also known as buggery.
- **Somnophilia**→Getting sexual arousal by fondling a stranger who is asleep.
- **Transvestism**→Sexual arousal from dressing in the clothes of the opposite sex. Also known as eonism.
- **Tribadism**→Same as lesbianism.
- **Troilism**→Intercourse between three people, either two females and a male or two males and a female. Another variation is when a person shares his wife/girl friend with another, and observes the act from a hidden place. Also known by various other names such as Triolism and *Ménage a trois*.
- **Undinism**→Same as Urolagnia.
- **Uranism**→Not to be confused with Urolagnia. Uranism is a general term given to the perversion of sexual instincts. Sexual gratification by fingering, fondling, licking also goes under the name Uranism.
- **Urolagnia**→Sexual excitation at the sight of urine, or people urinating. Also known as undinism and urophilia.
- **Urophilia**→Sexual arousal by urine.
- **Voyeurism**→Same as Peeping Tom; sexual arousal by observing nude individuals without their knowledge.
- **Zoophilia**→Sex with animals.

24. B.

25. A. ***Additional facts:*** *Zenanas* make their living through prostitution. Intercourse is offered via mouth or some other route. The student must also remember another term – *Hijrahs*, since this can also form a good MCQ. *Hijrahs* are males who have been castrated before puberty. When the wound heals, the scar invaginates, the local area resembling superficially that of the female. Due to the resulting hormonal imbalance they also develop feminine characters such as high pitched voice, female distribution of hair etc. They also act as prostitutes. Both *Hijrahs* and *Zenanas* are genetically males; *zenanas* have their genitals intact while *hijrahs* have them removed.

> *Hijras* include men, who castrate themselves *willingly*. Why they do it is debatable, but some of them sacrifice their genitalia to a goddess in return for the power to confer fertility on newlyweds and newborn children. While they are respected for this ritual role, they at the same time, are stigmatized for their ambiguous sexuality.

MULTIPLE ANSWER TYPE (PGI, CHANDIGARH PATTERN)

26. A,B,D,E.

27. A,B,C,D. Section 376(2) of IPC prescribes punishment for some special cases. Note that here the minimum sentence is ten years *and it is rigorous. Simple imprisonment can not be given under this section.* Under section 376 (1), which prescribes punishment for general cases of rape, the nature of imprisonment could be simple or rigorous and is also lesser in quantum (minimum 7 years).

All the tour cases mentioned under choices A, B, C and D come under this section. There are additional three situations (a total of seven special situations) inviting same punishment, which are as follows:

i. A public servant taking advantage of his official position commits rape on a woman in his custody (e.g. asking his secretary to stay late in office for dictation and then raping her when she is alone).

ii. A person being on the management or on the staff of a jail, remand home, or a women's or children's institution takes advantage of his official position and commits rape on any inmate.

iii. A person being on the management or on the staff of a hospital takes advantage of his official position and commits rape on a woman in that hospital.

28. A,B,E. The exact statement of section 375 of IPC is as follows:

375. Rape—A man is said to commit "rape" who, except in the case hereinafter excepted, has sexual intercourse with a woman under circumstances falling under any of the six following descriptions:

First—Against her will.

Secondly—Without her consent.

Thirdly—With her consent, when her consent has been obtained by putting her or any person in whom she is interested in fear of death or of hurt.

Fourthly—With her consent, when the man knows that he is not her husband, and that her consent is given because she believes that he is another man to whom she is or believes herself to be lawfully married.

Fifthly—With her consent, when, at the time of giving such consent, by reason of unsoundness of mind or intoxication or the administration by him personally or through another of any stupefying or unwholesome substance, she is unable to understand the nature and consequences of that to which she gives consent.

Sixthly—With or without her consent, when she is under sixteen years of age.

Explanation—Penetration is sufficient to constitute the sexual intercourse necessary to the offence of rape.

Exception—Sexual intercourse by a man with his own wife, the wife not being under fifteen years of age, is not rape.

STATE AMENDMENT

Union Territory of Manipur:

a. In clause sixthly, for the word "sixteen" substitute the word "fourteen"; and

b. in the Exception, for- the word "fifteen" substitute the word "thirteen".

It is important to appreciate that legislature has separated "will" and "consent" in two separate clauses. This means that it is possible for a woman to be "willing but not consenting" and "consenting but not willing". The difference between the two may not be very apparent to a student.

"Will" is more a psychological thing, while "consent" is more a legal concept. A girl below 16 years may psychologically want to have a sexual intercourse (i.e. she may be willing), but legally she can not be said to have consented. This is a case where the will is there, but consent is not there.

The opposite case (i.e. where the woman has legally consented but not willing) is more difficult to conceptualize. Here is an example:

A head of a company asks his subordinate to send his wife to him for intercourse if he wants a promotion. The subordinate coaxes his wife to go and have sexual intercourse with his boss, so he may get a promotion. The wife does not agree to this. At this stage, she is neither willing nor consenting: Later due to coaxing of her husband, she agrees to spend a night with his boss. When she reaches the boss' home she also repudiates him for resorting to such activities, but nevertheless spends a night with him, because her husband has coaxed her to do so. This is a case, where the legal consent is there, but there is no will. Such a case would also amount to rape.

26 Abortion

DEFINITIONS

1. **Which of the following statements concerning abortion is NOT correct?**
   A. Legally speaking abortion is the expulsion of the products of conception at any period of gestation before full term
   B. The distinction between abortion, miscarriage and premature labor are NOT recognized in Indian Law
   C. Abortion can be either natural or artificial
   D. Natural abortion occurs in about 0.5% of all pregnancies
2. **Which of the following is the CORRECT definition of abortion legally?**
   A. Termination of pregnancy before 28 weeks of pregnancy
   B. Termination of pregnancy AFTER the woman has become 'quick' with the child
   C. Termination of pregnancy any time before full term
   D. Termination of pregnancy after 24 weeks of pregnancy
3. **Which of the following is the CORRECT definition of abortion medically?**
   A. Premature expulsion of fetus/products of conception at ANY time before full term
   B. Premature expulsion of fetus/products of conception before 12 weeks
   C. Premature expulsion of fetus/products of conception between 12 and 20 weeks
   D. Premature expulsion of fetus/products of conception before 28 weeks
4. **MTP Act was passed in:**
   A. 1951
   B. 1970
   C. 1971
   D. 1973
5. **What is the age at which a woman can give a valid consent for MTP under the MTP Act 1971?**
   A. 12 years
   B. 16 years
   C. 18 years
   D. No age has been defined
6. **Injection of fluid into the uterus causes abortion due to:**
   A. Reflex stimulation of the uterine nerves causing it to expel contents
   B. Detachment of parts of the amniotic sac and placenta from the uterine walls
   C. Uterine atony
   D. Escape of liquor amnii from the uterus
7. **An ecbolic:**
   A. Increases uterine contractions
   B. Increases the flow of menstrual blood
   C. Causes uterine atony
   D. Increases the flow of urine

8. An emmenagogue:
A. Decreases uterine contractions
B. Decreases the flow of menstrual blood
C. Increases the flow of menstrual blood
D. Causes uterine atony

9. Diachylon, once commonly used to procure criminal abortion mainly contained:
A. Juice of *Semecarpus anacardium*
B. Lead oleate
C. Oil of pennyroyal
D. Mercuric nitrate

10. "Utus paste" was once commonly used to procure criminal abortion. Which was its main component responsible for causing abortions?
A. Iodine or some salt of iodine such as potassium iodide
B. Oil of pennyroyal
C. Borax
D. Some salt of lead

11. "Interruptin", once widely used for procuring criminal abortion contained
A. Mercuric nitrate
B. Borax
C. A mixture of Colocynth and Aloes
D. Elemental iodine

12. A 24 weeks pregnant woman goes to a quack and requests him to conduct an abortion. The quack takes a written consent. He then tries some unscientific procedure on her following which the woman dies. The quack can be successfully prosecuted under which of the following sections?
A. S 302 IPC
B. S 312 IPC
C. S 313 IPC
D. S 314 IPC

MULTIPLE ANSWER TYPE (PGI, CHANDIGARH PATTERN)

13. Under the MTP Act 1971, a doctor having which of the following training/experiences is qualified to conduct an MTP up to 20 weeks of pregnancy?
A. One who has holds a post-graduate degree or diploma in gynaecology and obstetrics
B. One who has assisted a registered medical practitioner in the performance of 25 cases of termination of pregnancy
C. One who has completed 6 months of house surgency in gynaecology and obstetrics
D. One who has had an experience at any hospital for a period of not less than one year in the practice of obstetrics and gynaecology
E. One who holds an MS in surgery and then has assisted a registered medical practitioner in the performance of 25 cases of MTP

14. Which of the following facts about the "abortion stick" are correct?
A. It is a thin wood or bamboo stick around 12-18 cm long (about half a foot) long
B. It is beaten on the abdomen to procure abortion
C. It is the twig of an irritant plant, which is cut in pieces and given to the pregnant woman to eat to cause an abortion
D. One end of this stick is wrapped with a rag soaked with juices of marking nut, calotropis, jequirity, asafoetida or paste made up of irritant salts such as arenious oxide and red lead
E. One end of this stick is introduced into the vagina up to the level of os and retained there till contractions begin

ANSWERS

DEFINITIONS

1. **D.** ***Related fact:*** The rate is about 10 to 15%.
2. **C.** ***Related fact:*** The definition of abortion in a LEGAL SETTING is required ONLY when there is a charge on someone that he has done criminal abortion on a woman. The word "abortion" as such is NOWHERE defined in Indian law, neither in IPC, nor in MTP. The word that comes closest to abortion in Indian law is "miscarry", and it is defined in section 312 I.P.C. This is taken as equivalent of abortion. According to Section 312 I.P.C. if abortion is done in an "illegal manner" *any time* before full term, the abortionist would be held liable.

   This question can be changed slightly and asked like this→Legally "abortion" is termination of pregnancy (a) before 6 weeks (b) before 16 weeks (c) before 26 weeks (d) before full term. The answer is (d).
3. **D.** ***Related fact:*** If the fetus was expelled AFTER 28 weeks of pregnancy, it would be called stillbirth, if it was alive just before delivery but did not show any signs of life after being born.
4. **C.** Although MTP Act was passed in 1971, it came into force from April 1, 1972.
5. **C.** ***Related fact:*** Three ages that are very important from a medicolegal angle, and which are quite often confused together are 12 years, 16 years and 18 years. Please remember the following facts:

   12 years: Age of consent for general physical examination.

   16 years: Age of consent for a girl for sexual intercourse.

   18 years: Age of consent for MTP.

   This leaves a few legal dilemmas though:

   i. A 17-year-old girl (in fact any girl between 16-18 years) can give a valid consent for sexual intercourse, but if she becomes pregnant as a result, she can not give a valid consent for MTP.

   ii. A 14-year-old girl (in fact any girl between 12-16 years) can have voluntary sexual intercourse with her boy friend. If the girl's parents want to sue the boy by asserting that it was a case of statutory rape, the girl can always refuse physical examination.
6. **B.**
7. **A.**
8. **C.**
9. **B.** Diachylon is in fact plaster originally composed of the juices of several plants, but now made of lead salts and oil. It essentially consists of glycerin mixed with lead salts of the fatty acids (e.g. lead oleate). This plaster was often scraped to recover the metallic lead and ingested. Though abortion did occur sometimes, illness and death with acute and subacute poisoning was commoner.
10. **A.** "Utus paste" is a mixture of soap, myrrh resinoid and potassium iodide, where the iodide acted as an irritant causing abortion. It was once used for legitimate abortions as well, but soon became popular with criminal abortionists. It was particularly useful in late abortions. This paste is injected into the cervix from a collapsible tube (much like a modern toothpaste tube) with a uterine applicator. It was a hazardous method of procuring abortion, death occurring chiefly due to

necrosis, infarction of the uterine wall, poisoning, air or fat embolism (note the paste contained soap also).

11. **D.** Like "Utus paste", interruptin was also a paste used exactly in a similar manner. It contained elemental iodine which acted as an irritant. The risks were the same as with "Utus paste".

12. **D.** Section 314 I.P.C. deals with death of mother caused by an act done with intent of miscarriage with or without the consent of the woman. The student should remember following sections related to abortion:

S 312→Causing miscarriage *with* woman's consent: Woman herself can be charged under this section if she tries miscarriage on herself. If she was not quick with the child, punishment is 3 years and fine; if quick the punishment is 7 years and fine.

S 313→Causing miscarriage *without* woman's consent: The punishment is life imprisonment with fine whether or not the woman was quick with the child or not.

S 314→Death caused by act done with intent to cause miscarriage: Remember that in both s 312 and s 313, death of mother is *not* caused. If however the death is caused the person will be charged under this section. Punishment is 10 years and fine, if the woman had given consent for miscarriage, and life imprisonment and fine, if the woman had not consented.

S 315→Act done with intent to prevent child being born alive or to cause it to die after birth: The person carrying out miscarriage is liable to be prosecuted under this section if the pregnancy was greater than 28 weeks. By this time the child becomes viable and by trying this procedure, he is preventing the child to be born alive.

S 316→Causing death of quick unborn child by act amounting to culpable homicide: This is rather complex. The best example is this→A person attacks a pregnant mother with knife. The mother is quick with the child. The person had no intention to cause miscarriage. His intention was to kill mother. He stabs the mother. The knife enters the uterus and kills the child. The mother is subsequently saved. The attacker can not take defense that he had no intention to cause miscarriage. He would be charged under this section (Fig. 26.1).

The students may fruitfully go through the Table 26.1 for a bird's eye view of various IPC Sections related to criminal abortion.

MULTIPLE ANSWER TYPE (PGI, CHANDIGARH PATTERN)

13. **A,C,D.** Choice (B) is not correct for two reasons. Section 4 of *The Medical Termination of Pregnancy Rules, 2003* gives qualifications of a doctor qualified to do MTP under the MTP Act 1971. Qualifications

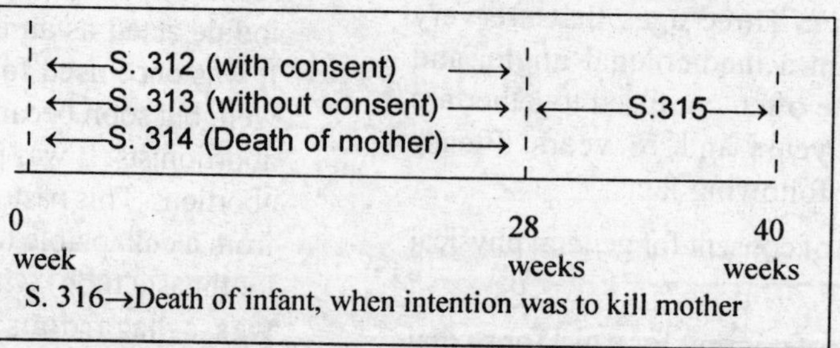

Fig. 26.1: Sections of IPC related to criminal abortion

Table 26.1: Table illustrating various IPC sections related to criminal abortion. Remember that as we go from left to right of the table or from top to bottom, the offence become graver and more serious

		Consent Yes	Consent No
Death No	Not quick	S312→3 years or fine or both *plus* fine	S313→imprisonment for life or for 10 years
	Quick	S312→7 years *plus* fine	
Death Yes	Quick or not quick	S314→ 10 years *plus* fine	S314→imprisonment for life or for 10 years *plus* fine

mentioned under choices (A), (C), and (D) are given here. Regarding assisting a registered medical practitioner in conducting 25 MTPs, the rule says that a doctor is qualified if he has assisted a registered medical practitioner in the performance of 25 cases of medical termination of pregnancy *of which at least five have been performed independently in a hospital established or maintained, or a training institute approved for this purpose by the Government.* Even if a doctor fulfils this qualification, he can do MTPs only upto 12 weeks, and NOT upto 20 weeks. Doctors holding qualifications only under choices (A), (C) and (D) can perform MTPs upto 20 weeks.

14. A,D,E.

27 Infanticide Including Battered Baby Syndrome

1. **Which of the following facts regarding infanticide is NOT correct?**
   A. Infanticide has not been defined in the Indian Penal Code
   B. Infanticide is punishable under section 302 I.P.C.
   C. In a case of infanticide the mother is NOT punishable in India
   D. In a case of infanticide a post mortem examination is a must

2. **Which of the following facts about the *Infanticide Act of England*, 1938 is incorrect?**
   A. It deals with killing of a child under 12 months of age
   B. It applies only to the mother
   C. It applies to everyone who kills a child below 12 months of age
   D. In India, there is no equivalent Act

3. **Filicide is:**
   A. Sudden infant death syndrome
   B. Stabbing of a child by a metal file
   C. Beating of a child by its parents
   D. Killing of a child by its parents

4. **Neonaticide is killing of a child within:**
   A. 1 hour of its birth
   B. 24 hours of its birth
   C. 15 days of its birth
   D. One month of its birth

5. **All of the following facts about stillbirth are correct *except*:**
   A. The child is born before 28 weeks of pregnancy
   B. After being born it did not show any signs of life
   C. The child was alive in utero
   D. The child dies during the process of birth

6. **Autolytic decomposition of the dead foetus in an aseptic environment, as in the uterus is known as:**
   A. Putrefaction
   B. Adipocere
   C. Mummification
   D. Maceration

7. **Spalding's sign is seen in:**
   A. Live born premature child
   B. Dead born child
   C. Still born child
   D. Both (B) and (C) above

8. **Robert's sign is a sign of:**
   A. Down's syndrome in the fetus
   B. Gonadal agenesis in the fetus
   C. Intrauterine growth retardation
   D. Intrauterine death

9. **Spalding sign is diagnostic of:**
   A. Prematurity
   B. Postmaturity
   C. Fetal death
   D. Hydrocephalus

10. Macerated fetus indicates:
A. A dead born child
B. A stillborn child
C. A live born child
D. Intra Uterine Growth Retardation

11. According to Indian law, which of the following constitutes birth of a living child?
A. If any part of the child has been brought forth from the birth canal, even though the child may not have breathed or been completely born
B. If any part of the child has been brought forth from the birth canal, and the child has shown signs of respiratory efforts
C. The child must have been completely brought forth from the birth canal, respired and the umbilical cord has been severed
D. Nowhere does Indian law define the birth of a living child

12. Hydrostatic test is done to:
A. Differentiate between a stillborn and a dead born child
B. Differentiate between a live born and still born child
C. Assess the time interval for which the child survived after birth
D. Assess if the child was capable of being born alive or not

13. Hydrostatic test is based on the following fact:
A. Weight of liver increases after birth, because portal vein brings in more blood
B. Specific gravity of the lungs decreases after birth due to respiration
C. Umbilical arteries obliterate after birth
D. Umbilical veins obliterate after birth

14. For hydrostatic test to be positive at all stages, the following must be present inside lung alveoli:
A. Residual air
B. Tidal air
C. Exudates and tidal air
D. Amniotic fluid

15. Hydrostatic test is also known as:
A. Fodere's test
B. Ploucquet's test
C. Wreden's test
D. Raygat's test

16. Aerated lungs may sink in hydrostatic test in following conditions:
A. Presence of an alveolar duct membrane
B. Complete absorption of air from the lungs
C. Both (A) and (B) above
D. Aerated lungs always float in hydrostatic test

17. Unaerated lungs may float in hydrostatic test in following conditions:
A. When gases have been released as a result of putrefaction
B. When artificial respiration has been given
C. Unaerated lungs never float in hydrostatic test
D. Both (A) and (B) above

18. Which of the following refers to Fodere's test?
A. There is air in the stomach and intestine
B. There is air in the middle ear
C. The weight of both lungs (combined) is about 30-40 g before respiration and about 60-70 g after respiration
D. Before respiration, both lungs together form about 1/70 of the total body weight of the infant. After respiration they weigh about 1/35 of the total body weight

19. If the baby is born alive, the combined weight of lungs will be 1/x of the total body weight. What is the value of x here?
A. 3.5
B. 7.0
C. 35
D. 70

20. Breslau's second life test for the presence of air in:
A. Stomach and intestines
B. Lungs
C. Middle ear
D. Anal canal

21. Testing for the presence of air in the middle ear is:
A. Fodere's test
B. Ploucquet's test
C. Breslau's second life test
D. Wreden's test

22. *Vagitus uterinus* is a condition when:
A. Uterus is atrophied and is imperceptibly merged with vagina
B. Uterus protrudes out of vagina, making it medico legally impossible to differentiate between live born and dead born child
C. Child cries when still in uterus
D. The uterine outlet fails to relax, making it difficult for child to be born, causing it to die within the uterus

23. *Vagitus vaginalis* is:
A. An infection of vagina
B. An infection of uterus
C. A cry of unborn baby while within vaginal canal
D. Combined infection of both vagina and the uterus

24. Which of the following is the earliest to close?
A. Umbilical artery
B. Umbilical vein
C. Ductus venosus
D. Ductus arteriosus

25. In India, what is usually taken as the age of viability of a child?
A. 24 weeks (168 days)
B. 28 weeks (196 days)
C. 210 days
D. 280 days

26. Legal age in India by which fetus is capable of independent existence is:
A. 180 days
B. 210 days
C. 220 days
D. Not defined in Indian law

27. All the following facts about concealment of birth by secret disposal of dead body are correct *except*:
A. It is punishable u/s 318 of IPC
B. The maximum punishment for this crime is 7 years
C. The crime is punishable irrespective of the fact whether the child had died before, during or after birth
D. It is applicable not just to parents but to anyone who conceals birth in this way

28. Caffey's syndrome is another name for:
A. Secondary drowning of infants in amniotic fluid
B. Munchausen's syndrome by proxy
C. Battered baby syndrome
D. Sudden infant death syndrome

29. Violent shaking of a child is most likely to produce:
A. Rupture of the spleen
B. Fracture of long bones
C. Subdural haematoma
D. Fracture of the orbital plates of the skull

30. Exposure and abandonment of child under twelve years by his parents may lead to their prosecution under section:
A. 301 I.P.C.
B. 317 I.P.C.
C. 318 I.P.C.
D. 363 I.P.C.

31. All of the following signs indicate live birth, *except*:
A. Presence of air in the middle ear
B. Presence of milk in the stomach
C. Diaphragm at the level of 6th or 7th rib
D. Presence of vernix caseosa over the body

MULTIPLE ANSWER TYPE (PGI, CHANDIGARH PATTERN)

32. Hydrostatic test is not necessary in which of the following conditions?
- **A.** When the stomach contains milk
- **B.** When the baby is a monster
- **C.** When the baby is born with polydactyly
- **D.** When the baby is born with Down's syndrome
- **E.** When cicatrization of the umbilical cord has occurred

33. Medicolegal questions arising in cases of infant deaths are:
- **A.** Whether the child was stillborn or dead born
- **B.** Whether the child was male, female or intersex
- **C.** Whether the infant had attained the age of viability or not
- **D.** Whether the child was dolichocephalic, mesaticephalic or brachycephalic, indicating its racial origin
- **E.** What was the cause of his death?

34. Which of the following lung features indicate that the newborn was a live born baby?
- **A.** Lungs are more voluminous
- **B.** Right lung shows a depression of azygous vein
- **C.** Lungs are bluish-violet
- **D.** The margins of the lung are very sharp
- **E.** Lungs are harder in consistency

35. Which of the following changes in stomach indicate live birth?
- **A.** Milk in the stomach
- **B.** Rich arterial supply of stomach
- **C.** Air in stomach
- **D.** Closure of pyloric sphincter
- **E.** Closure of cardiac sphincter

36. Which of the following facts about exposure and abandonment of child by parent or person having its care is true?
- **A.** It is punishable only if the exposed child was under 12 years of age
- **B.** It is punishable u/s 318 of I.P.C.
- **C.** The maximum punishment for this crime is 7 years or fine or both
- **D.** It is applicable to any person who abandons a child irrespective of the fact whether he was his parent or whether the child was under his care or not
- **E.** It is applicable only to the father and mother of the child or any person having care of such child

ANSWERS

1. **C.**
2. **C.** Under the *Infanticide Act*, 1938, of England, killing of a child under 12 months of age by its mother is a crime which deserves leniency, because the mother's mental faculties may be disturbed (this is a known physiological fact). The *Infanticide Act*, 1938 provides a defence to mothers where "at the time of the act or omission the balance of her mind was disturbed by reason of her not having fully recovered from the effect of giving birth to the child or by reason of the effect of lactation consequent upon the birth of the child."

   This "special defence" is available only to mothers and not to anyone else. There is no such equivalent law in India. Hence if in India, a mother kills her child under effects of delivery or lactation, she would be charged under S. 302. She can take a defence under s.84 of IPC (unsoundness of mind), but it may prove difficult.

   Additional info: England has traditionally viewed infanticide as a "special crime" passing its first Infanticide Act in 1623 under the Stuarts and subsequently the Infanticide Acts of 1922 and 1938. Most recently England passed the Infanticide Act of 1978 which allows a lesser sentence for attempted infanticide.
3. **D.**
4. **B.**
5. **A.** For a death to be termed stillbirth, the child must be born *after* 28 weeks of pregnancy. Before 28 weeks, it is usually known as abortion.
6. **D.** ***Variant:*** A variant is often asked like this →Asceptic autolysis is seen in (a) Maceration (b) Mummification (c) Adipocere (d) Putrefaction. Answer is (a) Maceration.
7. **B.** Spalding's sign [named after Alfred Baker Spalding, American obstetrician and gynecologist, 1874–1942] is a radiological sign. It is overlapping of fetal skull bones seen on x-ray (or ultrasound) examination. It occurs due to shrinkage of cerebrum after intrauterine death.
8. **D.** Robert's sign is a sign of intrauterine fetal death usually seen radiologically or ultrasonographically during the 2nd and 3rd trimesters. Robert's sign is said to be positive, when air is seen in aorta, pulmonary vessels or abdomen. Robert's sign is the earlier sign to appear; it appears as early as 12 hours after intrauterine death. Spalding's sign appears as late as about 7 days after death.

   Major signs of intrauterine death (seen sonographically) are:
   - Absent cardiac activity.
   - Exaggerated curvature (hyperflexion) of the fetal spine.
   - Crowding of the ribs shadow with loss of normal parallelism.
   - Air in aorta, pulmonary vessels or abdomen (Robert's sign).
   - Overlapping skull bones (Spalding's radiographic sign).
   - Reduction of biparietal diameter by 5 mm at 4 days' interval.
   - Lack of all fetal motion during a 10-minute period of careful observation.
   - Fetal maceration.
9. **C.**

10. A.

11. A. The definition of live birth is different in different countries, and even in our own country different according to different statutes.

English law: According to the English law, live birth means that the child must be born completely external to the mother, irrespective of the attachment or severance of the cord, and manifesting some sign of independent life. Thus if the entire body of the child has issued forth from the mother, but one leg is still in the birth canal, and the child is crying, according to English law it would not be a live birth.

Indian law: In India, at least two different bodies of law define live birth.

i. Section 2(d) of The *Registration of Births And Deaths Act*, 1969 is more like the English law above. According to it, "live-birth" means the complete expulsion or extraction from its mother of a product of conception, irrespective of the duration of pregnancy, which after such expulsion or extraction, breathes or shows any other evidence of life, and each product of such birth is considered live-born.

ii. Explanation 3 of section 299 of I.P.C. defines live-birth completely differently. According to this explanation, a child may be called "live born", if any part of that child has been brought forth, though the child may not have breathed or been completely born.

Consider these three situations now:

Situation 1: The child has issued forth completely from the birth canal. The cord may or may not have been severed. It is live birth according to English law as well as both organs of Indian law mentioned above.

Situation 2: Most of the body of child has issued forth from the birth canal, and the child is respiring; but a part of it is still inside the birth canal, say a leg. This is NOT live birth according to English law or The Registration Of Births And Deaths Act, 1969 of India. But it is live birth according to Explanation 3 of section 299 of IPC. If such a child is killed, it would be considered equal to causing the death of a living child and not foeticide.

Situation 3: Only a part of the body, say an arm has issued forth from the birth canal. The situation is same as situation 2 above. Causing the death of such a child would not be considered foeticide; it would be considered equal to causing death of a living child.

12. B.

13. B. To be sure, the weight of lungs increases due to blood flowing in them. But at the same time their volume increases too because of inspirations. The increase in volume more than compensates for the increase in weight. The net effect is a decrease in specific gravity. The specific gravity of lungs before respiration is said to be 1.04 to 1.05, while after respiration it is 0.94. This causes the lungs to float in water (sp gr 1.00) in a live born child. In a child who has never respired after birth, the lungs would drown.

14. A. The capacity of the lungs is physiologically divided into three areas: (i) Residual air, which is air that is left in the lungs after full expiration (ii) Tidal air, which is the ebb and flow of normal breathing (0.5 Liters) and (iii) Vital capacity, which is the total amount of air that can be exhaled from full inspiration to full expiration (4 to 5 Liters).

Also remember that:

Vital capacity – tidal air volume = reserve volume.

Hydrostatic test is performed in following four stages:

1. Whole thoracic pluck consisting of both lungs and heart are placed in a bucket of

water. If the pluck floats, it indicates that the infant may have born alive. If the pluck sinks, move to second stage.

2. Each brochus is tied, and lungs severed above the ligature. Each lung is then placed separately in water. If either lung floats, it indicates that the infant may have born alive. If either lung sinks, move to third stage.
3. Cut each lung in 12-20 pieces, and then observe if they float. Same criteria applies as above.
4. Each piece is now taken out of water, wrapped in a piece of cloth and squeezed by putting a weight. This is an important step as *it removes the tidal air. Residual air* still remains within the alveoli, which can not be taken out by any means. If the pieces of lung still float, the live birth of the infant is said to have been established. If the lungs were earlier floating due to artefacts (such as gases introduced by artificial respiration), the pieces of lung would not continue to float till the last stage.

Additional info:

1. A piece of liver is also sunk in water as control. It must sink in normal conditions. If it floats, the test may be of dubious value.
2. Radiography of lungs may be done to see air within them.
3. At the third stage, when each lung has been divided into 12-20 pieces following two examinations may be done:
   i. Dip each piece under water and squeeze between thumb and finger and see if any bubbles are escaping.
   ii. Roll a piece of lung gently between a finger and thumb near the ear and see if there is a crackling crepitant noise.

15. D.

16. C. If the child has respired, one would expect the lungs to float, yet they may sink because of certain reasons. They are:

1. ***Diseases:*** Some diseases which cause consolidation, may cause even the aerated lungs to sink, leading to misinterpretation of the test. These diseases are pneumonia, and acute oedema.
2. ***Alveolar duct membrane:*** Normally this membrane is absent at the time of birth. But if it is present, it would prevent entry of air in the alveoli, even if violent efforts were made to inhale.
3. ***Feeble respiratory effort:*** If after the initial few normal respirations, the respiratory efforts become feeble, more air would be expelled during the expiration, than would be taken in during inspiration. This would cause all air to be expelled from the lungs eventually. By conducting hydrostatic test on such a child, one would tend to think that the child had never respired (and thus born dead) although the truth is otherwise.
4. ***Complete absorption of air from the lungs:*** It is well-known that the heart keeps beating even after respiration has stopped. If the heart beats for an unusually long period after cessation of respiration, all air within the lungs would be absorbed by the circulation.

17. D. Not only do the aerated lungs sink, sometimes unaerated lungs may float giving one the impression that the baby had been born alive, while he was actually born dead. The conditions under which this happens are as follows:

1. ***Putrefactive gases:*** If the child has been dead for some time (enough for putrefactive changes to set in), putrefactive gases within the lungs would make them

lighter than water. This fallacy can be checked to some extent by simultaneously checking if the liver is also floating in water or not. Normally liver should sink in water. But if even the liver floats, it is a clear indication that putrefactive changes have set in. Liver should be floated in water only if there are no naked eye appearances of putrefaction. If naked eye changes of putrefaction, such as greenish discoloration of the body, and foul smell etc are present, it is a foregone conclusion, that the hydrostatic test is useless.

2. ***Artificial respiration:*** If the child was born dead, and efforts were made to revive him by giving forceful respiration (either mouth-to-mouth, or by a cannula), much air may reach the lungs, causing them to float.

18. **C.** Lungs increase in absolute weight after birth. This is the Fodere's test. The test referred to in choice (D) is the Ploucquet's test.

Variant: This question has also been asked as→Fodere's test is for (a) Homicide (b) Live birth (c) Mercury poisoning (d) Methanol poisoning. The answer is (b) Live birth.

19. **C.** This is the Ploucquet's test. Before respiration the lungs weigh 1/70 of the total body weight.

20. **A.** Breslau's second life test is another test to indicate whether the baby was born alive. During respiration, usually some air enters the GIT too. If the stomach and intestines are removed *en bloc*, their both ends tied and placed in water, they would float if there is air within the stomach. The test has been called the second test of life, because in mediaeval times, the test of primary importance was considered to be hydrostatic test, this (Breslau's test) being only a corroborative test. Thus if the stomach and intestines floated, it would mean that the child had been born alive.

21. **D.** During embryonic life, the middle ear contains gelatinous tissue. During efforts of breathing, some air enters the middle ear through the Eustachian tube. Thus if the air is found in the middle ear, it is quite reasonable to suppose that the child had been born alive. Named after **Roberto Wreden** of St. Petersburgh.

Note: This test is sometimes wrongly spelt as "Wredin's test".

22. **C.** Rarely after the early rupture of membranes, air may enter the uterus and the child may breathe and cry. This crying may even be heard by anxious relatives waiting outside the delivery room. They may believe that the baby has been born, and is alive and healthy. If this baby later dies within the birth canal for natural reasons, it could be extremely difficult to convince them that the child was never born alive in the first place. They would always believe that the child died because of medical negligence. If hydrostatic test is performed in these cases, it would indicate respiration further corroborating the doubts of the relatives.

A similar cry when the child is within the vagina is known as *vagitus vaginalis*. A related question is below.

23. **C.** For detailed explanation of this question, please see above.

24. **A.** ***Related fact:*** This is one of the most tricky questions students can face. Remember this mnemonic:

A→V→V→A→O

This stands for Arteries [umbilical, there are two of them), Veins (ductus venosus and umbilical vein (left umbilical vein; remember only left is left!), Arteriosus (ductus), Ovale (foramen)].

The position of Ductus venosus:

It is in the liver. It starts where umbilical vein joins the left branch of portal vein, and ends when it joins the left hepatic vein to immediately end in IVC.

Also remember Table 27.1:

Table 27.1: Various fetal structures, their closure periods and the final anatomical structures they transform into

Structure	Closure period	Final structure
Umbilical arteries	10 hours to 3 days	Medial Umbilical fold
Left Umbilical vein	3-5 days	Round ligament of liver (also known as ligamentum teres)
Ductus venosus	3-5 days	Ligamentum venosum
Ductus arteriosus	7-10 days	Ligamentum arteriosum
Foramen ovale	2-3 months	Fossa ovalis

Sometimes fossa ovalis can take longer to close, and sometimes remains open throughout life. In that case it may give rise to a condition, known as *morbus ceruleus*.

The peritoneum lining the lower part of the anterior abdominal wall is raised into five ridges. The one in the median plane extends from the apex of the urinary bladder to the umbilicus. It contains the urachus and is termed the *median umbilical fold*. Lateral to this are the medial umbilical folds, which contain the obliterated umbilical arteries, and still lateral to them are the lateral umbilical folds, which contain the inferior epigastric artery.

The spaces between the median and medial umbilical folds are called supravesical fossae. Space between medial and lateral umbilical folds is called the medial inguinal fossa. The space lateral to lateral umbilical fold is the lateral inguinal fossa.

25. C. Nowhere in Indian law has viability been defined as in the English law. It is however taken as 210 days (from LMP) by common consensus. In English law the age of viability has been defined. It is 24 weeks *[The Infant Life (Preservation) Act, 1929]*.

26. D. As stated earlier, age of viability of an infant is not defined legally in India. However by common consensus it is taken to be 210 days. At the age of viability, a special chemical, called the pulmonary surfactant appears in the alveoli of lungs. This chemical reduces the surface tension of the alveoli and they become able to inflate. When the pulmonary surfactant is deficient, neonatal respiratory distress syndrome (RDS, also called hyaline membrane disease) may result.

Additional info: Pulmonary surfactant is rich in disaturated phosphatidyl choline (lecithin). Lecithin synthesis in the lung increases dramatically as the lung matures and begins producing surfactant. Lecithin levels are generally expressed as a ratio against sphingomyelin, a non-pulmonary lipid whose concentration is relatively constant in amniotic fluid (Remember L for lung, and lecithin). Thus the lecithin level is generally expressed as a lecithin-to-sphingomyelin ratio or L/S ratio. L/S ratios of greater than 2 are rarely associated with RDS. L/S ratios of less than 2 indicate increased risk of RDS.

Phosphatidylglycerol (PG) is another lipid that shows a similar time course. It is also an indicator of lung maturity.

27. B. The maximum punishment for this crime is imprisonment of 2 years and/or fine. The complete statement of this section is as follows:

S 318. Concealment of birth by secret disposal of dead body—Whoever, by secretly burying or otherwise disposing of the death body of a child whether such child die before or after or during its birth, intentionally conceals or endeavours to conceal the birth of such child, shall be punished with imprisonment of either description for a term which may extend to two years, or with fine, or with both.

28. C.

29. C.

30. B. This question often appears wrongly in several MCQ books as→ Negligence on the part of the father towards the son can be punished under section (a)319 (b)317 (c) 315 (d)318. The intended answer is (b) 317, but this is a wrongly framed question.

31. D.

MULTIPLE ANSWER TYPE (PGI, CHANDIGARH PATTERN)

32. A,B,E. Hydrostatic test not necessary when their is a conclusive proof that the child was either born alive or dead.

Conclusive proof of life occurs under following conditions:

1. **The stomach contains milk:** This means the child has ingested milk. This is a conclusive proof that the child was born alive.
2. **Cicatrization of the umbilical cord:** This is a vital change, and occurs a few days after birth. This is also a sure proof that the child was born alive.

Conclusive proof of child having been born dead occurs under following conditions:

1. **Foetus less than 180 days of gestation:** When one determines the gestational age of the foetus and finds that it has been born before 180 days of gestation. Age of viability in India is generally taken to be 210 days, but a child born before 180 days (30 days before the usually accepted period of viability) can certainly be said to be non-viable and thus born dead.
2. **Monster:** When the foetus is a monster, is anencephalic, double headed, or shows any other gross anomaly which is incompatible with life.
3. **Macerated foetus:** We have seen that maceration takes about 4-5 days to occur. Thus it means that the foetus was already lying dead in the womb for some time.

33. A,C,E. Medico-legal questions arising in a case of infanticide are:

1. Whether the child was stillborn or deadborn?
2. Whether the infant had attained the age of viability or not?
3. Whether the child was born alive?
4. If born alive, how long did the child live after birth?
5. What was the cause of his death?
6. Whether the dead infant really belonged to the mother?
7. Has the mother charged with infanticide recently delivered?

34. A. Following lung features are usually seen to differentiate a live born from a still born baby.

1. **Volume:** Lungs are more voluminous after breathing has taken place. They also completely cover the heart. Unrespired lungs do not cover the heart completely.
2. **Margins:** Before respiration, the margins are sharp. After respiration, they are more rounded.
3. **Consistency:** Before respiration, the lungs are harder in consistency; they are more like liver in consistency. After respiration they trap air within them. This causes them to become much softer in consistency.
4. **Colour:** Before respiration, the lungs are bluish-violet, but after respiration they become light red, due to blood rushing in.

5. **Weight of the lungs:** The weight of the lungs increases after respiration because of the blood rushing in. The weights of the lungs may be determined in two ways, either in terms of their absolute weight, or in terms of a fraction of the whole body weight.

35. A,C. Milk in the stomach is a conclusive indication that the child had been born alive, so much so that in its presence, even hydrostatic test is not conducted.

36. A,C,E. This crime is punishable u/s 317 of I.P.C. However if the child dies as a result of abandonment or exposure, the culprit will also have to face the charges of murder or culpable homicide, as the case may be. This section is completely stated as follows:

S 317. Exposure and abandonment of child under twelve years, by parent or person having care of it: Whoever being the father or mother of a child under the age of twelve years, or having the care of such child, shall expose or leave such child in any place with the intention of wholly abandoning such child, shall be punished with imprisonment of either description for a term which may extend to seven years, or with fine, or with both.

***Explanation*:** This section is not intended to prevent the trial of the offender for murder or culpable homicide, as the case may be, if the child die in consequence of the exposure.

6 FORENSIC PSYCHIATRY

28 Forensic Psychiatry

DEFINITIONS AND GENERAL ASPECTS

1. **Psychiatric diseases are currently classified according to:**
   A. DSM-III
   B. DSM-IV
   C. DSM-IV-TR
   D. DSM-V

2. **"Waxy flexibility" is typically seen in:**
   A. Catatonic type schizophrenia
   B. Paranoid type schizophrenia
   C. Disorganized type schizophrenia
   D. Residual type schizophrenia

3. **A false belief in something which is not a fact is called:**
   A. Illusion
   B. Delusion
   C. Delirium
   D. Hallucination

4. **An aerial root is dangling from a tree and it is perfectly visible as such to normal people. However a psychiatric patient perceives it as a snake. This is an example of:**
   A. Illusion
   B. Delusion
   C. Hallucination
   D. Fugue

5. **A psychiatric person hears sounds of daggers being sharpened, while normal people around him do not hear anything. This is an example of:**
   A. Illusion
   B. Obsessive compulsive behavior
   C. Hallucination
   D. Fugue

6. **Clérambault-Kandinsky syndrome is an example of:**
   A. Illusion
   B. Hallucination
   C. Delusion
   D. Alcoholic neurosis

7. **A disorder in which a person suffers a bout of amnesia and then flees his home and forgets his identity is known as:**
   A. Abreaction
   B. Impulse
   C. Affect
   D. Fugue

8. **An hallucinatory or dream-like state caused by such conditions as prolonged deprivation of sleep, sensory isolation, or drugs is known as:**
   A. Oneirophrenia
   B. Somnolentia
   C. Semisomnolence
   D. Lucid interval

9. A psychoanalytical technique of curing patients, whereby long forgotten and other traumatic experiences or repressed emotions are revived and brought into consciousness is known as:
A. Fugue
B. Empathy
C. Oneiroid state
D. Abreaction

10. Pseudodementia is seen in:
A. Anxiety neurosis
B. Schizophrenia
C. Manic states
D. All of the above

11. *Mens rea* refers to:
A. Guilty action
B. Guilty mind
C. Civil responsibility of the insane
D. Sleep walking

12. According to the old system of classification of the mentally retarded, an idiot was one, who had an IQ:
A. Below 20
B. Between 20-49
C. Between 50-69
D. Between 70-80

CRIMINAL RESPONSIBILITY OF THE INSANE

13. Indian lunacy act was passed in:
A. 1804
B. 1881
C. 1912
D. 1921

14. The Mental Health Act in India was passed in:
A. 1912
B. 1974
C. 1987
D. It is still lying in Parliament for approval

15. Which of the following sections of the Indian law incorporates the McNaughten's rule?
A. Section 44 I.P.C.
B. Section 84 I.P.C.
C. Section 87 I.P.C.
D. Section 84 Cr.P.C.

16. A person is suffering from delusions of infidelity. Under a false delusion that his wife is infidel, he kills his wife and her supposed paramour. Which of the following options applies best to his case?
A. He can get relief under section 84 I.P.C.
B. He can get relief under section 85 I.P.C.
C. He can get relief under McNaghten's rule
D. He is not entitled to any relief

17. Which of the following has been used as the rule for the criminal responsibility of the insane?
A. McNaughten's rule
B. Durham's rule
C. Curren's rule
D. All of the above

18. Lucid interval is seen in:
A. Insanity
B. Malignant disease
C. Electric shock
D. Syphilis

MENTAL HEALTH ACT, 1987

19. Which of the following facts regarding voluntary admission in a psychiatric hospital or psychiatric nursing home is INCORRECT?
A. Under section 15 of the Act, any mentally ill person can himself get admitted in a psychiatric hospital or psychiatric nursing home, without the opinion of any relative or friend
B. In case of a minor who is mentally ill, only a guardian can make an application

for his admission in a psychiatric hospital or psychiatric nursing home

C. When a person wants to get admitted in a psychiatric hospital or psychiatric nursing home, the medical officer in charge of the hospital or nursing home MUST admit him within a period of 24 hours

D. The request for discharge by a patient who has got admitted on a voluntary basis, can be made by himself

20. Which of the following facts regarding the discharge of a voluntarily admitted patient is INCORRECT?

A. A voluntarily admitted patient can get a discharge whenever he likes, and the medical officer in charge has absolutely no control over this matter

B. If a minor who was admitted by his guardian attains majority while in hospital, it is the duty of the medical officer in charge to inform him as soon as possible that he has attained majority

C. If a minor was admitted on a voluntary basis by his guardian, and he has attained majority while in the hospital, he must make a request for his continuance as an inpatient within one month, if he wants to continue as an inpatient

D. If a medical officer in charge has received an application of discharge from a voluntarily admitted patient, he can make a Board consisting of 2 doctors, and if the opinion of the Board is that the patient needs further treatment, the medical officer in charge can deny discharge to him

21. If a wandering, dangerous or cruelly treated mentally ill person is brought before a magistrate for a reception order, the magistrate may order the detention of the person in an observation ward for enabling a doctor to certify him as mentally ill. How long can such a person be detained by a single magisterial order?

A. 5 days

B. 10 days

C. 30 days

D. There is no such limit

22. A person accused of murder alleges that by reason of unsoundness of mind, he did not know the nature of the act he committed. On whom lies the burden of proving that he was of unsound mind at the time of committing the act?

A. Police

B. Magistrate

C. On person himself

D. On all of the above

MULTIPLE ANSWER TYPE (PGI, CHANDIGARH PATTERN)

23. McNaughten rule is concerned with:

A. Litigation of the insane

B. Criminal responsibility of the insane

C. Rape of an insane woman

D. Suicide of an insane person

E. Civil responsibility of the insane

24. Which of the following are examples of impulse control disorders?

A. Kleptomania

B. Trichotillomania

C. Capgras syndrome

D. Mutilomania

E. Fugue

25. Which of the following facts regarding tendering of evidence by a mentally ill person are correct?

A. A mentally ill person can not tender evidence at all

B. A mentally ill person can tender evidence during periods of lucid interval

C. A mentally ill person can tender evidence if he is above 18 years

D. A person suffering from delusions can tender evidence if he is able to tell what he has seen, and who also understands the obligations of an oath

E. A mentally ill person can tender evidence if he is has a valid degree in medicine and surgery

26. Morbid jealousy may be seen in:

A. Paranoid schizophrenia

B. Acute Dhatura poisoning

C. Alcoholism

D. Acute charas poisoning

E. Cocaine addiction

ANSWERS

DEFINITIONS AND GENERAL ASPECTS

1. C. ***Related fact:*** DSM or "The Diagnostic and Statistical Manual of Mental Disorders" was published by the American Psychiatric Association first in 1952, mainly to bring a uniformity in the naming of psychiatric disorders, many of which were haphazardly named before this date. Same disease was often called by different names in different cultures making a meaningful communication between psychiatrists a near impossibility. The first edition of this manual was called **DSM-I** and it contained about 60 different disorders.

   Subsequently this manual has been revised a number of times. **DSM-II** was published in 1968, **DSM-III** in 1980, **DSM-III-R** (Revised) in 1987, **DSM-IV** in 1994 and finally **DSM-IV-TR** (Text Revision) in 2000. Work on **DSM-V** has already begun and it will be published in 2011.

2. A. ***Additional info:*** Schizophrenia is a mental illness characterized by disordered thinking, delusions, hallucinations, emotional disturbance, and withdrawal from reality. Some experts view schizophrenia as a group of related illnesses with similar characteristics, typified by (i) 'positive symptoms' [presence of symptoms which should *not* be there e.g. delusions and hallucinations], (ii) 'negative symptoms' [absence of behaviors/traits, which should be there[1] e.g. inappropriate emotion, poverty of speech (alogia), and lack of motivation (avolition), absence of normal social and interpersonal behaviors] and (iii) 'disorganized symptoms' [consisting of thought disorders like knight's move thinking[2], and disorganized behavior[3] and speech].

[1]Sometimes called 'deficit' symptoms

[2]Knight's move thinking (or derailment) is said to occur when the patient moves from one train of thought to another which has no apparent connection to the first ("I was going from Mumbai to .... where did you buy that tie?"). The name apparently takes its name from the chess piece that moves two steps forward and one to the side.

[3]Such as unnecessary, repetitive movements.

The condition affects between one-half and one percent of the world's population, occurring with equal frequency in males and females (although the onset of symptoms is usually earlier in males).

Historically, schizophrenia was classified into catatonic, hebephrenic, and paranoid, but now this classification is obsolete. DSM-IV-TR (please see answer to an earlier question) now classifies schizophrenia into five subtypes[4]:

[4]To make matters somewhat confusing, ICD-10 (International Classification of Diseases, 10th Revision), uses nine subtypes: These are:
F20.0 Paranoid schizophrenia
F20.1 Hebephrenic schizophrenia
F20.2 Catatonic schizophrenia
F20.3 Undifferentiated schizophrenia
F20.4 Post-schizophrenic depression
F20.5 Residual schizophrenia
F20.6 Simple schizophrenia
F20.8 Other schizophrenia
F20.9 Schizophrenia, unspecified

(A short note on International classification of Diseases: ICD-10 was endorsed by the Forty-third World Health Assembly in May 1990 and came into use in WHO Member States as from 1994. This classification had its origins in the 1850s. The first edition, known as the *International List of Causes of Death*, was adopted by the International Statistical Institute in 1893. WHO took over the responsibility for the ICD at its creation in 1948 when the Sixth Revision, which included causes of morbidity for the first time, was published. ICD-10 is the latest in this series. Unlike DSM-V, which is slated to appear in 2011, there are no immediate plans to develop an ICD-11.

While ICD-10 attempts to classify *all* diseases, DSM-IV-TR classifies *only* psychiatric illnesses. Unfortunately ICD-10 and DSM-IV-TR (the two major "disease classification indices" in existence today) do not always agree on the classification of psychiatric illnesses. However for classification of psychiatric illnesses, DSM-IV-TR is by and large considered the Bible).

i. Disorganized type (295.1) [earlier known as hebephrenic schizophrenia].
ii. Catatonic type (295.2).
iii. Paranoid type (295.3).
iv. Undifferentiated type (295.9).
v. Residual type (295.6).

[The numbers within brackets refer to the numerical codes which DSM gives to these subtypes.]

Major diagnostic criteria of each type are as below:

- In **disorganized type**, thought disorder (e.g. knight's move thinking) and flat or inappropriate emotions (incongruous grinning and grimacing) are present together. Behavior and speech are disorganized; they often burst out laughing for no apparent reason. Their contact with reality is extremely poor. Their behavior is best described as silly or fatuous. These are the typical "*paagal*" patients as a common man understands it.
- In **catatonic type**, marked peculiarities of posture or movement are present. These may comprise waxy flexibility, where the patient's limbs can be 'molded' into a position and they would remain fixed in that position for long periods of time.[5] Disorganized and catatonic schizophrenia affect a very small percentage of people.

[5]Other major motor symptoms seen in catatonic schizophrenia are (i) Echopraxia (automatic imitation of another person's movements even when asked not to) (ii) Negativism (motiveless resistance to instructions and attempts to be moved, or doing the opposite of what is asked) and (iii) Posturing (adoption of inappropriate or bizarre bodily posture continuously for a substantial period of time without tiring)

- In **paranoid type**, delusions and hallucinations (most commonly auditory, but may also be visual) are present. It is the most prevalent type, found in some 40% of affected persons.
- In **undifferentiated type**, the patient meets the basic criteria for schizophrenia, but cannot be classified as either paranoid, disorganized, or catatonic types. It forms the second largest group after paranoid type.
- In **residual type**, the patient at one time met criteria for catatonic, disorganized, paranoid or undifferentiated schizophrenia. But currently the patient no longer has pronounced catatonic behavior, delusions, hallucinations or disorganized speech or behavior. The patient however is still ill, as indicated by either (i) Negative symptoms such as flattened affect (emotions), reduced speech output or lack of volition, or (ii) An attenuated form of at least 2 characteristic symptoms of schizophrenia, such as odd beliefs (related to delusions), distorted perceptions (hallucinations), odd speech (disorganized speech) or peculiarities of behavior (disorganized behavior).

Several variants can be asked on this question based on the above information. One frequently asked question is→Most common hallucinations seen in schizophrenia are (a) visual (b) auditory (c) tactile (d) olfactory. The answer is (b) auditory.

3. **B.**

4. **A.** ***Related fact:*** False perception of a stimulus (an aerial root or a rope), which has a real existence is called illusion. A variant of this question may be asked like this→The false perception of a stimulus, which has a real existence is called (a) delusion (b) illusion (c) fugue (d) hallucination. The answer is (b) illusion.

5. **C.** ***Related fact:*** Conditions where there is no real stimulus, yet the person perceives them are termed hallucinations. Any sense organ may be involved; visual hallucinations involve sight (someone seeing snakes dangling from a branch when there is absolutely nothing dangling from there; not even aerial roots as in the previous question), auditory hallucinations involve hearing (as in the above example) and tactile hallucinations involve sense of touch (someone feeling ants crawling underneath his skin). Gustatory and olfactory hallucinations are less common.

   A variation of the question may be asked like this→The false perception in the absence of any stimulus is called (a) delusion (b) illusion (c) fugue (d) hallucination. The answer is (d) hallucination.

6. **C.** ***Related facts:*** Clérambault-Kandinsky syndrome (also known as Kandinsky-Clérambault syndrome) is a clinical entity in which the patient believes his mind is being controlled by someone else or external forces. Since it is a false belief in something which is not a fact, it is a kind of delusion. Several types are recognized. In one form – known as command automatism – activities are carried out without conscious knowledge on the part of the subject, with automatic obedience to any command or suggestion.

   The syndrome is named after a French physician **Gaëtan Gatian de Clerambault** (1872-1934), and the Russian psychiatrist **Victor C. Kandinsky** (1825-1889) who described this syndrome.

   Additional info: de Clerambault's name has been applied to yet another syndrome known as de Clerambault's syndrome or simply Clerambault's syndrome. This is the delusion that one is loved by another person, usually of higher social status or celebrity.

7. **D.** The word "fugue" comes from the Latin *fuga* (flight) and *fugere* (to flee). Also known as dissociative fugue or psychogenic fugue, it is a curious disorder in which a person suffers a bout of amnesia and then flees his home and forgets his identity. Often the person will travel far away from his home, assume a new identity, and live as a different person until he "snaps out" of his amnesic state. A fugue state is often triggered by stress.

   Fugue state is important in forensic psychiatry because a person who commits a crime under the fugue state may claim defence under section 84 of the I.P.C.

8. **A.** ***Related facts:*** The term comes from the Greek words "*oneiros*" (dream) and "*phrenos*" (mind). Also known as "oneiroid state", it has some of the characteristics of simple schizophrenia, such as a confusional state and clouding of consciousness. Persons affected by oneirophrenia have a feeling of dream-like unreality which in its extreme form may progress to delusions and hallucinations. Therefore, it is considered an schizophrenia-like acute form of psychosis. A person doing a criminal act during an oneiroid state may not be held responsible for his criminal actions.

9. D. ***Related facts:*** The term abreaction has a long history in psychiatry and has its origins in psychoanalysis. Many psychiatrists believe that patients repress their past traumatic experiences (such as childhood sexual abuse) into their subconscious. This may give rise to several psychological disorders. If somehow these traumatic experiences are brought at their conscious level, their psychological symptoms will disappear. Many techniques including drugs (e.g. barbiturate-assisted interviewing) are used for this. This is known as abreaction. An abreaction is typically an unpleasant state; sometimes a client will cry after experiencing it.

   Abreaction is used rarely and only by a minority of consultants. Future psychiatrists are unlikely to be skilled in the use of abreaction and its use will decline. Abreaction is still used in Asia and the US.

10. B. ***Related facts:*** Dementia is significant loss of intellectual abilities such as memory capacity, severe enough to interfere with social or occupational functioning. Dementia is more frequent with increasing age. Alzheimer's disease is the most common form of dementia. Among other causes are medical conditions (thyroid disease, drug toxicity, thiamine deficiency with alcoholism, and others), brain injury, strokes, multiple sclerosis, infection of the brain (such as meningitis and syphilis), HIV infection, hydrocephalus, Pick's disease, and brain tumors.

    Pseudodementia (false dementia) is an extreme condition of general apathy simulating dementia, possibly with no actual defect of intelligence. It is seen in organic brain disease, epilepsy or schizophrenia.

11. B. ***Related facts:*** Legally speaking, a crime is said to consist of two components – a guilty mind or *mens rea* and a forbidden act or *actus reus*. If either of the two is missing, criminal responsibility is diminished or absent.

    The concept of *mens rea* is central to forensic psychiatry. Insane people may commit a forbidden act (say murder), but they do not have a guilty mind, as they do not know what they are doing. So they are exempt from punishment.

12. A. ***Related facts:*** Old system of classification of mental retardation used three terms – idiot, imbecile and moron. These terms have become so stigmatized today that they are no more used by psychiatrists. Unfortunately questions continue to be asked on these, so it is useful to remember this older classification:

    Idiot: IQ below 20. Their mental age is below a three year old child; they are clumsy, awkward, untidy and require constant supervision in the performance of the simplest requirement of living.

    Imbecile: IQ between 20-49. They may attain a mental level of six or seven years. Imbeciles can generally talk with a very crude vocabulary, can be taught simple manual tasks.

    Moron: IQ between 50-69. The moron ranges in mental accomplishment between the eight-year level and the lower adult normal which is ordinarily reached at about the fifteenth year.

    Borderline deficiency: IQ between 70-80. As stated above, these terms are now largely obsolete and mental deficiency is now generally called *mental retardation.*

    Table 28.1 shows the currently used classification of mental retardation in the USA:

Table 28.1: Classification of various subnormal IQs

IQ Range	*Classification*
Below 20	Profound
20-34	Severe
35-49	Moderate
50-69	Mild

It would be interesting to note the classification of individuals with higher IQs too. Cognitive psychologist Lewis Madison Terman (1877-1956) of US classified higher intelligence as follows (Table 28.2):

Table 28.2: Classification of various supernormal IQs

IQ Range	Classification
90-110	Normal or average intelligence
110-120	Superior intelligence
120-140	Very superior intelligence
140 and over	Genius or near genius

CRIMINAL RESPONSIBILITY OF THE INSANE

13. C. ***Related fact:*** This Act has now been repealed, and has been replaced by the *Mental Health Act.*

14. C.

15. B.

16. D. While applying section 84 I.P.C. one cannot get a blanket relief if he is suffering from delusions or some other mental disorder. The rule of the thumb is to see, what should have been the course of action of a normal person, if the delusions were deemed to be true. No one is entitled to kill his wife, even if she is *actually* infidel. At most he is entitled to divorce her, but not kill her. So a person who kills even under delusions of infidelity is not entitled for an exception under section 84 of I.P.C.

17. D. A variant of this question is→All of the following are related to legal responsibility of an insane person except (a) McNaughten's rule (b) Durham's rúle (c) Rule of nine (d) Curren's rule. The answer is (c).

18. A. Lucid interval means "a clear interval". In several forms of insanity, a person may be completely normal between two bouts of insanity. This normal period between two bouts of insanity is known as "lucid interval".

Lucid interval, or a clear period is also seen in head injury. Here lucid interval refers to a period of consciousness between two successive periods of unconsciousness. First the person falls unconscious due to concussion immediately after he gets a head injury. He then recovers, but after sometime becomes unconscious once again due to slowly developing extradural hematoma.

Sometimes there is a delay (or lucid interval) between trauma involving multiple fractures and cerebral fat embolism. This occurs after fat is released from the fatty bone marrow and then embolized in the brain. This may be clinically confused with the development of extradural haematoma.

MENTAL HEALTH ACT, 1987

19. C. ***Related facts:*** *The Mental Health Act 1987* makes the following provisions regarding voluntary admission of patients:

- Any major can make an application for admission if he thinks that he is mentally ill (under section 15 of the Act), but it is *not* mandatory for the doctor to admit him.
- If the mentally ill person is a minor (below 18 years), he can not make an application on his own behalf. The application must be made by his guardian (Section 16 of the Act).
- It is important to note that if an application is made under section 15 or 16 of the Act, the medical officer in charge of the hospital is NOT BOUND to admit such patient. Section 17 of the Act empowers him to make such enquiries as he may deem fit, to find out if he indeed is mentally ill. If he finds that the applicant is NOT mentally ill, he may not admit him (he must however make such enquiries within 24 hours of receipt of application.

In other words, the medical officer incharge may admit the patient or reject admission; either action has to be taken within 24 hours of the receipt of application). Hence choice (C) is the intended choice.

20. A. ***Related facts:*** It is an interesting fact that although a person can get himself voluntarily admitted in a psychiatric hospital, he can not get a discharge at his own will. Some interesting facts relating to discharge are:

21. **B.** Whenever a wandering, dangerous or cruelly treated mentally ill person is brought before the magistrate for a reception order, the procedure is that the magistrate will examine the person himself and cause him to be examined by the medical officer. However if it appears to the medical officer that such a person is feigning insanity (perhaps if he has committed a crime), he may need to watch him for an extended period of time. To enable him to do so, the magistrate can pass an order to detain the allegedly mentally ill person for a period of 10 days [section 28 (1) of *Mental Health Act*]. If more period of detention is required, further orders for detention have to be passed. However any single order can not be for more than 10 days, and the total detention period can not be more than 30 days [section 28(2)].

This fact is quite often wrongly asked as this→**For diagnosis of lunacy a person can be kept under observation at a stretch for (a) 2 days (b) 7 days (c) 10 days (d) 30 days.** The intended answer here is (c), but it is important to appreciate that this is not a correct question. A period of detention of 10 days in one order, and 30 days in total is prescribed *only* under Section 28 (1) and 28 (2), which deal with wandering, dangerous or cruelly treated mentally ill persons.

Such is not the case with, say, a voluntary patient. If he requests the medical officer incharge for admission (u/s 15), the medical officer must dispose of his application (by either admitting him, or refusing admission) within 24 hours of such request. In other words, in this case, the medical officer has to diagnose mental illness within 24 hours!

22. **C.** Section 105 of *Indian Evidence Act* clearly states that in the above case the burden of proof lies on the accused person himself and not on any other person.

MULTIPLE ANSWER TYPE (PGI, CHANDIGARH PATTERN)

23. **B.**

24. **A,B,D.** Kleptomania is an irresistible desire to steal; trichotillomania an irresistible desire to pull hair out; and mutilomania an irresistible desire to mutilate and kill others. People with trichotillomania repetitively pull their hair out at the root from places like the scalp, eyebrows, or eyelashes, sometimes causing baldness. Other impulse control disorders commonly encountered in MCQs are **pyromania** – an irresistible desire to set fire to buildings and other things, and **dipsomania** – an irresistible desire to drink alcohol.

Capgras syndrome is a psychiatric disorder, but it is NOT an impulse control disorder. Victims of Capgras syndrome often cannot recognize their own image, say in a mirror. Also known as "mirror self-misidentification" it is named after French psychiatrist **Jean Marie Joseph Capgras**, who described this syndrome for the first time.

25. **B,D.** Section 118 of the *Indian Evidence Act* clearly states who can testify. There is an explanation appended at the end of this section. This explanation states, "*A lunatic is not incompetent to testify, unless he is prevented by his lunacy from understanding the questions put to him and giving rational answers to them*". Note that this explanation

still uses the word "lunatic", although this term has completely been banished from the *Mental Health Act 1987.*

26. A,C,E. ***Related facts*:** Morbid jealousy is known by several names – The Othello syndrome, Othello psychosis, delusional jealousy, erotic jealousy syndrome, or sexual jealousy. The term refers to the delusion of infidelity of a spouse or partner. Morbid jealousy affects males and, less often, females. It is characterized by recurrent accusations of infidelity, searches for evidence, repeated interrogation of the partner, tests of their partner's fidelity, and sometime stalking. The syndrome may appear by itself or in the course of paranoid schizophrenia, alcoholism, or cocaine addiction. As in *Othello*, the tragedy by Shakespeare, the syndrome can be highly dangerous and result in disruption of a marriage, homicide and suicide. (In the Shakespearean play "*Othello*", the main character Othello thinks that his wife Desdemona is infidel and strangles her. He then kills himself with a sword!). The term "Othello syndrome" for this disorder was coined by the English psychiatrist **John Todd** (1914-1987) in a paper he published in 1955.

7 FORENSIC SCIENCE

29 Forensic Examination of Biological Fluids, Stains, Trace Evidence and Other Material (Hair Etc.)

GENERAL

1. **Barberio's test is done for:**
   - **A.** Blood
   - **B.** Urine
   - **C.** Saliva
   - **D.** Semen
2. **Edmond Locard is known for:**
   - **A.** System of personal identification using the body measurements
   - **B.** Study of fingerprints
   - **C.** Formula for estimation of stature
   - **D.** Principle of exchange
3. **When two objects come in contact, a mutual exchange of material takes place between them. This principle is known as:**
   - **A.** Galton exchange principle
   - **B.** Locard exchange principle
   - **C.** Bertillion system
   - **D.** The rule of Haase
4. **Disputed paternity or maternity can be solved by using all the following *except:***
   - **A.** Blood grouping
   - **B.** HLA typing
   - **C.** Precipitin test
   - **D.** DNA profiling
5. **Christmas tree stain may be used to detect:**
   - **A.** Spermatozoa in vaginal swabs
   - **B.** Y-chromosome in mucosal cells
   - **C.** Urine stains
   - **D.** Occult blood

BLOOD

6. **The following tests are used for a blood stain *except*:**
   - **A.** Benzidine test
   - **B.** Florence test
   - **C.** Guaiacum test
   - **D.** Leucomalachite Green test
7. **Kastle-Mayer test is also known as:**
   - **A.** Benzidine test
   - **B.** Precipitin test
   - **C.** Phenolphthalein test
   - **D.** Haemochromogen test
8. **Takayama test detects:**
   - **A.** Seminal stains
   - **B.** Saliva stains
   - **C.** Blood stains
   - **D.** Urine stains

9. Takayama reagent is used in:
A. Guaiacum test
B. Kastle-Meyer test
C. Haemin crystal test
D. Haemochromogen crystal test

10. In Takayama test, which of the following is seen under microscope?
A. Yellowish to brownish rhomboid crystals
B. Yellow needle shaped crystals
C. Pink feathery structures
D. Spherical granules

11. Which of the following tests can best be used to determine the human origin of a blood stain?
A. Precipitin test
B. Benzidine test
C. Haemin crystal test
D. Any of the above

12. Test for detection of old blood stain is:
A. Gel diffusion
B. Precipitin
C. Absorption elution
D. Benzidine

13. Child's own gamma globulin begins to form from:
A. Third month of intrauterine life
B. Birth
C. Third month of extra uterine life
D. Second year of extra uterine life

14. Both mother and father have AB blood group. The blood group of the children can be:
A. A only
B. A and AB only
C. B and AB only
D. A,B or AB

15. In old blood stained fibre, blood grouping is done by:
A. Benzidine test
B. Acid elution test
C. Precipitin test
D. Hemin crystal test

16. Invisible blood stains at a scene of crime can be made visible by one of the following agents:
A. O-tolidine
B. Benzidine
C. Phenolphthalein
D. Luminol

17. Guaiacum test gives .... color in the presence of blood:
A. Pink
B. Deep blue
C. Bright green
D. Yellowish brown

18. Hydrogen peroxide is used in all of the following tests for blood *except*:
A. Benzidine test
B. Orthotolidine test
C. Luminol test
D. Teichmann's test

19. Which of the following is usually employed as a screening test for blood?
A. Takayama test
B. Teichmann test
C. Kastle –Meyer test
D. Spectrophotometry

SEMINAL STAINS

20. Which of the following facts about normal semen is NOT correct?
A. The quantity of seminal fluid in a single emission is 2-5 ml
B. There are about 60 to 150 million sperms per ml of semen
C. There are about 60 to 150 million sperms in any one emission
D. Spermatozoa constitute about 10% of the volume of semen

21. All of the following are tests for seminal stains *except*:
A. Takayama test
B. Barberio's test
C. Florence test
D. Acid phosphatase test

22. Which of the following facts about seminal stains is NOT correct?
- **A.** Seminal stains fluoresce with a bluish-white color, when examined under filtered ultraviolet light
- **B.** Fluorescence of seminal stains depends on choline portion of semen
- **C.** Fluorescence of seminal stains is very specific as other albuminous materials do not fluoresce
- **D.** Fluorescence of seminal stains is masked by blood and disappears if the stain is soaked in water.

23. Acid phosphatase activity in semen is......
- **A.** 500-1000 times lesser than in any other normal bodily fluid
- **B.** 50-100 times lesser than in any other normal bodily fluid
- **C.** 50-100 times greater than in any other normal bodily fluid
- **D.** 500-1000 times greater than in any other normal bodily fluid

24. Prostate specific antigen is found in:
- **A.** Seminal plasma
- **B.** Male urine
- **C.** Male blood
- **D.** All of the above

25. Florence test detects:
- **A.** Bilirubin
- **B.** Urine
- **C.** Semen
- **D.** Blood

26. Florence solution used in Florence test is composed of:
- **A.** Potassium iodide, iodine and water
- **B.** A saturated aqueous or alcoholic solution of picric acid
- **C.** Sodium hydroxide, pyridine and glucose
- **D.** Sodium chloride and glacial acetic acid

27. Spermine in semen is detected by:
- **A.** Barberio test
- **B.** Florence test
- **C.** Takayama test
- **D.** Ammonium Molybdate test

OTHER BIOLOGICAL STAINS

28. Edelman test is done to detect:
- **A.** Bile stains
- **B.** Fecal stains
- **C.** Urine stains
- **D.** Saliva stains

29. Jaffe reaction would detect the presence of:
- **A.** Urine
- **B.** Bile
- **C.** Milk
- **D.** Saliva

MULTIPLE ANSWER TYPE (PGI, CHANDIGARH PATTERN)

30. Which of the following tests indicate that the blood was menstrual in origin?
- **A.** It is lower in pH than the ordinary arterial or venous blood
- **B.** It contains distinctive vaginal or decidual cells
- **C.** Menstrual blood coagulates immediately
- **D.** It is more fluid than ordinary blood
- **E.** It contains five lactate dehydrogenase isoenzymes instead of the usual three

ANSWERS

GENERAL

1. D.
2. D. *Related facts:* **Edmond Locard** (1877 - 1965) was a French criminalist, who is known for two main contributions (i) his principle of exchange, widely known as *Locard's principle of exchange* and (ii) Poroscopy. Briefly stated, his principle of exchange says that when two things come in contact with each other, there is always a mutual transfer of material between them. This principle is very helpful in criminal investigation. For instance if a person has raped a female, according to this principle, some public hair from the male would transfer to those of the female and vice-versa.
3. B.
4. C. Precipitin test is used to determine the species origin of blood. All other tests can be used to solve disputed paternity or maternity. With DNA profiling, it can be done in 100% cases, but with blood grouping and HLA typing it is useful in select cases.
5. A. ***Related facts:*** Christmas tree stain is a very common staining technique used to detect spermatozoa. It uses two dyes - Nuclear Fast Red dye and Picroindigo-carmine (PIC). The former (Nuclear Fast Red dye) stains nuclear material red while the latter (Picroindigocarmine) stains most other cellular material (e.g. epithelial cells) various shades of green. It is called Christmas tree stain because red and green are traditional Christmas colors (the appearance is much like red ornaments on a green Christmas tree).

BLOOD

6. B.
7. C.
8. C.
9. D. ***Related fact:*** Takayama reagent is used in Haemochromogen crystal test. The crytals are of salmon pink color. Shape is feathery. No heating is required. Slide is examined under the microscope just in five minutes. Test is of more value than Teichmann test or Haemin crystal test.

Mnemonic for the tests:

- Teich**mann**→Haem**in**→**min**imum value →Described earlier (in 1853 by Ludwig Teichmann of Kracow, Poland).
- Takayama→Haem**o**chromogen→ **More** value→Described later (in 1912 by Masaeo Takayama, Japan).

Related facts for Teichmann test (of less value).

- Test consists of heating dried blood in the presence of glacial acetic acid and a halide (usually chloride) to form a hematin derivative.
- Place a sample of suspected blood on a microscope slide, add a small amount of chloride-containing glacial acetic acid, and heat.
- Crystals formed are **Hemin** or **Ferri-protoporphyrin chloride**.
- Crytals formed are observed micro-scopically; brown, rhombic.

- Stain age is not a problem in experienced hands.
- Greatest difficulty in performing the test is controlling the heating of sample. Very easy to overheat or underheat the preparation, resulting in failure of crystals to form.
- This problem is removed by Takayama, in which no heating is required (watch out for this fact, as this can form a good MCQ question).

Related facts for Takayama test (of more value):

- Principle: If heme is gently heated with pyridine uner alkaline conditions in the presence of a reducing sugar such as glucose, crystals of **Haemochromogen** or **Pyridine ferroprotoporphyrin** are formed. Note that though heating is not essential (unlike in Teichmann test), gentle heating at 37°C in an incubator, especially in cold weather will hasten reaction.
- This reaction was examined in detail by Takayama. According to him, the mixture that gives best results is:
    - o Water: Saturated glucose solution: Sodium hydroxide (10%): pyridine = 2:1:1:1.
    - o This fact can be asked in an MCQ like this→Which of the following tests for blood uses saturated glucose solution and sodium hydroxide? (a) benzidine (b)Takayama (c) Teichmann (d) Spectroscopy→Answer of course is (b) Takayama.
    - o Another related MCQ could be→ Which of the following is **NOT** a constituent of Takayama reagent? (a) Sodium chloride (b) Glucose (c) Sodium Hydroxide (d) Pyridine → The answer is (a) Sodium chloride. Remember→Sodium chloride is used in Teichmann test, NOT in Takayama test.
    - o A related MCQ on Teichmann test could be→Which of the following reagents is NOT used in Teichmann test? (a) Glacial acetic acid (b) Sodium chloride (c) Sodium hydroxide (d) Both (a) and (c)→The correct answer is (c) Sodium Hydroxide.
- How the Takayama test is conducted?
    - o Place dried stain extract, or powdered material scrapped from the stain on a glass slide and cover with a cover slip.
    - o The cover slip is generally very small (2 millimeters square or even smaller). This allows the test to be carried out on a small stain quantity.
    - o Two or three drops of Takayama's reagent solution are allowed to run in under the cover slip and saturate the sample.
    - o Slide is examined under the microscope after five minutes.
    - o Pink feathery crystals are seen, which confirm presence of hemoglobin.
- The test is effective on aged stains.
- The test gives positive results.
- Most recent improvement of Takayama test has been offered by **A.L.Hatch** in 1993. It is known that oxygen and pyridine compete for the same binding site on the heme molecule. Hatch used Cleland's reagent (dithiothreitol) to reduce this competition and shift the reaction in favor of pyridine. This increases the rate at which hemochromogen crystals are formed.
- Related MCQ on this could be→ Cleland's reagent could be used to accelerate which of the following tests? (a) Teichmann's

test (b) Ammonium molybdate test (c) Florence test (d) Takayama test→ The correct answer is (d) Takayama test.

10. C.

11. A. ***Related fact:*** Benzidine test is merely used for screening of blood. It does not confirm blood. Haemin crystal test confirms blood, but does not give the species. It is the precipitin test which gives the species.

12. D. ***Related facts:***

- Benzidine test is also known as Adlers test, because much of the early forensic work with benzidine was done by Adlers as early as in 1904.
- Color developed is blue, which may eventually turn to brown.
- Occupational Safety and Health Administration (OSHA) recognized benzidine as a carcinogen in 1974, and is thus seldom used in forensic laboratories today.
- O-tolidine is a closely related compound. It is a 3,3′ dimethyl derivative of benzidine. It was also once used as a screening test for blood, but like benzidine, it is also found to be carcinogenic and thus its use has also been stopped now. Since 1992, tetramethylbenzidine (TMB), a 3,3′,5,5′ tetramethyl derivative of benzidine is being used (Figs 29.1 to 29.3).

13. C. ***Related fact:*** At birth newborn has all gamma globulin from his mother. As such Gm and Inv studies are useful in cases of mix up or exchange of babies in hospitals.

14. D. A number of other permutations and combinations of this question may be asked. Inheritance of ABO blood groups can be recapitulated by following table (Table 29.1).

To help solve such questions also remember the following three laws (often known as *Bernstein's laws*):

i. Agglutinogen A or B can not be present in the blood of the child, unless it is present in the blood of one or both its parents.
ii. Parents belonging to group O can not beget a child belonging to group AB and parents belonging to group AB can not beget a child of group O.
iii. If an individual is homozygous for a blood group gene, its product must appear in the blood of *all* his children.

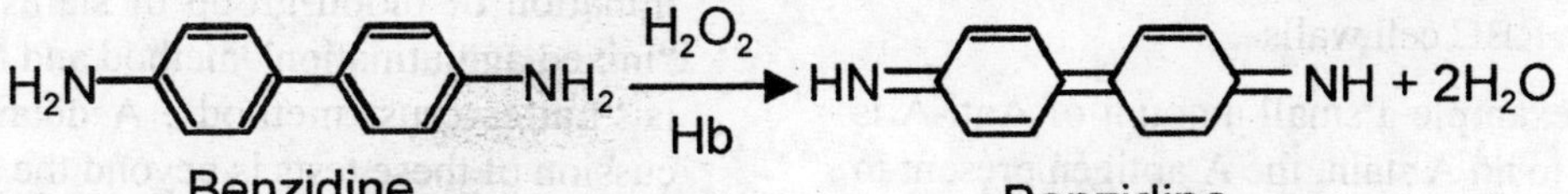

Benzidine (Reduced)

Benzidine (Oxidized)

Fig. 29.1: Benzidine oxidation in the presence of blood

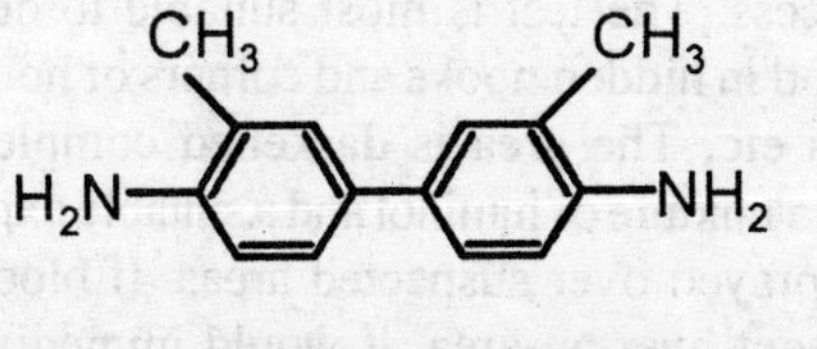

Fig. 29.2: Orthotolidine

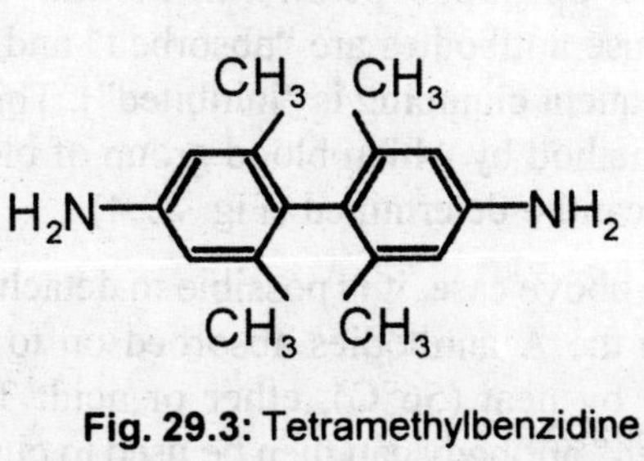

Fig. 29.3: Tetramethylbenzidine

Table 29.1: Blood groups of parents and the possible and impossible blood groups of their children

Blood group of parents		*Blood group of children*	
First parent	*Second parent*	*Possible blood groups*	*Impossible blood groups*
O	O	O	A, B, AB
O	A	O,A	B,AB
O	B	O,B	A,AB
O	AB	A,B	O,AB
A	A	O,A	B,AB
A	B	O,A,B,AB	None
A	AB	A,B,AB	O
B	B	O,B	A,AB
B	AB	A,B,AB	O
AB	AB	A,B,AB	O

Related question: A related question is often asked like this→Bernstein's laws are concerned with (a) Cephalic index (b) Blood groups (c) Dental maturity (d) Postmortem changes. The answer is (b) Blood groups.

15. **B.** When blood dries to form a stain, blood cells – like other cells – dehydrate and their structures are damaged. Since the RBCs are broken in stains, it is not possible to do their blood grouping by conventional methods. Staining is done by indirect methods utilizing the fact that antigens are still sticking to the broken RBC cell walls.

If for example a small amount of Anti-A is added to an A stain, the A antigen present in the broken RBC walls would "absorb" Anti-A, making Anti-A ineffective for subsequent clumping of known group A blood. This is known as "absorption inhibition" test (because antibodies are "absorbed" and the subsequent clumping is "inhibited"). This is one method by which blood group of blood stain can be determined (Fig. 29.4).

In the above case, it is possible to detach (or elute) the A antibodies absorbed on to the stain, by heat (56°C), ether or acid. This "eluted" antibody can then be used to clump known A cells. This is known as "absorption elution" or "acid elution" test. This is the second method of determination of blood group of stains (Fig. 29.5).

By repeating the above two tests by different antisera (Anti A, Anti B and Anti H), blood group of any stain can be determined. Acid elution method is considered to be the best method for determining blood group of stains.

There are two more methods for determination of blood group of stains. One is "mixed agglutination" method and the other is "Lattes crust method". A detailed discussion of these tests is beyond the scope of this book.

16. **D.** ***Related facts:*** Luminol (3-aminophthalhydrazide) has a property of luminescing after oxidation in acid or alkaline solution. Heme group of blood is known to accelerate this process. The test is most suitable to detect blood in hidden nooks and corners of houses, cars etc. The area is darkened completely and a mixture of luminol and a suitable oxidant is sprayed over suspected areas. If blood is present over an area, it would immediately start glowing with a blue-white light. The

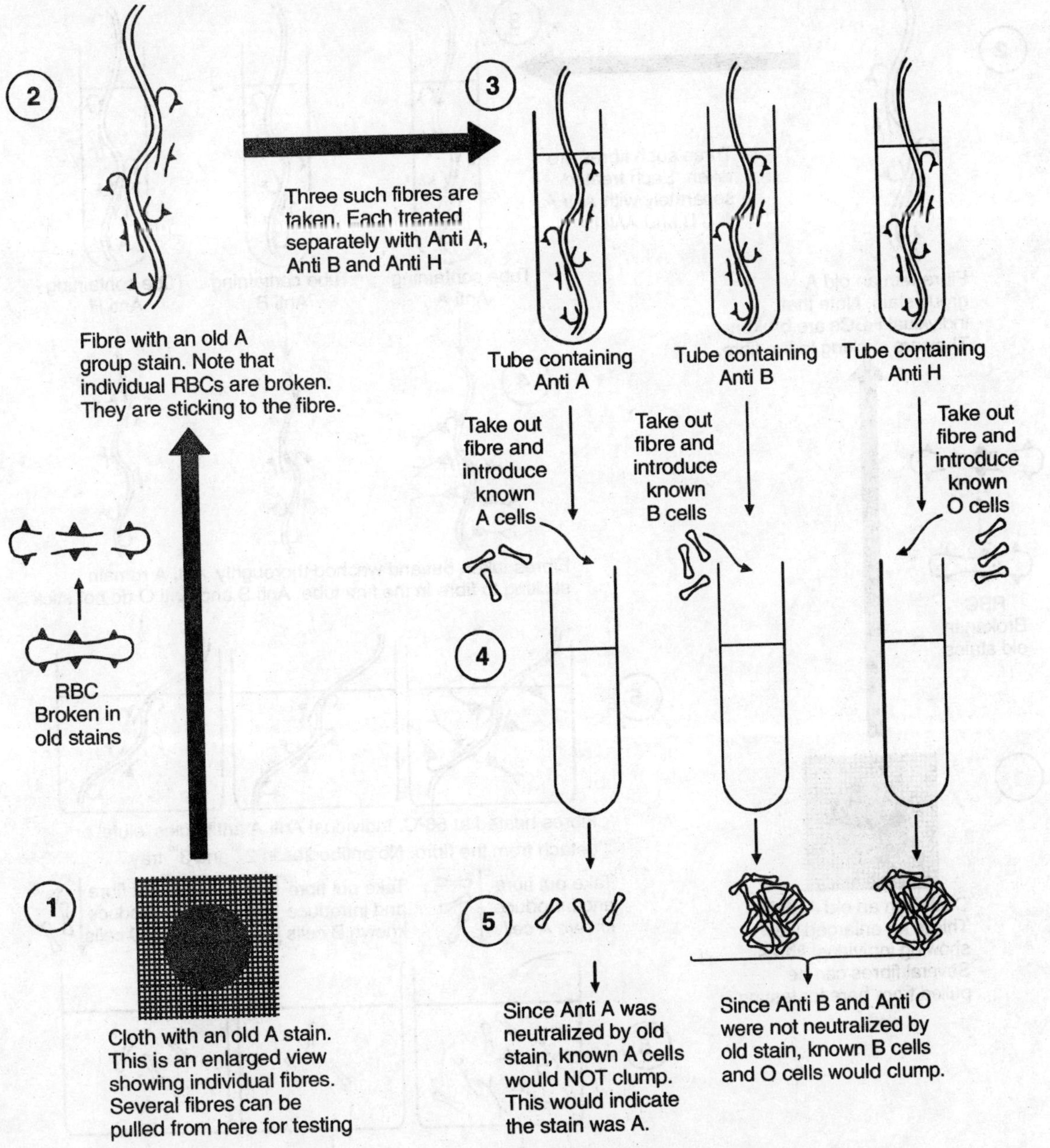

Fig. 29.4: Principle of absorption—inhibition test

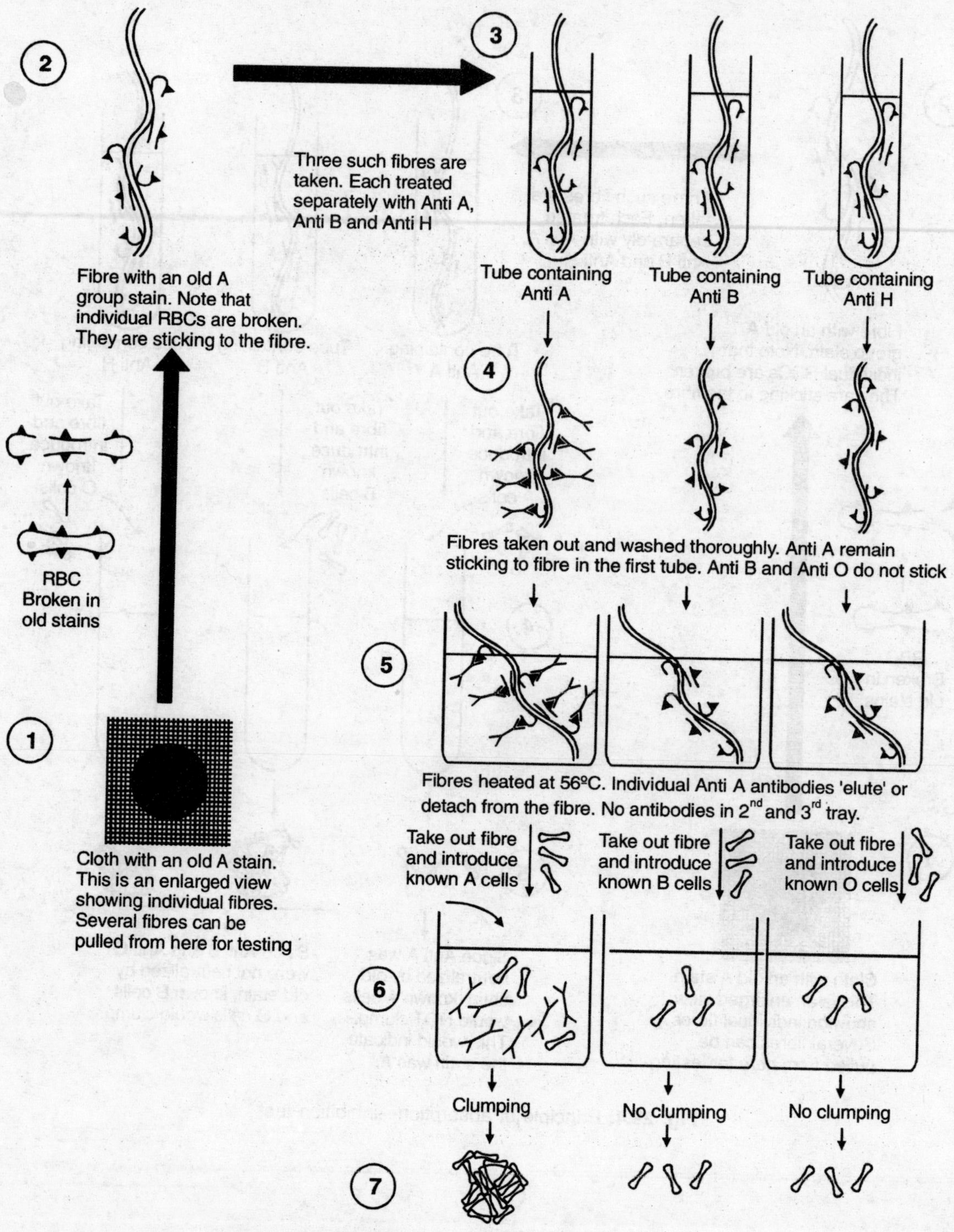

Fig. 29.5: Principle of absorption elution test

test is so sensitive that blood in a dilution of 1 in 5,000,000 can be detected. Thus if the criminal has so thoroughly washed the area, that blood is not visible to the naked eye, luminol test would still show the presence of blood. Since the glow is transient in nature, it is important to record the luminol reaction with photography.

Note: Many students confuse the test with "Luminal". "Luminal" is the trade name of the sedative phenobarbital. Medical students – especially those in forensic medicine – have to remember both terms. The mnemonic to remember them is:

Lumin**a**l : Phenobarbit**a**l.

Lumin**o**l : Bl**o**od.

17. B. ***Related facts:*** Six color tests have been traditionally used by forensic scientists to detect blood stains. All these tests use the peroxidase like activity of heme to knock a nascent oxygen atom off hydrogen peroxide. This nascent oxygen atom brings about a color change in various reagents. These color changes have often been asked in examinations. Here are all color changes (Table 29.2):

Table 29.2: Various screening tests for blood and the colors they give

S.No	Reagent	Color change
1.	**B**enzidine	Intense **B**lue
2.	Ortho-tolidine	blue green
3.	Tetramethylbenzidine (TMB)	Green or blue green
4.	**P**henolphthalein (Kastle –Meyer test)	**P**ink
5.	Leucomalachite green	Bright green
6.	Guaicum	Deep blue

Mnemonic: Remember **B** both for **B**enzidine and **B**lue. Ortho-tolidine and TMB are both related to benzidine so the color is similar (blue green). Remember **P** both for **P**henolphthalein and **p**ink.

Note:

i. Guaicum impregnated paper is also used to detect occult blood in stool. The principle is same.

ii. All color tests mentioned above use hydrogen peroxide.

18. C. ***Note:*** This rather confusing question has stumped students since long. As noted above both benzidine and orthotolidine tests are color tests, which involve hydrogen peroxide. Teichmann's test as such does not use hydrogen peroxide. It involves formation of haemin crystals with glacial acetic acid and sodium chloride. However similar crystals may be obtained from indigo dyed fabrics. To differentiate these from true haemin crystals, a drop of hydrogen peroxide is added, when true haemin crystals will give off bubbles of gas, but false crystals will not. This is because heme group in blood has a peroxidase like activity and it knocks off an oxygen atom from hydrogen peroxide. Luminol test does not use hydrogen peroxide at any stage.

Variant: In some interesting variants of this question—possibly to confuse students—the choices given are like this (a) Benzidine test (b)Phenolphthalein test (c) o-toluidine test (d)Teichmann's test. In this variation (c) o-toluidine becomes the right answer (Note the different spellings of this compound). o-toluidine is a test for chloride ions in water and not for blood. This test does not use hydrogen peroxide and is of no particular interest to forensic scientists.

19. C. The correct answer is Kastle-Meyer test – also known as the Phenolphthalein test. All other tests are confirmatory tests.

Additional info: Students may want to know more about screening tests and confirmatory tests. To understand these tests, the concept of "sensitivity of a test" and "specificity of a test" need to be appreciated.

The **sensitivity of a test** determines the ability of the test to detect blood at very minuscule concentrations. If a test is able to detect blood at extremely low concentrations, it would be called a test with a HIGH SENSITIVITY.

The **specificity of a test** has nothing to do with detection at low concentrations; instead it signifies the ability of the test to come positive ONLY WHEN BLOOD IS PRESENT. If, for example, we take 100 suspicious stains of blood of which the stain was truly of blood only in, say, 63 cases, a test with a very high specificity would be positive only in those 63 cases; in all other cases, it would be negative. A test with lesser specificity may come positive when the stain was other than blood (false positive) or may come negative when the stain was really blood (false negative). In other words a test with a high specificity should ideally have a 0% false positive and a 0% false negative rate.

Tests that are used for screening purposes usually have high sensitivity (99 percent) even at the expense of a low specificity, since once a test result is negative, further testing is usually not done.

Benzidine, Ortho-tolidine, Tetramethylbenzidine (TMB), Phenolphthalein (Kastle–Meyer test), Leucomalachite green and Guaicum tests are *screening tests* of blood, i.e. they are able to detect blood at very low concentrations. They do not have a very high specificity, i.e. they may come positive even when the stain was not really blood.

On the other hand tests like Takayama and Teichmann have a very high specificity (even though they may have a low sensitivity), i.e. they are *confirmatory tests* of blood. These tests come positive ONLY when the stain is that of blood. We of course must know the reason why this is so – because they make crystals of hemoglobin.

A look at the Table 29.3 may also be helpful.

It must be appreciated that for every test **True positive + False negative** is always 100%. Similarly **False positive + True negative** is also always 100%.

A good screening test must have a very high true positive rate, say 99.9%, i.e. it must almost always be able to detect blood when it is present. It is quite possible that such a test may have a high false positive rate also, but that does not really matter, as our main interest is in the fact that true blood stains may not be missed.

A good confirmatory test must have a very low false positive rate, say 0.1%, i.e. it must almost never say the stain is blood, when it actually is not.

An ideal test for blood must have a 100% true positive and a 0% false positive rate. None of the tests mentioned above fulfill these criteria. Such tests are indeed rare.

Table 29.3: The concept of sensitivity and specificity of a test. Refer text for details

	Test says the stain is blood	*Test says the stain is not blood*
The stain is truly of blood	True positive	False negative
The stain is not of blood, but looks like that of blood (say it is a stain of tomato sauce)	False positive	True negative

SEMINAL STAINS

20. C.

21. A. Takayama test is for confirmation of blood.

22. C. Other albuminous materials and even detergents are known to fluoresce under UV light, so fluorescence of seminal stains is NOT specific.

23. D.

24. D. ***Related fact:*** Prostate Specific antigen is also known as PSA or p30 (because it has a molecular weight of about 30 Kilo Daltons). It was identified by Sensabaugh in 1978 as a suitable marker for semen.

It is a glycoprotein with protease activity. PSA is unique to prostatic tissue and is located in the cytoplasm of the prostatic ductal epithelium and in secretions of the ductal lumina. Its concentration in semen varies from 300 to 4200 micrograms per ml with a mean of 1200 micrograms per ml.

Elevated serum PSA concentrations have been associated with prostate cancer and benign prostatic hypertrophy.

It is found in seminal plasma, male urine and male blood, but in **none** of the female tissues or fluids. That is why detection of p30 in the vagina is a reliable indicator of semen.

PSA can be detected by a number of techniques. Main among these are (i) Thin layer immunoassay (ii) Commercially available enzyme linked immunosorbent assays.

25. C. ***Related facts:*** (i) Florence test is not proof of seminal fluid. It only indicates presence of some vegetable or animal substance (ii) Florence test detects choline, which originates from the seminal vesicles, but may originate from a number of other sources (iii) Crystals formed are of choline iodide (iv) Crystals of choline iodide formed in Florence test resemble haemin crystals, but are larger.

26. A.

27. A. ***Related fact:*** A saturated aqueous or alcoholic solution of picric acid when added to seminal fluid gives rise to yellow needle shaped crystals of spermine picrate. This is the Barberio test. It depends on the presence of prostatic secretion.

Florence test is to detect Choline. Dark brown rhombic crystals of choline iodide are formed in this test. Florence test is indicative of seminal fluid.

Following (Table 29.4) about the two most often asked tests of semen will be helpful.

OTHER BIOLOGICAL STAINS

28. B. ***Related facts:*** Edelman test is based on the fact that urobilinogen is present in fecal stains. First urobilinogen is oxidized to urobilin by alcoholic mercuric chloride. In the next stage alcoholic zinc chloride is added. If urobilin has been formed it would form a zinc-urobilin complex, which gives a green fluorescence.

Table 29.4: Two most commonly asked tests for semen

Test	*Reagent used*	*Chemical nature of crystals formed*	*Shape and color of crystals*	*Crystals are due to the presence of*
Florence test	Florence solution (Potassium iodide, iodine and water)	Choline iodide	Dark brown rhombic	Choline which comes from Seminal vesicles
Barberio test	A saturated aqueous or alcoholic solution of picric acid	Spermine picrate	Yellow needle shaped	Spermine from prostatic secretion

29. A. *Related facts:* Presence of urea, creatinine or amines is presumptive evidence of presence of urine. In the presence of picric acid and a weak base, creatinine would give a bright-red coloration. This is the so called Jaffe reaction.

MULTIPLE ANSWER TYPE (PGI, CHANDIGARH PATTERN)

30. A,B,D,E. *Related facts:* Sometimes in criminal investigations, it may become necessary to tell that a given stain was menstrual in origin. Alleged rape and sexual assaults, for example, may involve the question whether bloodstains were caused by menstruation bleeding or by injury. Following facts must be taken into account to determine this:

i. Menstrual blood is lower in pH, i.e. it is more acidic (owing to the presence of vaginal secretions).

ii. It contains vaginal, cervical and decidual cells.

iii. Menstrual blood does not coagulate. It is because it has already coagulated within the uterine cavity and has again become fluid. It contains fibrinolysins. Fibrinogen degradation products (FDP) are also present in relatively high concentration in menstrual blood. These can be detected immunologically by haemagglutination inhibition technique. If sheep RBC coated by fibrinogen are mixed with serum containing antifibrinogen they would agglutinate. But this reaction is inhibited if the antibody has already reacted with fibrinogen or fibrinogen degradation products (FDP), as in menstrual blood.

The concentration of FDP is also higher in postmortem blood. To differentiate between menstrual and postmortem blood myoglobin concentration may be done, which is higher in postmortem blood but lower in menstrual blood.

Table 29.5: Differentiation between peripheral blood, menstrual blood and post mortem blood

	FDP-D dimer concentration	Myoglobin concentration
Peripheral blood	Low	Low
Menstrual blood	High	Low
Postmortem blood	High	High

In general:

- The mean FDP-D dimer concentration in menstrual bloodstains is about 200 times higher than in peripheral bloodstains.
- The mean myoglobin content in postmortem bloodstains is about 4000 times higher than in menstrual bloodstains.

It must be realized that seminal fluid has fibrinolytic activity too. Thus the presence of seminal fluid in a blood stain must be excluded.

iv. Menstrual blood is more fluid than ordinary blood, because, during its trickling descent, it becomes mixed with uterine and vaginal mucus.

v. There are five isozymes of lactate dehydrogenase (LDH), namely LDH-1, LDH-2, LDH-3, LDH-4 and LDH-5. Venous blood primarily consists of just LDH-1, LDH-2 and LDH-3, while menstrual blood contains all five isozymes. Furthermore, menstrual blood shows far less amounts of LDH-1 and LDH-2 than blood from other sources.

vi. Matrix metalloproteinases (MMP) are present in endometrium, but not in peripheral blood. This fact has recently been exploited in determination of menstrual origin of blood. Matrix metalloproteinases are zinc-dependent endopeptidases involved in the breakdown of extracellular matrix components and expressed when tissue degradation and remodeling is required. This includes physiological conditions like menstruation, as well as pathological conditions like invasive tumor growth or wound healing.

vii. Large number of microorganisms may be found, which are not found in ordinary blood [e.g. *Trichomonas vaginalis*, monilia, Doderlein's bacillus (*Lactobacillus acidophilus*)]. It is important to realize that it is the latter that metabolizes glycogen (of vaginal epithelium) to lactic acid, giving an acidic pH to vaginal secretions, which in turn gives an acidic reaction to menstrual blood.

PART 2
TOXICOLOGY

8 GENERAL PRINCIPLES RELATING TO POISONS

30 Introduction and Law Relating to Poisons

1. The science that studies poisons in all its aspects is known as:
A. Poisonology
B. Venomology
C. Toxicology
D. All of the above

2. The word "toxicology" comes from:
A. An Egyptian word meaning "killing shrewdly"
B. A Roman word meaning "poisons"
C. A Greek word meaning a bow
D. A Sanskrit word meaning "bitter substance"

3. The use of toxicology to aid medicolegal investigation of death and poisoning is known as:
A. Clinical toxicology
B. Biotoxicology
C. Police toxicology
D. Forensic toxicology

4. The scientific analysis of the effects of toxic chemicals on cultured bacteria or mammalian cells is known as:
A. *In vitro* toxicology
B. *In vivo* toxicology
C. Mammalian toxicology
D. Bacterio-mammalian toxicology

5. Which of the following poisons was historically used as an "ordeal" poison?
A. Marking nut
B. Calabar bean
C. Ergot
D. Arsenic

6. Which of the following is usually regarded as the father of toxicology?
A. Hippocrates
B. Galen
C. Sushruta
D. Orfila

7. A toxin that is injected by an animal into its prey to produce a harmful effect is best known as:
A. Poison
B. Toxin
C. Venom
D. Toxalbumen

8. Toxinology is the study of:
A. Poisonous effects of insect stings
B. Poisonous effects of mushrooms and plants
C. Poisonous effects of venomous snakes
D. All of the above

9. The *Drugs and Cosmetics Act, 1940:*
A. Gives the power to the manufacturer to fix the maximum price of the drug
B. Bans advertisements of drugs having a profound sexual content

C. Controls the manufacture, sale and distribution of drugs
D. Prescribes very harsh punishment for illegally importing narcotic drugs

10. **Narcotic Drugs and Psychotropic Substances Act was passed in the year:**
A. 1981
B. 1983
C. 1985
D. 1986

11. **Under the *Drugs and Cosmetic Rules, 1945*, a schedule H drug means:**
A. Antibiotics, antihistaminics and other chemotherapeutic agents
B. Drugs and poisons to be sold only on the prescription of a registered medical practitioner
C. All vaccines and sera
D. All biological and special products

12. **The object of which of the following acts is to allow only the registered pharmacists to compound, prepare, mix or dispense medicines on the prescription of a medical practitioner?**
A. The Pharmacy Act 1948
B. The Drugs Control Act 1950
C. Narcotic Drugs and Psychotropic Substances Act 1985
D. The Drugs and Cosmetics Act 1940

13. **Which of the following Acts provides for the issue of cash memo for sale, marking of prices, and exhibiting list of prices of various drugs?**
A. Poisons Act 1919
B. The Drugs and Cosmetic Act 1940
C. The Pharmacy Act 1948
D. The Drugs Control Act 1950

14. **The object of which of the following acts is to ban advertisements which offend decency or morality?**
A. The Drugs and Cosmetic Act 1940
B. The Pharmacy Act 1948
C. The Drugs and Magic Remedies Act 1954
D. The Drugs Control Act 1950

15. **Salicylic acid is usually classified as:**
A. A mineral acid
B. A neurotic poison
C. A cardiac poison
D. An organic acid

16. **Which of the following class of poisons generates a strong desire to sleep?**
A. Inebriant poisons
B. Somniferous poisons
C. Deliriant poisons
D. Neurotic poisons
E. Spinal poisons

17. **Brown discoloration of the mucosa of the stomach is seen in poisoning with:**
A. Mercury
B. Nitric acid
C. HCN
D. Datura

18. **Extensive necrosis of proximal convoluted tubules (PCT necrosis) is seen in:**
A. Heavy metal poisoning
B. Chloroform
C. Oxalic acid
D. All of the above

19. **Odorless poisoning is due to:**
A. Phenol
B. Phosphorus
C. Cyanide
D. Calotropis

MULTIPLE ANSWER TYPE (PGI, CHANDIGARH PATTERN)

20. **Which of the following facts are correct about parasuicide?**
A. It is committing suicide after committing a murder
B. The most common mode of parasuicide is ingestion of drugs

C. It is a term applied when two or more persons commit suicide in a joint pact
D. It is not a true suicide, but just an apparent attempt at suicide
E. It is also known as "deliberate self harm"

21. Which of the following qualities must be present in an ideal homicidal poison?
A. It should have an attractive color
B. It should have no odor
C. It should produce its effect immediately
D. It should mimic the symptoms of a disease
E. It should be undetectable in the dead body

22. Which of the following poisons classically mimic the symptoms of a natural disease?
A. Strychnos nux vomica
B. Hydrochloric acid
C. Arsenic
D. Organophosphorus
E. White phosphorus

23. Which of the following are stupefying poisons?
A. Datura
B. Arsenic
C. Cannabis
D. Strychnos nux vomica
E. Chloral hydrate

24. Characteristics of ideal suicidal poison are:
A. It should produce painful death
B. Should be easily available
C. Should be cheap
D. Should be minimally toxic
E. Should be bitter in taste

25. Which of the following may be considered as ideal suicidal poisons?
A. Hydrochloric acid
B. Barbiturates
C. Strychnos nux vomica
D. Opium
E. Cannabis indica

26. Under the *Drugs and Cosmetic Act, 1940*, the definition of cosmetic includes:
A. Cleansing agent
B. Beautifying agent
C. Agent for promoting attractiveness
D. Soap
E. Nail polish

ANSWERS

1. **C.**

2. **C.** The word "toxicology" comes from the Greek word *toxon* which means a bow for shooting arrows. The word *toxeuma* meant an arrow. Since in ancient times, poisons were often used on the tips of arrows to render them more lethal, the word *toxicos* came to refer to such a poison. The Greek word *logos* means "the study of" or "the science of". Combining the two Greek words, we get the word *toxicology*.

3. **D.**

4. **A.** ***Additional info***: *In vitro* (literally 'in glass') testing methods are employed primarily to identify potentially hazardous chemicals and/or to confirm the lack of certain toxic properties in the early stages of the development of potentially useful new substances such as therapeutic drugs, agricultural chemicals and direct food additives. Most toxicologists believe that *in vitro* toxicity testing methods can be a useful, time- and cost-effective supplement to toxicology studies in living animals (which are termed "*in vivo*" or "in life" methods). However, it is generally accepted that the available *in vitro* tests are not presently adequate to entirely replace animal toxicology tests.

5. **B.** Calabar bean is the common name of *Physostigma venenosum*. It contains a deadly poison physostigmine. It was historically used as an "ordeal poison", i.e. to differentiate between a guilty and an innocent person. If a guilty person ate its bean, he would die, but if an innocent person took it, he would vomit and be saved. The reasoning is obviously flawed, yet the natives of Africa employ this bean for this purpose till date. They call it eséré. People were so confident in the accuracy of the test that suspects would voluntarily take an emulsion of the seed to prove their innocence.

6. **D.** ***Additional info***: His full name was Mathieu Joseph Bonaventure Orfila (1787-1853). He was a French toxicologist.

7. **C.** The important difference between a poison and a venom is that while a poison must be ingested to produce a harmful effect, a venom must be injected. A fish when ingested may be a cause of poisoning but may not have any poisonous apparatus to inject a venom into its enemy. Such a fish is poisonous but not venomous. On the contrary a fish may have a poisonous apparatus to inject venom into its prey, but may not be poisonous to eat. Such a fish is venomous but not poisonous. A fish can be both venomous and poisonous.

8. **D.** Toxinology is a subdiscipline of toxicology. It studies *biological exposures*, such as insect stings, poisonous mushrooms and plants, venomous snakes and aquatic life. In other words, it refers to the study of poisons produced by living organisms.

9. **C.** The *Drugs and Cosmetics Act, 1940* controls the manufacture, sale and distribution of drugs. This is specifically written in the Act itself in the beginning under the title "Comments".

10. **C.**

11. **B.** ***Additional info**: Under Drugs and Cosmetic Rules, 1945,* there are a total of 25 schedules (From Schedule A till Schedule Y). Each schedule gives some important legal information about drugs and cosmetics. A

few of these are important to medical personnel.

Schedule H drugs under the *Drugs and Cosmetic Rules, 1945* means drugs and poisons to be sold only on the prescription of a registered medical practitioner. Other choices fall under different schedules.

According to rule 97 (1) (b) of the *Drugs and Cosmetic Rules, 1945*, all Schedule H drugs have to be labeled with the symbol **Rx** and conspicuously displayed on the left top corner of the label and be also labelled with the following words:

Schedule H Drug – Warning: To be sold by retail on the prescription of a Registered Medical Practitioner only.

Some important drugs falling under schedule H are alprazolam, analgin, antibiotics, barbituric acid and its derivatives, cimetidine, dapsone its salts and derivatives, heparin and insulin etc.

Two other schedules (G and X) important from a medicolegal angle are:

Schedule G: All drugs mentioned under the schedule have to be labelled as follows:

Caution: it is dangerous to take this preparation except under medical supervision.

These words must be conspicuously printed and surrounded by a line within which there shall be no other words.

Some important drugs falling under schedule G are chlorpropamide and its salts, ethosuximide, glibenclamide and phenformin.

Schedule X: Schedule X contains drugs which though are used therapeutically, are also potential drugs of abuse. Some examples are amobarbital, amphetamine, ethchlorvynol, glutethimide, methaqualone, phencyclidine and phenometrazine.

According to rule 97 (1) (d) of the *Drugs and Cosmetic Rules, 1945*, all Schedule X drugs have to be labeled with the symbol **XRx** which shall be in red conspicuously displayed on the left top corner of the label and be also labeled with the following words:

Schedule X Drug – Warning: To be sold by retail on the prescription of a Registered Medical Practitioner only.

It is a general belief among students that only schedule H drugs have to be labelled like this. **This is not correct**. *Both schedule H and schedule X drugs have to be labelled as above*. In general, schedule X drugs are *more* dangerous than schedule H drugs.

An important MCQ based on this information may be asked as follows:

Qu: Under the *Drugs and Cosmetic Rules 1945*, drugs in which of the following schedules have to be labelled with the warning "To be sold by retail on the prescription of a Registered Medical Practitioner only"?

(a) Schedule G drugs (b) Schedule H drugs (c) Schedule X drugs (d) both (b) and (c) above.

Most students are likely to tick (b), but the correct choice is (d).

It is an important exercise for medical students to go to the hospital pharmacy (or a private pharmacist shop) and ask the pharmacist there to show him some schedule G, H and X drugs.

As this author found out during his student days, the pharmacist would be very happy to do this, and the student would gain important insights and practical information looking at the labels.

Some other important schedules are:

Schedule C: Biological and special products (e.g. insulin, pituitary extract).

Schedule E(1): List of poisonous substances under the Ayurvedic (including Siddha) and Unani system of medicine (e.g. *Datura, Abrus precatorius, Conium maculatum*).

Schedule F(1): This schedule containing vaccines, antisera and diagnostic antigens is of interest to veterinarians only. According to rule 78 of *Drugs and Cosmetic Rules 1945*, license to manufacture or sell these products would be given only under some special circumstances and if some particular conditions have been fulfilled. Schedule F(1) is divided in four parts (Parts I till Parts IV).

Part I mentions vaccines e.g. Rabies vaccine, Ranikhet disease vaccine (living)[1], Rinderpest lapinised vaccine (living)[2], Swine fever vaccine lapinised and canine hepatitis vaccine (living). As can easily be seen, **all** vaccines under this schedule are of interest to veterinarians only (the rabies vaccine meant in this part is meant for dogs). The schedule also gives detailed guidelines on the preparation, standards, storage and labelling of these vaccines. For instance, rabies vaccine (living) should be stored at 2° to 4° Celsius only.

Part II mentions antisera such as anti-anthrax serum and anti-fowl-cholera serum.

[1]Synonymous with Newcastle disease vaccine (Living). Ranikhet disease or Newcastle disease affects birds, and is caused by a Paramyxovirus. In 1926 a ship from the Far East docked at Newcastle-Upon-Tyne (England). Some leftovers from the ship containing chicken carcasses was fed to local chickens, which all died from the deadly new disease.
The disease was first reported from Java in 1926 but outbreaks were soon reported from Newcastle in Britain, Ranikhet in India and Colombo in Sri Lanka. It soon spread, either naturally or by being transported between countries in refrigerated meat. It now has world-wide distribution.

[2]Synonymous with Rabbit Adapted Cattle Plague Vaccine (living) Lapinised.

Part III mentions diagnostic antigens such as Brucella abortus plain antigen.
Just like vaccines, all antisera and diagnostic antigens mentioned under this schedule are meant for veterinarians only.

Part IV does not contain any products. Just gives some general comments about the drugs above.

Schedule J: List of diseases and ailments for the cure of which no drug should be advertised (e.g. AIDS, obesity, paralysis, leucoderma, premature ageing, improvement in vision).

12. A. It is useful to remember that this Act does not apply to the dispensing by a doctor for his own patients.

13. D.

14. C.

15. D. It is an organic acid. Some other organic acids are oxalic acid, carbolic acid and acetic acid.

16. B.

17. B.

18. D. Proximal Tubule (PT) consists of an initial convoluted portion (the proximal convoluted tubule or PCT) and a straight portion (the pars recta). The length of PT in humans is 14 mm (as compared to that of distal convoluted tubule which is just 1 mm). PCTs are physically located in the cortex. PCTs as well as the pars recta, are qualitatively differentiated from the remainder of the nephron and collecting duct by their lumenal brush border, which can be recognized in routine H&E stains.

Proximal tubular toxins frequently affect both convoluted (PCT) and straight segments (the pars recta). The injury is caused via three main mechanisms. The mechanisms along with the toxins are as follows:

1. **Direct perturbation of Cell or Subcellular Organelle Function**
   a. Aminoglycosides→Gentamicin
   b. Heavy Metals
      i. Cadmium
      ii. Mercury
      iii. Lead.
2. **Xenobiotics that cause Injury via Metabolic Activation with or without Organic Ion Transport.** Here the chemical introduced in the body is not toxic as such, but liberates toxic by products, usually via microsomal MFOs (Mixed Function Oxidases). That is why the toxicity of these chemicals is reduced by agents which inhibit MFOs (e.g. piperonyl butoxide) and increased by agents which stimulate MFOs (e.g. polybrominated biphenyls)
   a. Organohalides
      i. Chloroform
   b. Cephalosporins and other beta-lactam antibiotics
   c. Mycotoxins
      i. Ochratoxin A (incidentally Ochratoxin A is incriminated as the cause of Balkan nephropathy, which is an important syndrome in Eastern Europe)
      ii. Fumosin-B
   d. Halogenated Alkenes
      i. Hexachloro-1,3-butadiene
      ii. Tetrafluoroethylene
      iii. Chlorotrifluoroethylene
      iv. Trichloroethylene
      v. Dichlorovinyl cysteine
   e. Cisplatin
3. **Xenobiotics perturbing cellular, interstitial, or Lumenal Substrate**
   a. Phosphate
   b. Iron
   c. Zinc
   d. Ethylene glycol
   e. Oxalate/oxalic acid
   f. Amino acid toxicity—Lysinoalanine (usually found in processed foods meant for human consumption) and Lysine. An amino acid, which is of interest here is D-serine. It induces necrosis which is restricted to pars recta (PCT is not affected by D-serine, but is mentioned just for completeness).

19. D. ***Related facts*:** All other poisonings are associated with typical smell. Phenol has a characteristic sickly sweet smell, phosphorus has the garlic smell and cyanide has the odor of bitter almonds.

MULTIPLE ANSWER TYPE (PGI, CHANDIGARH PATTERN)

20. B,D,E. ***Related facts*:** Other names for parasuicide are *pseudocide* and "*suicidal gesture*". Parasuicide is an apparent attempt at suicide, in which the aim and intent is NOT death. It is aimed merely at frightening the relatives, as when they do not allow a teenager to marry a person of his/her choice. It can be 'a cry for help', the person feeling this is the only way that his/her level of distress is recognised. Most common method is ingesting a sublethal drug overdose, although wrist slash is also used often. Previous parasuicide is a predictor of suicide.

21. B,D,E. An ideal homicidal poison should be colorless, odorless and tasteless. It must produce its effect quite late, otherwise, the poisoner may be immediately under suspicion.

22. A,C,E. *Strychnos nux vomica* mimics tetanus; arsenic, cholera and white phosphorus, acute yellow atrophy of the liver.

23. A,C,E.

24. B,C. An ideal suicidal poison should produce a painless death. It should be highly toxic so that it kills rapidly. Although taste is of no consequence, an ideal suicidal poison should be tasteless or should have a pleasant taste.

25. B,D. Deaths with hydrochloric acid and *Strychnos nux vomica* are very painful, so these poisons are not preferred by suicides. *Cannabis indica* does not cause death, unless taken in extremely large quantities. Opium and barbiturates produce sleep early, so they may be considered as ideal suicidal poisons.

26. A,B,C,D,E. *All answers are correct.* Cosmetic is defined under section 3(aaa) of the Drugs and Cosmetic Act 1940. It means *any article intended to be rubbed, poured sprinkled or sprayed on, or introduced into, or otherwise applied to, the human body or any part thereof for cleansing, beautifying, promoting attractiveness, or altering the appearance, and includes any article intended for use as a component of cosmetic.*

Most texts taught in this country would have us believe that soap is *not* included in the definition of cosmetic (consequently many students are not likely to tick choice (D) and they would be wrong). Indeed, before 1982 soap was not included in the definition of cosmetic, but in that year by *Drugs and Cosmetics (Amendment) Act, 1982*, soap was also included. This amendment came into force on 13 November 1982.

31 General Principles of Treatment

1. Substances which oxidise poisons and thus render them inactive may be called:
- **A.** Mechanical antidotes
- **B.** Chelating agents
- **C.** Chemical antidotes
- **D.** Physiological antidotes
- **E.** None of the above

2. Which one of the following is a mechanical antidote?
- **A.** Animal charcoal
- **B.** Tannic acid
- **C.** Nalorphine
- **D.** BAL

3. The usual dose of activated charcoal, when used as an antidote for poisoning, is:
- **A.** 2-4 g
- **B.** 15-20 g
- **C.** 50-100 g
- **D.** 400-500 g

4. Which of the following facts regarding treatment of poisoning is NOT CORRECT?
- **A.** The most useful and harmless household emetic is a saturated solution of common salt
- **B.** Ipecac Fluid extract should NEVER be used for inducing emesis
- **C.** Syrup of Ipecac is the most useful household emetic
- **D.** Apomorphine as an emetic is NOT effective orally

5. The usual emetic dose of syrup of ipecac in the adults is:
- **A.** 2 ml
- **B.** 10 ml
- **C.** 30 ml
- **D.** 45 ml

6. Gastric lavage is contraindicated in .... poisoning:
- **A.** Kerosene
- **B.** Carbolic acid
- **C.** Alcohol
- **D.** Salicylate

7. Which of the following statements is not true?
- **A.** Apomorphine given as an emetic is NOT effective orally
- **B.** Syrup of Ipecac may be effective as an emetic even in antiemetic poisoning such as that by phenothiazines
- **C.** Syrup of Ipecac should NEVER be followed by a drink of water, as it may cause fulminant vomiting causing rupture of oesophagus
- **D.** Ipecac can produce toxic effects on the heart because of its content of emetine

8. The usual emetic dose of apomorphine in adults is:
- **A.** .06 mg

B. 0.6 mg
C. 6 mg
D. 60 mg

9. **Rumack-Matthew Nomogram is used in the evaluation of toxicity and planning of treatment in which of the following poisonings?**
A. Acetaminophen
B. Cyanide
C. Digitalis
D. Organophosphorus insecticides

10. **The usual fatal dose in terms of tablets of paracetamol (each weighing 500 mg) is:**
A. 10-20 tablets
B. 40-50 tablets
C. 70-80 tablets
D. 100-120 tablets

11. A female accidentally takes 100 tablets of paracetamol, and is brought 4 hours after ingestion. The most appropriate line of action would be
A. Immediate gastric lavage with activated charcoal
B. Administration of N-acetylcysteine
C. Hemodialysis
D. Forced alkaline diuresis

12. **Which of the following is the ideal tube for performing gastric lavage?**
A. Ewald's tube
B. Ryle's tube
C. Lavacuator
D. Foley's catheter

13. **In which of the following poisonings, hemodialysis may not be useful?**
A. Methanol
B. Diazepam
C. Aspirin
D. Paracetamol

14. **In which of the following poisonings, forced alkaline diuresis would NOT be helpful?**
A. Mecoprop
B. Chlorpropamide
C. Phenobarbitone
D. Amphetamine

15. **In which of the following poisonings, forced acidic diuresis would NOT be helpful?**
A. Phencyclidine
B. Methadone
C. Carbamates
D. Cocaine

ANTIDOTES

16. **Which of the following facts about BAL is INCORRECT?**
A. Lead is chelated extracellularly by BAL, but NOT intracellularly
B. In G-6-PD-deficient patients BAL may induce hemolysis
C. BAL cannot be given to persons with known allergy to peanuts
D. BAL should never be administered simultaneously with medicinal iron as the combination is toxic

DUTIES OF MEDICAL PRACTITIONERS

17. **In a case of homicidal poisoning, the first duty of a doctor is to:**
A. Inform the police
B. Call the magistrate to record dying declaration
C. Treat the poisoning
D. Inform the relatives

18. **Medical practitioner should inform the police, if the poisoning is:**
A. Homicidal
B. Accidental
C. Suicidal
D. All of the above

19. The doctor should preserve the following pieces of evidences in cases of suspected poisoning:
- **A.** Suspected articles of food, vomit, excreta etc.
- **B.** Any recent stains on bedclothes, furniture etc.
- **C.** Full or empty bottles, paper packets, unused capsules or liquids lying around
- **D.** All of the above

20. In a case of suspected poisoning when the doctor decides to do stomach wash, the first washing should always be done with:
- **A.** The specific antidote
- **B.** Plain water
- **C.** Potassium permanganate
- **D.** Hydrogen peroxide

MULTIPLE ANSWER TYPE (PGI, CHANDIGARH PATTERN)

21. Which of the following poisons are NOT well adsorbed by activated charcoal?
- **A.** Alcohols
- **B.** Aspirin
- **C.** Caustics
- **D.** Barbiturates
- **E.** Lithium

22. General principles of management of poisoning include:
- **A.** Removal of unabsorbed poison from the body
- **B.** Administration of antidotes
- **C.** Administration of analeptic agents
- **D.** Elimination of absorbed poison by enhanced excretion
- **E.** Administration of carbon dioxide to stimulate respiratory centre, which may be depressed due to poison

23. Elimination of poison by enhanced excretion is achieved by:
- **A.** Extracorporeal Bone marrow clearance
- **B.** Peritoneal dialysis
- **C.** Charcoal haemoperfusion
- **D.** Silicate haemoperfusion
- **E.** Whole bowel irrigation

24. Which of the following facts about gastric lavage are TRUE?
- **A.** Gastric lavage must be undertaken irrespective of the fact whether the patient has ingested a toxic or a non-toxic agent
- **B.** Endotracheal intubation must be done prior to gastric lavage in a comatosed patient
- **C.** The length of the tube to be inserted is 100 cm
- **D.** Gastric lavage must be performed even if the patient does not give consent
- **E.** The preferred route of insertion is nasal

25. Coma cocktail consists of:
- **A.** Thiamine
- **B.** Physostigmine
- **C.** Dextrose
- **D.** Picrotoxin
- **E.** Naloxone

26. Which of the following are duties of a medical practitioner in a case of suspected poisoning?
- **A.** Inform neighbors about the poisoning
- **B.** Carefully observe and record symptoms in relation to food
- **C.** Preserve suspected articles, excreta and stomach wash
- **D.** Preserve stomach wash only, as other evidences are not permissible in law
- **E.** Request the patient to go to police and lodge an FIR, and start treatment only after that

27. Which of the following drugs may be helpful in a case of paracetamol ingestion?
- **A.** Methionine
- **B.** Aspirin
- **C.** N-acetylcysteine
- **D.** Ethyl alcohol
- **E.** Cysteamine

ANSWERS

1. C.
2. A.
3. C. ***Related fact:*** Activated charcoal is a fine, black powder that is odorless, tasteless, and nontoxic. It is often given after gastric lavage (and not before). It is considered to be the single most effective agent available today. The usual adult dose 50-100 g mixed in about 8 ounces of water (this is about the volume of one average bottle of cold drink. 1 ounce is 30 ml). The pediatric dose is 1 g/kg.

   Activated charcoal is not the same thing as burnt toast as many students believe. It is prepared by a special technique – destructive distillation of such substances as wood, pulp, bone, starch, petroleum, lactose, sucrose and coconut shells.

   (Destructive distillation is a process by which organic substances such as these are decomposed by heat in the *absence of air* and distilled to produce useful products such as oils and gases. These portions are collected separately as they are driven off. Wood, for example, when treated in this way yields acetic acid, methyl or wood alcohol, charcoal, and a number of hydrocarbons. Coal yields coal gas, coal tar, ammonia, and coke).

   This process opens up millions of tiny pores between the carbon atoms.

   Activated charcoal is good at trapping other carbon-based impurities ("organic" chemicals), as well as single molecules like chlorine. Many other chemicals are not attracted to carbon at all – e.g. sodium, nitrates, etc. – so they pass right through. This property is incidentally exploited in industry in charcoal based filters. An activated charcoal filter will remove certain impurities while ignoring others. Once all the bonding sites are filled, an activated charcoal filter stops working. At that point one must replace the filter.

   Surface area of activated charcoal is very large (about 1000 squre meters/g) allowing it to *adsorb* (not absorb) large quantities of poisons on its surface. Super-activated charcoal (Super-Char) has a surface area of about 2500-3000 square meters/g. Compare this with the area of a soccer field, which is about 7300 square meters.

   The word *adsorb* is important here. When a material adsorbs something, it attaches to it by *chemical attraction* (absorption on the other hand is *physical* in nature). The huge surface area of activated charcoal gives it countless bonding sites. When poisons pass next to the carbon surface, they attach to the surface and are trapped.
4. A. ***Related fact:*** Saturated solution of common salt can cause hypernatremia and is considered very dangerous to use as an emetic. There is a difference between **Ipecac Fluid Extract** and **syrup of Ipecac.** Ipecac Fluid extract is 14 times more potent and may cause fatalities. It (Ipecac Fluid extract) is NEVER used as an emetic. Apomorphine is **NOT** effective orally and must be given parenterally, usually by the subcutaneous route.
5. C. ***Related fact:*** In children from 6 months till 12 years, it is 15 ml.
6. A. ***Related facts:*** Gastric lavage in kerosene poisoning may cause aspiration of kerosene in the respiratory tract setting up fulminant chemical pneumonitis. Other contraindications of gastric lavage are:
   - Corrosives except carbolic acid (because stomach wall becomes thick and leathery in carbolic acid). This is

the only absolute contraindication; rest all are relative contraindications.

- Children→relative contraindication, because stomach wash tube is too thick.
- Hypothermia→relative contraindication, because body temperature would need careful attention.
- Comatose conditions→because it can cause aspiration. Can be done with a cuffed endotracheal tube in place.
- Convulsive poisonings (e.g. strychnine)→because it can exacerbate convulsions. Convulsions need be controlled first.
- Volatile poisons→Can cause aspiration pneumonitis.

7. C. ***Related fact:*** Apomorphine is indeed not effective orally. It has to be given parenterally, usually by the subcutaneous route. Syrup of Ipecac acts both on CTZ, as well as on gastric mucosa, so it may be useful in antiemetic poisoning. Syrup of Ipecac is usually followed by by a drink of water because emesis may not occur when the stomach is empty.

8. C. ***Related fact:*** In the children it is 0.06 mg/kg.

9. A. ***Related fact:*** Acetaminophen is a para-aminophinol derivative. Also known as Paracetamol in India. In USA, more often known as acetaminophen. This nomogram plots plasma concentration on the Y-axis and "hours after ingestion" on the X-axis. The X-axis scale is linear, while Y-axis scale is logarithmic. There is slope from upper left to lower right (Fig. 31.1). Patients falling on the upper right half have a chance of hepatotoxicity and hence should be treated with the antidote N-acetyl cysteine (NAC). Patients falling in the lower left half are safe. Figure 31.1 shows that NAC is started as soon as the

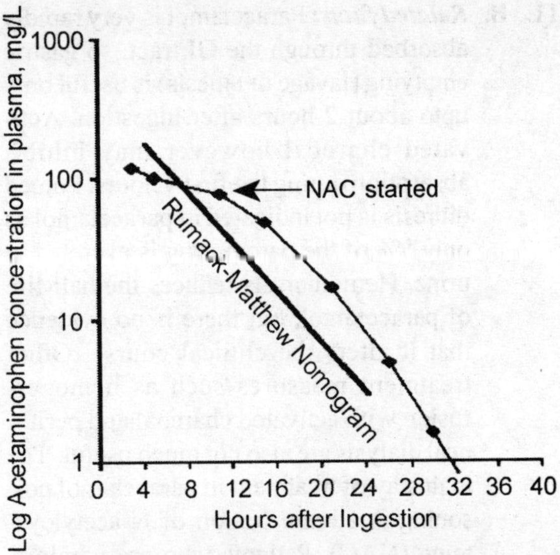

Fig. 31.1: Rumack Matthew nomogram

plasma concentration of acetaminophen crosses over to the right side of the nomogram.

10. B. ***Related info:*** The usual fatal dose is 20-25 g. Remember the following additional facts:

- Paracetamol is more dangerous in alcoholics, so they succumb at lower doses
- 20 tablets in normal persons may produce severe hepatotoxicity
- Children under the age of 10 years appear more resistant to toxic effects of paracetamol.
- Paracetamol produces liver toxicity by producing the metabolite N-acetyl-p-benzoquinoneimine (NAPQI), which is a strong oxidising agent. It binds covalently to hepatocytes, causing liver necrosis and occasionally to renal cells causing renal damage. It is normally detoxified by conjugation with reduced glutathione and excreted in the urine as mercapturic acid and cysteine conjugates.

11. B. ***Related facts:*** Paracetamol is very rapidly absorbed through the GI tract, so gastric emptying (lavage or emesis) is useful only upto about 2 hours after ingestion. Activated charcoal however may inhibit absorption during the first 4 hours. Forced diuresis is not indicated in paracetamol as only 5% of the parent drug is excreted in urine. Hemodialysis reduces the half-life of paracetamol, but there is no evidence that it alters the clinical course. Other treatment measures such as hemoperfusion with activated charcoal and peritoneal dialysis are also not much useful. The mainstay of treatment in paracetamol poisoning is administration of N-acetylcysteine (NAC). Patients who are administered NAC within 8-10 hours fair very well.

Remember following additional facts about N-acetylcysteine (NAC):

- It is available as MUCOMYST and MUCOSIL.
- NAC is effective orally as well as intravenously.
- NAC has a foul smell and taste. Thus if desired to be given orally it must be diluted with soft drinks to make a 5% solution. The solution must be consumed within one hour of preparation.
- Oral loading dose is 140 mg/kg, followed by the administration of 70 mg/kg every 4 hours for 17 doses (total 18 doses over 72 hours).
- NAC prevents paracetamol toxicity by following mechanisms:
  - o Prevents binding of NAPQI to hepatocytes (see explanation of previous question).
  - o Directly binds to NAPQI.
  - o Enhances synthesis of additional glutathione.
  - o Acts intracellularly as a glutathione substitute.
  - o Reduces NAPQI back to paracetamol.

12. C. ***Related fact:*** Lavacuator is a double lumen stomach lavage/evacuator tube made up of special PVC which reduces risk of trauma to mucosal surface (note that the name lavacuator comes from "lavage" and "evacuator"). The double lumen allows for the simultaneous introduction of lavage solution under pressure and evacuation. Large elliptical eyes allow partially dissolved tablets or small clots to be removed (Figure 31.2). The main lumen is meant for intermittent evacuation. The secondary lumen is for rapid lavage under pressure. The tube is manufactured 48" in length and in 5 French sizes, 18, 22, 28, 32, and 36 from transparent polyvinyl chloride (Each unit on the French scale equals 0.3 mm. Thus the diameter of a 36 French size Lavacuator is 10.8 mm, or a little more than 1 cm). Depth markings appear on the body of the tube at 18", 22", 26", and 30" from the closed distal tip. Lavacuator tubes are available from Nellcor, USA. In India however the common Ewald or Boas tube is still very commonly used.

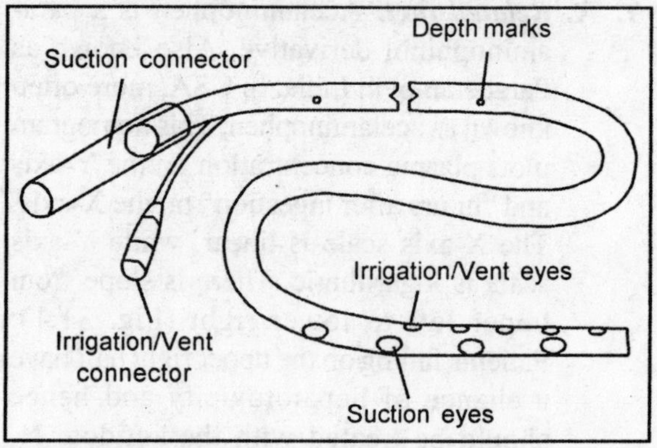

Fig. 31.2: A Lavacuator

13. B. ***Related fact:*** Toxins most amenable to enhanced elimination by dialysis are those

which (i) Have a low molecular mass (<500 Daltons) (ii) High water solubility (iii) Low protein binding (iv) Small volume of distribution (<1 Litre/kg body weight. Normal 0.6 Litres/Kg. 42 L/70 Kg) (v) Prolonged elimination (long half life) (vi) High dialysis clearance relative to total body clearance.

Hemodialysis should be considered in:

- All Alcohols (Methanol, Ethanol, Ethylene Glycols, Isopropyl alcohol).
- Amphetamine.
- Barbiturates.
- Bromide.
- Carbon monoxide.
- Chloral hydrate.
- Isoniazid.
- Meprobamate.
- Paracetamol.
- Paraldehyde.
- Paraquat.
- Salicylates.
- Single small molecules (Lithium, Heavy metals such as As, Hg etc.).
- Snake bite.

Note that most sedatives and hypnotics are included in this list, but not benzodiazepines!

Hemodialysis may not be useful at all in poisons having a high volume of distribution, or having a high proteing binding. Examples:

- Chloroquine (116-285 L/kg).
- Digitoxin (41 L/kg).
- Heroin (25 L/kg).
- Benzodiazepines such as diazepam. All benzodiazepines are bound to plasma proteins to the extent of 70-99%. It is interesting to note that diazepam has quite a low V_d (0.7-2.6 L/kg), yet its poisoning is not amenable to treatment with hemodialysis, because of its high protein binding.

Variant: A variant that has been asked is→Hemodialysis is done in all except (a) Barbiturates (b) Salicylates (c) Kerosene (d) Alcohol. The answer is (c) Kerosene.

14. D. ***Related fact:*** Forced alkaline diuresis would be helpful in all weakly acidic drugs/chemicals. They are mainly 8 in number. These are:

i. **Phenobarbitone** (remember this and related compounds are derivatives of barbituric acid).
ii. **Salicylates** (derivatives of salicylic acid).
iii. **2-4 D** (also commonly known as 2-4, dichlorophenoxyacetic acid. It is a hormone type herbicide. Plant growth regulator).
iv. **Mecoprop** (It is a phenoxypropionic acid herbicide. Basically a rung higher than 2-4 D, otherwise almost the same. Commonly known as MCPP also. It is also a hormone type herbicide).
v. **Chlorpropamide** (Oral hypoglycaemic agent. Sulfonylureas group. Trade name–Diabenese).
vi. **Diflunisal** (Difluorophenyl derivative of Salicylic acid, Available as DOLOBID. 3-4 times more potent than aspirin in treatment of osteoarthritis and musculoskeletal strains or sprains).
vii. **Fluoride.**
viii. **Methotrexate.**

In amphetamine poisoning, **forced *acidic* diuresis** is useful.

15. C. ***Related fact:*** Forced acidic diuresis would be helpful in all weakly alkaline drugs/chemicals. The procedure is LESS commonly employed than forced alkaline diuresis, because it is potentially hazardous. It is helpful mainly in the following 8 drugs/chemicals:

i. **Amphetamine.**
ii. **Phencyclidine (PCP).**
iii. **Methadone.**
iv. **Cocaine.**
v. **Quinine.**
vi. **Quinidine.**
vii. **Sympathomimetics.**
viii. **Strychnine.**

ANTIDOTES

16. A. ***Related facts:*** Choice (A) is the intended answer. Lead is chelated BOTH intracellularly as well as extracellularly by BAL. Two molecules of BAL combine with one atom of lead to form a complex that is excreted in the bile and urine. BAL can not be given to persons allergic to peanuts, because it comes as a suspension in arachis oil (which is another name for peanut oil!). Another fact that is useful to remember is that BAL is available in 3-mL ampules. Each ml contains 100 mg of BAL, 200 mg of benzyl benzoate and 700 mg of peanut oil (10% BAL and 20% benzyl benzoate in arachis oil). The combination of BAL with benzyl benzoate and arachis oil protect it against oxidation, and thus act as preservatives.

Other important facts to remember about BAL:

- BAL is highly lipid soluble but has limited water solubility.
- Other names for BAL are dithiol-2,3-dimercaptopropanol and dimercaprol.
- Essentially it is a molecule of propanolol, with two hydrogen atoms replaced by –SH groups. While the formula for propanolol is C_3H_7OH, for BAL it is $C_3H_5(SH)_2OH$. The antihypertensive PROP**R**ANOLOL (Please note the extra "R") has absolutely no strcutural similarity with BAL. Structure of BAL is given below:

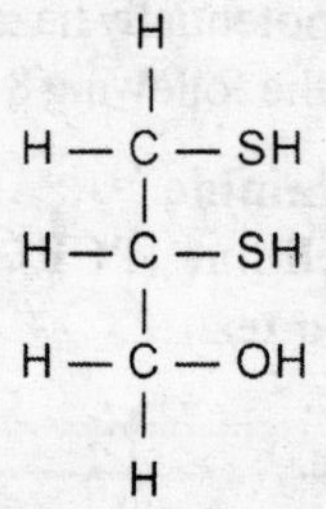

Fig. 31.3: Chemical structure of BAL

- BAL is a relatively colorless liquid with a strong nauseating sulfurous odor. In fact so nauseating is it, that it is supposed to be one of the reasons of patients being unable to tolerate it well.
- Two most common reasons cited for patients being unable to tolerate BAL are (i) extremely painful injections and (ii) strong nauseating sulfurous odour.
- BAL is a colorless liquid with a sulfur odor, similar to rotten eggs.
- BAL injections can ONLY be given deep IM. Remember it comes as a suspension in peanut oil. Injecting it IV may cause fat embolism.
- BAL as well as all other metal chelators are rather non-specific in chelating metallic ions. Essential ions such as copper and zinc are also chelated. This is one of the reasons why therapy with these chelators (especially EDTA), should not be carried out for more than 5 days at a stretch. Repeat courses if necessary may be given after a 2-5 day recovery period.
- Dissociation of the BAL-metal chelate takes place in an acidic urine. Therefore it is desirable to maintain an alkaline urine during BAL therapy. It may protect kidneys from damage.
- While BAL is indicated in elemental and inorganic mercury poisoning, it is CONTRAINDICATED in organic mercury poisoning. Reason→It leads to increased neurotoxicity.
- BAL is particularly useful in patients who have ingested mercuric salts (mercuric chloride). In these patients, patients usually don't tolerate oral antidotes well (mercuric salts being corrosive in nature).
- BAL is contraindicated in Liver dysfunction. Other contraindications to BAL include preexisting renal disease, pregnancy (except in life-threatening circums-

tances; BAL is teratogenic in animal models) and concurrent use of medicinal iron (BAL and iron together form a complex that is very toxic).

- BAL administration to patients on gold therapy for rheumatoid arthritis may lead to an exacerbation of the arthritis.

DUTIES OF MEDICAL PRACTITIONERS

17. C.

18. D. ***Additional info and food for thought:*** The usual answer which is expected from students is (A). And the reasoning which is forwarded is that since section 302 IPC (homicide) is included in section 39 of Cr.P.C. (this section prescribes crimes which the general public must inform to the nearest magistrate or police officer) and section 309 IPC (attempt to commit suicide) is not, the doctor is not bound to inform the police in suicidal poisonings.

But this is not a correct reasoning, because such important sections as 304 B (dowry death), 319 (hurt), 320 (grievous hurt), 375 (rape) and 498 A (husband or relative of a woman subjecting her to cruelty) of IPC are also not covered in section 39 Cr. P.C., and we all know that the doctor routinely informs all such cases to the police. Ideally a doctor should inform all cases of poisoning to the police, whether homicidal, accidental or suicidal. Suicidal poisoning is definitely a crime (u/s 309 IPC), and not reporting this crime to police may amount to collusion on the part of the doctor. Similarly cases of accidental poisoning may be due to careless handling or negligent conduct of some person in relation to that poison (for instance if some maid kept a bottle of acid on the shelf negligently and a member of the house drank that acid taking it to be water). Such negligent conduct of a person with respect to any poisonous substance is punishable under section 284 of IPC, and once again not reporting this incident may amount to collusion on the part of the doctor. Thus the doctor is legally bound in all these cases to inform the police.

Furthermore, section 176 of IPC clearly states that when a doctor who is legally bound to give information to police, omits to give this information would be punished with a maximum sentence of six months or with a fine of Rs. 1000.

This still leaves us with the provisions of section 39 Cr.P.C. and it may be argued whom it is meant for. Let us examine section 39 Cr.P.C. in original:

39. Public to give information of certain offences.- (1) Every person, aware of the commission of, or of the intention of any other person to commit, any offence punishable under any of the following sections of the Indian Penal Code (45 of 1860) namely:

i. Sections 121 to 126, both inclusive, and section 130 (that is to say, offences against the State specified in Chapter VI of the said Code);
ii. Sections 143, 144, 145, 147 and 148 (that is to say, offences against the public tranquillity specified in Chapter VIII of the said Code);
iii. Sections 161 to 165A, both inclusive (that is to say, offences relating to illegal gratification);
iv. Sections 272 to 278, both inclusive (that is to say, offences relating to adulteration of food and drugs, etc.);
v. Sections 302, 303 and 304 (that is to say, offences affecting life);
vi. Section 382 (that is to say, offence of theft after preparation made for causing death, hurt or restraint in order to the committing of the theft);
vii. Sections 392 to 399, both inclusive, and section 402 (that is to say, offences of robbery and dacoity);

viii. Section 409 (that is to say, offence relating to criminal breach of trust by public servant, etc.);

ix. Sections 431 to 439, both inclusive (that is to say, offences of mischief against property);

x. Sections 449 and 450 (that is to say, offence of house-trespass);

xi. Sections 456 to 460, both inclusive (that is to say, offences of lurking house-trespass); and

xii. Sections 489A to 489E, both inclusive (that is to say, offences relating to currency notes and bank notes), shall, in the absence of any reasonable excuse, the burden of proving which excuse shall lie upon the person so aware, forthwith give information to the nearest Magistrate or police officer of such commission or intention.

(2) For the purposes of this section, the term "offence" includes any act committed at any place out of India which would constitute an offence if committed in India.

As can be seen, the title of section 39 Cr.P.C. itself clearly mentions that it is meant for *general public* and *not for doctors*. Thus a member of general public is *NOT legally obliged* to give information to the police if he sees, say, a rape going on in the vicinity of his house, but this may not be necessarily true of a doctor to whom such a victim is brought for treatment. He is bound to report this crime to the police. We do know that a doctor sitting in casualty routinely informs the police officer as soon as a case of 375 IPC comes to him. If he were indeed guided by the provisions of section 39 Cr.P.C. there would have been no need for him to inform even rape to the police.

It is often argued that since the doctor is also a member of the public, he is guided by section 39 Cr.P.C., but this again is not true. *A doctor has a greater responsibility than the general public*. If he imagines that since section 375 is not included in section 39 Cr.P.C., he need not inform the police, he would actually be committing a serious legal error. There is important medicolegal evidence on the body of the the accused (such as pubic hair of the accused sticking to his genitalia) and the victim (such as semen of the accused). If he fails to inform the police and deliver this medical evidence to it, he can be charged under section 201 I.P.C. (causing disappearance of evidence of offence).

A further argument in this case is regarding confidentiality. It has been argued that if a doctor informs the police where he need not inform, he may be breaking his commitment to professional secrecy. It is also argued that if a doctor reports a case of suicidal poisoning to the police, the patient may sue him for breaking his commitment to professional secrecy. But this is also not true, as all these cases would be treated under privileged communication, i.e. the doctor is in a privileged position to make such communications to the police.

It is also argued sometimes that while a doctor *incharge of a government or public hospital* must inform all cases of poisoning (suicidal, homicidal or accidental) to the police, *a private practitioner need inform only cases of homicidal poisoning*. There is no legal basis under this assertion and this is also an incorrect statement.

Variant: A variant of this question is often asked like this→If the poisoning is homicidal in nature, the doctor is bound by law to inform the police under which of the following sections

(a) Section 302 IPC (b) Section 39 Cr.P.C.
(c) Section 39 IPC (d) Section 300 IPC.

The expected answer is (b) Section 39 Cr.P.C. But of course in the light of above discussion, the student must appreciate this is not a correctly framed question.

19. D.

20. B. This is necessary, since a sample of ingested poison need be sent to the chemical laboratory. Using any chemical listed in other choices, may chemically react with the poison making the chemical analysis useless.

MULTIPLE ANSWER TYPE (PGI, CHANDIGARH PATTERN)

21. A,C,E. ***Related facts and mnemonics***: Remember CLIME for agents which are NOT WELL ADSORBED by activated charcoal. C→Caustics, carbamates, L→ Lithium; I→Iron; M→Methyl alcohol, metals; E→Ethanol, Ethylene glycol.

 Remember that "C" above *does not* stand for cyanide, which is adsorbed well by activated charcoal. Many books would have us believe that cyanide is poorly adsorbed by activated charcoal, but this is not so. 1 g of activated charcoal binds about 35 mg of cyanide. Considering that lethal dose of cyanide is between 100-200 mg, administration of cyanide is quite beneficial in cyanide poisoning. Furthermore, prophylactic administration of superactivated charcoal in animals who received fatal doses of cyanide improved their chances of survival!

 Substances well adsorbed by activated charcoal include aspirin, acetaminophen, barbiturates, glutethimide, phenytoin, theophylline, cyclic antidepressants and most inorganic and organic materials.

22. A,B,D. Analeptic agents are no more used in poisoning. Even in earlier times, these agents were used only in CNS depressants and not in any general poisoning. Carbon dioxide is never administered in poisoning cases.

23. B,C,E. There are no such term as "Extracorporeal Bone marrow clearance" and "Silicate haemoperfusion".

24. B. Since gastric lavage is essentially a traumatic procedure, it must not be used when the patient has ingested a non-toxic agent or a non-toxic dose of a poisonous agent. The length of the tube to be inserted is 50 cm in adults and 25 cm for a child. Performing gastric lavage without consent may amount to assault u/s 351 of I.P.C. The preferred route of insertion of gastric lavage tube is oral and NOT nasal.

 Endotracheal intubation must be done prior to gastric lavage in a comatosed patient to prevent the possibility of aspiration.

25. A,C,E. Coma cocktail consists of (i) Thiamine (Vitamin B_1) 100 mg (ii) Dextrose 100 ml of 50% solution (50 g) (iii) Naloxone 2 mg. This cocktail should be administered IV in all cases of unknown poisonings which present as coma.

 Rationale of giving this treatment is that a very high proportion of poisoned comatose patients are subequently found to have ingested either (i) Alcohol (ii) Hypoglycaemic agents or (iii) Opioids. Thiamine, dextrose and naloxone take care of each of these poisons respectively.

 Thiamine is administered to treat and/or avoid Wernicke-Korsakoff syndrome in comatose patients. This strategy is not well supported by the literature, and few patients regain consciousness following thiamine infusion. Still, routine use of thiamine is safe, inexpensive, and prevents the possibility of delayed deterioration secondary to nutritional deficiency. Thiamine is particularly important in the nutritionally deplete alcoholic.

 Coma may be due to hyperglycaemia (rather than hypoglycaemia). But since administration of dextrose to hyperglycemic patients is unlikely to cause harm, it is administed routinely.

Naloxone rapidly reverses coma, respiratory depression, and hypotension induced by opioids. An initial dose of 0.2 to 0.4 mg is administered IV (or endotracheally).

If there is no response after 2 to 3 min, an additional 1 to 2 mg can be administered and repeated up to 10 mg as required.

Using a higher dose up front may precipitate large cardiovascular changes in opioid dependent patients. Several opioids such as meperidine, propoxyphene, diphenoxylate, methadone, and pentazocine require large doses of naloxone, but lack of response to 10 mg of naloxone generally excludes opioid toxicity. Opioid antagonism with naloxone lasts 1 to 4 h requiring repeat doses or continuous infusion in significant intoxication.

Coma may be due to anticholinergic excess, and one may be tempted to administer physostigmine. But it is not recommended as it can produce serious convulsions. Its use is advocated only if it is KNOWN that the coma is due to anticholinergic poisoning.

Older analeptics such as picrotoxin, amphetamine, doxapram, nikethamide and caffeine are now not recommended as they can do more harm than good (agitation and convulsions).

26. **B,C.**

27. **A,C.** ***Related facts:*** Methionine acts as a glutathione precursor and may be useful, but is both less reliable than NAC and unsafe if given late in the overdose. Cysteamine was once popular but is no more recommended today. In fact in the US, Cysteamine is not even available commercially. In some countries (most notably Norway and Finland) paracetamol preparations are sold as a paracetamol/methionine combination making the job of potential suicides almost impossible!

9 CORROSIVE POISONS

32 Acids

1. **In dilute solutions, most corrosives act as:**
   A. Irritant poisons
   B. Somniferous poisons
   C. Delirious poisons
   D. Inebriant poisons
2. **Oil of vitriol is:**
   A. Nitric acid
   B. Hydrochloric acid
   C. Sulfuric acid
   D. Citric acid
3. **The actions of corrosive acids are characterized by:**
   A. Extraction of water from the tissues
   B. Coagulation of cellular proteins
   C. Conversion of hemoglobin into hematin
   D. All of the above
4. **Which one of the following is the systemic action of oxalic acid poisoning?**
   A. Hepatic failure
   B. Hypoglycaemia
   C. Hypercalcemia
   D. Renal failure
5. **Which one of the following poisonous substances, although known as an acid, does not turn blue litmus red and has no acid reaction?**
   A. Hydrochloric acid
   B. Nitric acid
   C. Carbolic acid J
   D. Oxalic acid
6. **Carbolic acid is readily absorbed from:**
   A. Alimentary tract
   B. Respiratory tract
   C. Intact skin
   D. All of the above
7. **Xanthoproteic reaction is seen in poisoning with:**
   A. Hydrochloric acid
   B. Nitric acid
   C. Sulfuric acid
   D. Both (A) and (B) above
8. **Which poisonous acid is present in rhubarb leaves, sorrel, spinach and tomato?**
   A. Phenol
   B. Oxalic acid
   C. Citric acid
   D. Muriatic acid
9. **"Boiled lobster syndrome" is seen in poisoning with:**
   A. Hydrochloric acid
   B. Boric acid
   C. Oxalic acid
   D. Chromic acid

10. Paresthesias, tetany, hyper-reflexia, muscle twitches and muscle cramps are typical symptoms of poisoning with:
A. Sulphuric acid
B. Nitric acid
C. Oxalic acid
D. Citric acid

11. Which one of the following is contraindicated in corrosive poisonings?
A. Analgesics
B. Gastric lavage
C. Neutralization of acid or alkali
D. Milk by mouth

12. Which of the following acids is also known variously as acid of sugar, acid of sorrel or salt of sorrel?
A. Picric acid
B. Oxalic acid
C. Nitric acid
D. Hydrochloric acid

13. The fatal dose of oxalic acid is:
A. 15-30 mg
B. 1.5-3.0 g
C. 15-30 g
D. 200-300 g

14. Which of the following is the best antidote for oxalic acid poisoning?
A. BAL
B. Animal charcoal
C. Calcium gluconate
D. Magnesium sulphate

15. *Aqua fortis* is another name for:
A. Acetic acid
B. Sulphuric acid
C. Nitric acid
D. Carbolic acid

16. Ochronosis is seen in .... poisoning:
A. Mercury
B. Phenol
C. Datura
D. Copper sulphate

17. Carboluria is seen in acute poisoning with:
A. Nitric acid
B. Sulphuric acid
C. Oxalic acid
D. Phenol

18. Aromatic odor to the breath is seen in poisoning with:
A. Oxalic acid
B. Tartaric acid
C. Carbolic acid
D. All of the above

MULTIPLE ANSWER TYPE (PGI, CHANDIGARH PATTERN)

19. Which of the following facts about phenol are CORRECT?
A. It is an aromatic hydrocarbon derived from coal tar
B. In poisoning by phenol stomach tube can not be passed
C. Common synonyms for phenol include carbolic acid, hydroxybenzene, phenic acid, phenolum, and phenyl hydrate
D. Phenol has antiseptic properties
E. It is used in chemical face peels, nerve injections, and topical anesthesia for skin and mucous membranes

20. Which of the following are synonyms of Hydrochloric acid?
A. Oil of vitriol
B. Salt of sorrel
C. Muriatic acid
D. Aqua fortis
E. Spirit of salts

ANSWERS

1. A.
2. C.
3. D.
4. D.
5. C.
6. D.
7. **B.** Nitric acid, a strong oxidizing agent, reacts with the organic matter (principally proteins) of the skin to form 2,4,6-trinitrophenol (xanthoproteic acid or picric acid), which is yellow in color. Nitrogen monoxide is released in this reaction.

   Xanthoproteic reaction is used in biochemistry to detect proteins. Concentrated nitric acid is added to the solution to be tested and the mixture warmed cautiously. A yellow colour results if the solution contains proteins. After thoroughly cooling the mixture under the tap, a little amount of strong ammonia is added, when the colour is intensified to orange.

   You can do a simple demonstration of xanthoproteic reaction at home. Take egg white from an egg and mix concentrated nitric acid with it. After two minutes, egg white turns yellow. This does not happen if egg white is mixed with any other acid, say hydrochloric or sulphuric acid.
8. **B.** It is present in the form of calcium oxalate. Oxalates may also be produced by several common molds. *Penicillium* and *Aspergillus* molds can convert sugar into calcium oxalate at very high yields.

   Variant: This question has been asked the other way round too, in this way→The leaves of which of the following plants contains large amounts of oxalates: (a) *Ricinus communis* (b) Rhubarb (c) Aconite (d) Prickly poppy. The answer is (b) Rhubarb.
9. **B.** In boric acid poisoning, the major symptom is erythema, desquamation and exfoliation. The skin of the patient looks like a boiled lobster.
10. **C.** ***Additional information:*** All the symptoms mentioned are typical of hypocalcemia. Oxalic acid causes hypocalcemia by combining with calcium in the plasma to form insoluble calcium oxalate. Precipitation of calcium oxalate in the proximal tubules of the kidney may lead to local necrosis of the tubular epithelium, producing kidney dysfunction and electrolyte imbalance.
11. **B.**
12. **B.**
13. **C.**
14. **C.** Calcium gluconate combines with oxalic acid to form insoluble oxalates and thus prevents its absorption. Both calcium gluconate and calcium lactate are effective. The dose is 150 mg/kg orally. Electrocardiogram with serum calcium monitoring are also required. Renal failure (due to deposition of calcium oxalate crystals in proximal tubules) may require hemodialysis.
15. **C.** ***Related facts***: This term is now almost obsolete. In Latin "*aqua*" means water. This word gives rise to many words interesting to scientists—*aqua tepida* (warm water), *aqua fortis* (literally "strong water" referring to nitric acid), *aqua regia* or *aqua regis* (literally "water of the king", a mixture of concentrated nitric and hydrochloric acids capable of dissolving the "royal metal" gold) and *aqua vitae* (literally, "water of life" or concentrated aqueous ethanol, C_2H_5OH).

There is an interesting limerick on *aqua fortis*, which may perhaps help you remember its meaning.

Aquavit, taken neat, makes one placid.
Have too much, though, and you may go flaccid.
And avoid aqua fortis—
You'll get rigor mortis!
It's commonly called nitric acid.

Additional fact: Other terms for nitric acid are **Engraver's acid** and **azotic acid.**

16. B. ***Related facts:*** Ochronosis is the deposition of dark pigment in connective tissues (especially the ear cartilage and the ocular tissue). This disorder is most often seen with alkaptonuria, a metabolic disorder. However ochronosis can also occur occasionally from exposure to some noxious substances, such as phenol, trinitrophenol, resorcinol, mercury, picric acid, benzene, hydroquinone, and antimalarials.

In alkaptonuria the dark pigment deposited is **homogentisic acid (HGA)** which can not be catabolized because there is a deficiency of **homogentisic acid oxidase.** In chronic phenol poisoning, the pigments that are deposited are metabolic products of phenol such as hydroquinone and pyrocatechol.

Ochronosis was first defined by Virchow who histologically described the connective tissue in alkaptonuria. He gave this name because he found that under the microscope the hue of the cartilage appeared ochre or yellow.

17. D. ***Related facts*****:** Carboluria is the presence of phenol (also known as carbolic acid) and its metabolic products, catechol (pyrocatechol or 1,2-Dihydroxybenzene) and quinol (hydroxyquinone or 1,4-dihydroxybenzene) in urine (Fig. 32.1).

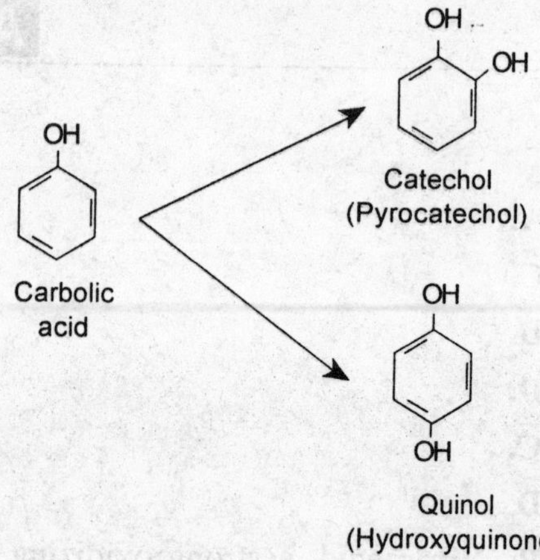

Fig. 32.1: Conversion of phenol to its metabolic products, catechol and quinol in the body, giving rise to yellow brown or even greenish urine

Pyrocatechol is colorless while hydroxyquinone is colored. Depending on its concentration, it varies in color from yellow-brown to green. On exposure to air it can turn dark green or even black.

Metabolism of benzene: In humans, phenol (hydroxybenzene), catechol and quinol are the major end products of benzene metabolism. Thus yellow brown or greenish urine can form in benzene poisoning as well.

Other useful facts to remember about phenol:

- Phenol has antiseptic, germicidal and anesthetic properties, and is useful in disinfectants and preservatives.
- In molecular biology research it is used to denature and remove protein from preparations of DNA and RNA. In fact it is its binding nature to protein that proves fatal to humans; its binding to hepatic and renal proteins leading to hepatic and renal failure.

- It can be absorbed through all routes. However most obnoxious route is inhalation.
- Cigarette smoke contains phenol.
- Due to anaesthetic properties of phenol, initial exposure may not be painful.
- Long skin exposure can progress to gangrene.
- Fatal dose is one gram.

[*Additional info:* In the plant world, hydroxyquinone acts as an antibiotic, which is often found at the site of plant injury. Think of a half eaten apple, which turns brown after some time. This brown color is due to hydroxyquinone.]

18. C. In carbolic acid poisoning, a small amount of carbolic acid may be eliminated through the lungs unchanged. This may give rise to an aromatic odor to the breath.

MULTIPLE ANSWER TYPE (PGI, CHANDIGARH PATTERN)

19. A,C,D,E. In phenol poisoning stomach tube can be passed because it hardens the stomach walls, and there is no danger of rupture of stomach.

20. C,E.

33 Alkalis

1. **In which of the following poisoning do the mucus membranes swell, and become translucent and soap like?**
   A. Hydrochloric acid poisoning
   B. Nitric acid poisoning
   C. Oxalic acid poisoning
   D. Caustic soda poisoning
2. **The following poisons are corrosive alkalies *except*:**
   A. Potassium oxalate
   B. Potassium carbonate
   C. Ammonia
   D. Potassium hydroxide
3. **"Spirits of Hartshorn" refers to which of the following alkali?**
   A. Potassium hydroxide
   B. Ammonia
   C. Sodium hydroxide
   D. Calcium hydroxide
4. **Self-inflating automotive airbags can cause accidental burns by:**
   A. Ammonia
   B. Calcium hydroxide
   C. Sodium hydroxide
   D. Potassium hydroxide
5. **Liquor ammoniae fortis is:**
   A. Hydride of ammonia
   B. Nitrite of ammonia
   C. Saturated Solution of ammonia in water
   D. Carbide from of ammonia
6. **The usual fatal dose of ammonia is:**
   A. 2-3 ml
   B. 20-30 ml
   C. 200-300 ml
   D. 500-750 ml

MULTIPLE ANSWER TYPE (PGI, CHANDIGARH PATTERN)

7. **Chemical burns can be produced by prolonged contact with:**
   A. Cement
   B. Hydrocarbons such as gasoline
   C. Mercury
   D. Phosphorus
   E. Phenol
8. **Which of the following facts about alkalies are CORRECT?**
   A. Alkalis penetrate tissues more than acids
   B. Alkalis classically produce coagulation necrosis
   C. Lye is an example of alkali
   D. The pH of alkalis range between 0 and 7
   E. Strong alkalis are very good antidotes for strong acids

9. Which of the following facts about Lye are correct?

A. It is a solution of approximately 95% NaOH

B. It is a solution of approximately 95% KOH

C. It is a solution of calcium chloride

D. It was once used as a domestic cleaning fluid

E. It is commonly used in soap making

10. Which of the following facts about alkalies are correct?

A. With fats they form soaps

B. With proteins they form gel like alkaline proteinates

C. Alkaline burns are far less dangerous than acidic burns

D. Salt of tartar is an alkali

E. Sal Volatile is an alkali

ANSWERS

1. **D.** The soapy feeling is because the alkali combines with the body fat to give rise to soaps.
2. **A.** Carbonates of sodium and potassium are alkalies.
3. **B.** ***Related facts:*** Hartshorn is a preparation of ammonia (chiefly ammonium bicarbonate) used as smelling salts. It is called so because a hart's (male of red deer) horns were at one time the chief source of ammonia. "Spirits of Hartshorn" refers to ammonia.
4. **C.** Most modern cars now have self-inflating bags, which protect the driver from forces of collision. Inside these airbags is a gas generator mixture containing NaN_3 (sodium azide), KNO_3, and SiO_2. When the car undergoes a head-on collision, there is intense deceleration. The signal from the deceleration sensor ignites this mixture by an electrical impulse, creating high-temperature. High temperature causes sodium azide to decompose, liberating the nitrogen gas which fills the airbag. The purpose of the KNO_3 and SiO_2 is to remove the sodium metal (which is highly reactive and potentially explosive) by converting it to a harmless material.

   Normally the temperatures generated are not sufficient to cause sodium azide to ignite. The temperature is just sufficient to produce nitrogen only. However when sodium azide (NaN_3) is inadvertently ignited, it breaks down to sodium hydroxide, which can cause facial and hand burns if the airbag breaks. Such patients should also be evaluated for the presence of corneal abrasions. Even Rescuers can sustain burns from released sodium hydroxide.
5. **C.** ***Related fact:*** Liquor ammoniae fortis contains 32.5% of ammonia. It is a colorless liquid having a very pungent characteristic odor. The solution is largely used for domestic purposes as paint, oil and dirt remover.
6. **B.**

MULTIPLE ANSWER TYPE (PGI, CHANDIGARH PATTERN)

7. **A,B,D,E. Cement** can indeed cause burns. Wet portland cement is approximately 64% calcium oxide (also called lime) and 21% silicon oxide with a pH of approximately 12.5 (This is very strong alkaline, considering that pH scale is logarithmic. Please note that pH of normal human skin is 5.5).

   Cement burns are common in construction workers who are exposed to cement. In these workers prolonged contact with wet cement allows the alkaline calcium oxide to penetrate and cause tissue destruction through liquefactive necrosis. The burn is complicated by the coarse texture of the cement, which causes abrasions in the skin, allowing penetration of the cement.

   The most frequently affected areas include the knees, the calves, and the feet (areas of the body coming in contact with wet cement most often; for example a construction worker may kneel in it or wet cement may fall into a boot). Often the initial contact does not produce pain, thereby allowing prolonged contact with the skin.

   Cement burns often take months to heal, and in extreme cases will need skin grafts or can even lead to amputation. Serious chemical burns to the eyes can also be caused following a splash of cement.

Additional facts on cement: Incidentally cement also contains hexavalent chromium which may be responsible for severe chromium allergies in cement workers (chromium is not added intentionally to cement; it comes from various sources during its manufacture. Among the sources blamed are volcanic rock used as a component, the scrapings from the refractory lining of the kiln, the steel balls used in the grinding mills, the different tools used for crushing and grinding the raw materials and the clinker). Cement typically contains about 50 parts per million (ppm) of chromium in its hexavalent state.

Since hexavalent chromium is also a carcinogen, its presence in cement is coming under increasing scrutiny. Scandinavian countries have by law limited the amount of hexavalent chromium allowed in portland cement.

Phosphorus: After exposure to air, white phosphorus spontaneously ignites and is rapidly oxidized to phosphorus pentoxide. This oxidation is an exothermic reaction which is responsible for phosphorus burns. Mere contact with phosphorus can also produce burns as it is extremely lipid soluble and readily penetrates the dermal layers. As skin penetration progresses, white phosphorus continues to be oxidized.

Phenol: When contact first occurs with phenol, the patient may experience a partial-thickness chemical burn accompanied by a strong pain sensation, swelling, and redness. Phenol may have some local anesthetic properties, which allow extensive damage to occur before the patient feels pain.

8. **A,C.** Alkalis classically produce liquefactive necrosis, and that is why they penetrate tissues deeper. Acids produce coagulation necrosis, in effect producing a tough eschar. This prevents the further penetration of acids, hence classically acids do not penetrate the tissues as deep as alkalies. In general, acids with a pH lower than 2 cause coagulative necrosis, while alkalis with a pH higher than 11.5 cause liquefactive necrosis.

   Strong alkalies are contraindicated in ingestion of strong acids, as they can damage tissues on their own.

9. **A,B,D.** Lye is a caustic solution of the chemical sodium hydroxide (soda lye) or (less commonly) of potassium hydroxide (potash lye).

10. **A,B,D,E.** ***Explanations and Additional info***: Alkalis form soaps with fats (saponification of the tissue lipids) and alkaline proteinates with tissue proteins. In fact, these two reactions help it penetrate the tissues much more deeply and cause more damage than the acids. In one report, calcium oxide mistakenly used to line a football field led to second- and third-degree burns in most of the players who were exposed. Salt of tartar is another name for potassium carbonate. Sal Volatile is another name for ammonium carbonate. Both of these are alkalis.

10 IRRITANT POISONS

34 Non-Metallic Irritants

1. Which of the following poisons occurs as translucent, waxy, luminous cylinders?
A. Ammonium bromide
B. Yellow phosphorus
C. Iodine
D. Spanish fly

2. The usual fatal dose of white phosphorus is:
A. 2 mg
B. 20 mg
C. 120 mg
D. 1500 mg

3. Garlic like odor is present in breath and excreta in poisoning by:
A. Cyanide
B. Lead
C. Copper
D. Phosphorus

4. The initial symptoms of phosphorus consisting of nausea, vomiting and diarrhea last for:
A. 5-10 minutes
B. 5-6 hours
C. 1-2 days
D. 1-2 weeks

5. The usual fatal period from poisoning by yellow phosphorus is about:
A. 6-7 minutes
B. 6-7 hours
C. 6-7 days
D. 6-7 weeks

6. Antidote once advocated in phosphorus poisoning was:
A. Copper sulphate
B. Dimercaprol
C. Potassium ferrocyanide
D. E.D.T.A

7. Smoking stool syndrome is seen in poisoning with:
A. Red phosphorus
B. Yellow phosphorus
C. Chlorine
D. Iodine

8. Asterixis is seen in:
A. Arsenic trioxide
B. Arsenic phosphide
C. Red phosphorus
D. Yellow phosphorus

9. Poisoning by irritants may be mistaken for:
A. Peritonitis
B. Gastroenteritis
C. Enteric fever
D. Intestinal obstruction

10. Glass jaw is caused by chronic poisoning with:

A. Chlorine
B. Bromine
C. Phosphorus
D. Silicates

MULTIPLE ANSWER TYPE (PGI, CHANDIGARH PATTERN)

11. Which of the following statements regarding phosphorus are TRUE?

A. Red phosphorus is extremely toxic
B. Yellow phosphorus when exposed to atmosphere gives off dense white fumes of phosphoric and phosphorus acids with a strong odor or garlic
C. Red phosphorus is more luminous than yellow phosphorus
D. White phosphorus turns yellow on exposure to sunlight
E. Yellow phosphorus mixed with powdered glass is used on the side (striking surface) of match boxes

12. Following symptoms are seen in first stage of acute phosphorus poisoning?

A. Phossy jaw
B. Faint fumes rising from the stools
C. Jaundice
D. Stools which are luminous in the dark
E. Foetor hepaticus

13. Substances used on the side of a safety match box include:

A. Powdered glass
B. Yellow phosphorus
C. Red phosphorus
D. Potassium chlorate
E. Antimony sulfide

14. Yellow phosphorus:

A. Is a completely different form than white and red phosphorus
B. Is white phosphorus that contains small quantities of red phosphorus
C. Is non poisonous in nature
D. Is non-metallic
E. Acts as a cellular poison by uncoupling oxidative phosphorylation

ANSWERS

1. **B.**
2. **C.** The range is usually considered as 60-120 mg (or 1 mg/kg). Recovery has however been recorded after 360 mg. The smallest recorded fatal dose in modern literature is 8 mg for an adult. It is interesting to compare it with the fatal dose of potassium cyanide, which is usually considered a very fatal poison. The fatal dose of potassium cyanide is 200-300 mg, almost twice the fatal dose of phosphorus!
3. **D.** ***Related facts:*** Poisons which cause a garlic like smell in breath are arsenic, dimethyl sulfoxide, phosphorus, selenium and tellurium.
4. **C.** ***Related fact:*** The symptoms of phosphorus poisoning are classically described in three stages (i) First stage reflects the severe irritative effects of phosphorus on the GIT. This includes nausea, vomiting, diarrhoea and abdominal pain. This stage begins in about 2-6 hours of ingestion and lasts for about 1-2 days. (ii) The second stage is symptom free. This is also known as the latent stage. Patient feels well and if hospitalized earlier, wants to go home. This stage lasts for a further 2-3 days. (iii) Symptoms return with a vengeance after this period. This stage is characterized by hepatic failure, renal insufficiency and recurrent involvement of the central nervous system. Jaundice is the major symptom seen at this stage.
5. **C.** ***Related fact:*** The usual fatal period in phosphorus poisoning is 6-7 days. However if there is very fulminant poisoning, the victim may die from collapse within 24 hours. Since in this question the *usual* fatal period is asked, choice (C) is the correct choice.
6. **A.** ***Related fact:*** At one time copper sulphate was advocated as an antidote to phosphorus, because it combines with phosphorus to form insoluble cupric sulphide, which can not be absorbed. However now, copper sulphate is no more used for phosphorus poisoning. Nowadays, the standard treatment of phosphorus poisoning is gastric lavage with potassium permanganate (1:5000 solution) or with 2% hydrogen peroxide to convert the phosphorus to harmless oxides.
7. **B.** ***Related fact:*** During the first stage of phosphorus poisoning, faint fumes (of phosphorus) may emanate from stools. This is referred to as the "smoking stool syndrome".
8. **D.** ***Related fact:*** Asterixis is the name given to flapping tremor of the hands. It is seen in third stage of acute phosphorus poisoning.
9. **B.** ***Related fact:*** This is because vomiting and diarrhoea are the major symptoms in both.
10. **C.** ***Related fact:*** Glass jaw is more commonly known as phossy jaw. The question may not mention the phrase "phossy jaw", because that might immediately give away the answer. The symptoms of glass jaw or phossy jaw start with toothache and lead upto necrosis and osteomyelitis of lower jaw (for some obscure reason, upper jaw is never involved[1] !). Anorexia, weakness, and anemia are also seen. The condition is thought to result from fumes of phosphorus pentoxide

---

[1]A good MCQ can be asked on this interesting piece of information like this→Phossy jaw involves (a) only upper jaw (b) only lower jaw (c) either or both jaws (d) either or both jaws and rarely a long bone too. The correct answer is (b) only lower jaw

to which match workers in olden times were exposed. Legend has it that match workers used to get phossy jaw, because they were required to suck matches during their manufacture, but this is probably not true.

Phossy jaw was first described in 1862 by the British physician **John Syer Bristowe** (1827–1895).

In sports, the term glass jaw is jocularly applied to a boxer with a weak jaw. The term is thus an oblique reference to a diseased and weak jaw produced by chronic phosphorus poisoning.

MULTIPLE ANSWER TYPE (PGI, CHANDIGARH PATTERN)

11. B, D. Red phosphorus is non toxic unless contaminated with yellow phosphorus. Red phosphorus is non-volatile, non-luminous, odorless and amorphous. It is the yellow phosphorus, which gives off garlic like smell. It is the red phosphorus (and not yellow phosphorus), which is used along with powdered glass on the side of match boxes. This fact may be asked as a separate MCQ also (see below).

Additional info: The tip of the match stick contains a mixture of potassium chlorate and antimony sulphide. Potassium chlorate is the oxidizing agent which is necessary to keep the flame lit. In some of the older brands lead oxide, lead chromate or manganese dioxide are employed for the same purpose. On burning, the safety match gives off sulfur dioxide in small quantities. Older "Lucifer matches" containing yellow phosphorus were not only dangerous (prone to ignite by themselves), but even gave off irritating oxides of phosphorus on burning. It caused every one around to cough and wheeze!

12. B, D. Phossy jaw is seen only in chronic phosphorus poisoning. Jaundice and foetor hepaticus is seen in third stage of phosphorus poisoning. Foetor hepaticus is the name given to a mousy odor to the breath. Remember the breath odors in the various stages of acute phosphorus poisoning:

First stage→Garlic smell.

Second stage→No particular smell.

Third stage→Foetor hepaticus (mousy odor).

13. A, C. ***Related facts:*** Yellow phosphorus is no more used in match industry now, as it causes phossy jaw. Potassium chlorate and antimony sulfide are used on the tip of match sticks and NOT on the sides of match boxes. It is important to differentiate between the two types of matches: safety matches and "strike anywhere" matches.

A safety match – commonly used in households – can only light when someone strikes it against the striking surface on the side of the match box. A "strike anywhere" match – much more difficult to get – can be lit by striking the match on anything solid. A "strike anywhere" match works in a similar way as a safety match, but instead of phosphorus being on a striking surface, it is added to the head of the match. The composition of the head of "strike anywhere" match is 6% phosphorus sesquisulfide (which is non toxic), 24% potassium chlorate, and small quantities of zinc oxide, red ochre (a pigment), powdered glass, glue and water.

14. B, E. ***Related facts:*** Phosphorus has only three "real" allotropes: white, red and black – others are all mixtures of these in various proportions. Red phosphorus is formed by heating white phosphorus to 250°C (482°F) or by exposing white phosphorus to sunlight. Red phosphorus is not poisonous and is not as dangerous as white phosphorus; frictional heating is enough to change it back to white phosphorus.

Black phosphorus is also formed by heating white phosphorus, but a mercury catalyst and a seed crystal of black phosphorus are required. Black phosphorus is the least reactive form of phosphorus and has no significant commercial uses.

Two other colors in which phosphorus is seen are yellow and violet. Yellow phosphorus is NOT a different allotrope of phosphorus, but just white phosphorus that contains small quantities of red phosphorus. White phosphorus turns yellow on exposure to sunlight because some of the white phosphorus turns into red phosphorus and the mixture appears yellow. Violet phosphorus is a mixture of the red and black allotropes.

Additional info: Phosphorus was first isolated in 1669 by Hennig Brand, a German physician and alchemist, by boiling, filtering and otherwise processing as many as 60 buckets of urine. This has incidentally been called the most disgusting method of discovering an element!

35 Insecticides and Weed-Killers

ORGANOPHOSPHORUS COMPOUNDS AND CARBAMATES

1. Organophosphorus insecticides exert their action by:
A. Producing methemoglobin
B. Hemolysing R.B.C.s
C. Inhibiting cholinesterase
D. Inhibiting carbonic anhydrase

2. The usual fatal dose of zinc phosphide is:
A. 5 micrograms
B. 5 milligrams
C. 50 milligrams
D. 5 grams

3. Tik 20 is an example of:
A. Alkyl phosphates
B. Aryl phosphates
C. Carbamates
D. Plant penicillins

4. Pralidoxime is contraindicated in:
A. Carbaryl poisoning
B. Malathion poisoning
C. Parathion poisoning
D. None of the above

5. Most specific test for organophosphorus poisoning is:
A. RBC Cholinesterase level
B. Plasma cholinesterase level
C. RBC uroporphyrin level
D. Measurement of serum levels of organophosphorus

6. Physostigmine, neostigmine and pyridostigmine are all examples of:
A. Organophosphates
B. Organochlorines
C. Carbamates
D. None of the above

7. The normal RBC cholinesterase levels, as measured in ΔpH/hour/0.02 ml red cells, are:
A. 0.075
B. 0.75
C. 7.5
D. 75

ORGANOCHLORINES

8. Which of the following insecticides is also known as "plant penicillin" because of its broad spectrum of activity against various insect pests?
A. DDT
B. Lindane
C. Toxaphene
D. Endrin

9. Which of the following is a polychlorinated hydrocarbon?

A. Malathion
B. Endrin
C. Parathion
D. Diazinon

10. When ingested, endrin is stored mostly in:
A. Brain
B. Liver
C. Bones
D. Fatty tissues

11. Which of the following statements best describes the fate of Endrin in the body?
A. It is completely metabolized
B. It is mainly excreted via urine
C. It gets concentrated in bile
D. It is excreted mostly in faeces

12. What is the average fatal dose for endrin?
A. 2-6 micrograms
B. 2-6 milligrams
C. 2-6 grams
D. 20-60 grams

13. What is the averaǥe fatal dose for DDT?
A. 15-30 micrograms
B. 15-30 milligrams
C. 1.5-3.0 grams
D. 15-30 grams

14. Which of the following is the specific antidote for DDT and endrin poisoning?
A. Atropine
B. Pralidoxime
C. A combination of 50% atropine and 50% Pralidoxime
D. None of the above

HERBICIDES AND WEED-KILLERS

15. Cacodylic acid contains which of the following?
A. Arsenic
B. Lead
C. Mercury
D. Nitric acid

MULTIPLE ANSWER TYPE (PGI, CHANDIGARH PATTERN)

16. Pseduocholinesterase is found in:
A. Red blood cells
B. Plasma
C. White matter of the brain
D. Liver
E. Gray matter of the brain

ANSWERS

ORGANOPHOSPHORUS COMPOUNDS AND CARBAMATES

1. **C.**
2. **D.**
3. **B.** It belongs to the group Aryl phosphates and is also known as Diazinon.
4. **A.** ***Related fact:*** Carbaryl is a carbamate and Pralidoxime (in fact all oximes) is contraindicated in all carbamates. Reasons —(i) Carbamates are weak inhibitors of cholinesterase, so cholinesterase reactivators are not required in the first place (ii) With oximes, carbamates form a "cabamate-oxime complex" which is a more potent cholinesterase inhibitor than carbamates alone. Thus it can nullify–or at least lessen—the action of atropine, which is the TRUE antidote in cases of carbamate poisoning.
5. **A.** ***Additional info:*** RBC cholinesterase levels are better indicators of acute or chronic organophosphorus poisoning than plasma cholinesterase levels, because RBC cholinesterase reflects the true cholinesterase levels. Plasma cholinesterase levels represent the pseudocholinesterase (which is a protein synthesized in liver) levels. Estimation of plasma cholinesterase levels suffers from following disadvantages:
   - It does not reflect true cholinesterase levels.
   - About 3% of general population suffers from congenital plasma cholinesterase deficiency.
   - Its levels may be reduced in severe liver disorders (since it is a liver protein) such as cirrhosis and also in neoplasia, malnutrition and infections.
   - Certain drugs such as morphine, codeine, lidocaine and succinylcholine can depress its activity.

   It might appear to some that direct measurement of serum levels of organophosphorus may be a better method, since it directly measures the "poison" in the system. However this is not a better method because:
   - Organophosphates are difficult to measure.
   - They are active at very low levels; these levels are different in different organophosphates.
   - Medical laboratories can readily measure the activities of enzymes. Because enzymes are catalysts, there is a multiplier effect that makes measurements of low molecular levels relatively easy.
   - The effect is the important thing, and is a true indicator of poisoning.
   - Because of genetic differences, some people are poisoned by lower levels of organophosphates than others.

   One thing to note, however, is that although RBC cholinesterase (or to be more specific, *decreases* in RBC cholinesterase) are the most sensitive indicator of organophosphate poisoning, it is significantly more difficult to measure than plasma cholinesterase. Plasma cholinesterase measurements are more convenient because of lower cost and wider availability. For this reason, RBC cholinesterase testing is normally done (in specialized laboratories) on a regular basis for agricultural workers (testing here has more relevance), whereas in cases of suspected acute organophosphorus poisoning, hospital laboratories will measure the plasma cholinesterase.

6. **C.** All these three compounds are examples of carbamates. Carbamates are derivatives of carbamic acid (NH_2COOH) (Figs 35.1 and 35.2).

7. **B.** ***Related facts:*** It may be useful to know how this level is calculated. Although cholinesterase activity in blood, serum and tissues can be measured by a number of methods, one of the most popular is the pH method of Michael, whereby a change in pH is measured, when cholinesterase acts on acetylcholine. The principle is that cholinesterase would hydrolyze acetylcholine producing acetic acid, which in turn would decrease the pH of the reaction mixture. Electrometric determination of the change in pH from 8.1 over a definite period of time (e.g. 1 hour) at a specific temperature (e.g. 25°C) represents the enzyme activity. Normal values of cholinesterase activity as measured by this method (in ΔpH/hour/0.02 ml red cells or plasma at 25°C, Mean ± SD) are as follows (Table 35.1):

Table 35.1: Normal RBC and Plasma cholinesterase activity in men and women (in ΔpH/hour/0.02 ml)

	Men	*Women*
RBC ChE	0.766 ± 0.081	0.750 ± 0.082
Plasma ChE	0.953 ± 0.157	0.817 ± 0.187

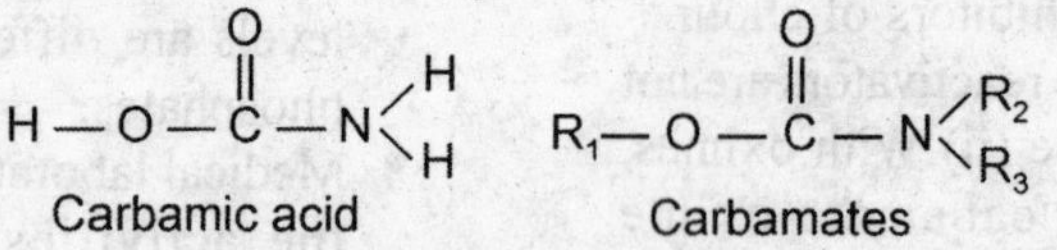

Fig. 35.1: Structure of carbamic acid and general structure of carbamates

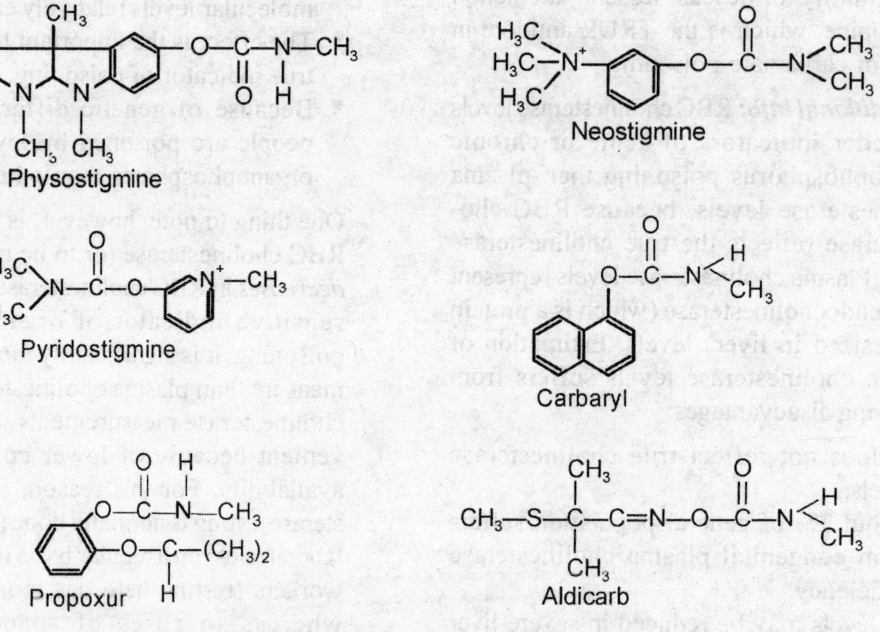

Fig. 35.2: Some common carbamates

In deaths due to organophosphorus insecticides the values will be much less than these. Twenty-five percent or greater depression of the red-cell cholinesterase level is a true indicator of poisoning. Death occurs when levels have decreased by more than 90%.

It is also useful to remember that the normal level of cholinesterase varies greatly between people. Therefore, when monitoring a person's cholinesterase level (e.g. farmers who are going to be exposed to organophosphorus pesticides), it is necessary to determine how much cholinesterase that person (the farmer) normally has. This is done by taking a blood sample at a time when the person has not been exposed to cholinesterase inhibitors for several months. A person's normal cholinesterase level is called the baseline. Once a person's baseline is established, it is used for comparison in future blood analyses to see if the person's level of cholinesterase has changed.

ORGANOCHLORINES

8. **D.**
9. **B. *Related facts to remember:*** All others are organophosphorus compounds (and not organochlorines).
10. **D. *Related facts:*** Because of this peculiar fact, in poisoning with endrin, samples of body fats (and blood) are taken for analysis. This can form another good question. For instance, the question may begin like this: **Question→**In which of the following poisonings, body fats must be taken for analysis? The correct answer should be a organochlorine (Aldrin, Dieldrin, Endrin, DDT etc.).
11. **D.**
12. **C.**
13. **D.**
14. **D. *Related fact:*** There is no known antidote of organochlorines. They are managed symptomatically. In some organochlorine poisonings *Cholestyramine*, a non-absorbable bile acid binding anion exchange resin is given. It is particularly useful in poisoning with Chlordecone. It makes use of the fact that most organochlorines have an enterohepatic circulation. It binds with the offending organochlorine molecule in the gut and prevents its reuptake, thus increasing its faecal excretion.

HERBICIDES AND WEED-KILLERS

15. **A. *Related fact:*** Cacodylic acid is $C_2H_7AsO_2$. Its structural formula is:

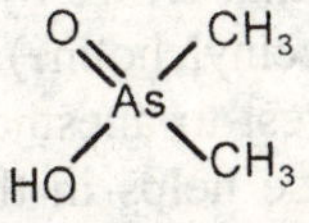

Fig. 35.3: Cacodylic acid

It is also called dimethylarsinic acid. Cacodylic acid is used as an arsenical herbicide.

MULTIPLE ANSWER TYPE (PGI, CHANDIGARH PATTERN)

16. **B,C,D. *Related facts:*** True cholinesterase is Acetylcholinesterase or AchE. Pseudocholinesterase is Butyrylcholinesterase or BchE or type 2 ChE. Levels of both are depressed in deaths owing to organophosphorus insecticides. The measurement of their levels can assist in the determination of the cause of death. In the absence of data on AchE inhibition, data on just the inhibition of BchE is more a reflection of exposure to organophosphorus insecticides than their true effect on the individual.

AChE is found mostly in RBC, motor end-plates and gray matter while BchE is found mostly in plasma, white matter and visceral organs such as liver, heart and pancreas.

The physiological function of BChE is unknown; there is no known physiological substrate for this enzyme. Postulated functions of BChE include a role in the transmission of slow nerve impulses, in lipid metabolism, a regulatory role in choline homeostasis, role in permeability of membranes, in the protection of fetus from toxic compounds, a role in the degradation of acetylcholine and in tumourigenesis. BuChE has also been called a "physiological flypaper" or "sink" in as much as it mops up some of the organophosphates (and other anticholinesterases) and thus offers protection against low doses of organophosphorus poisoning.

It is known that BChE hydrolyzes suxamethonium (succinylcholine) and for this reason it is of interest to anesthesiologists. Butylcholinesterase helps in the metabolism of exogenous choline ester drugs, and succinylcholine is one such drug. Other drugs which are metabolized by BchE are mivacurium, procaine, and cocaine. A congenital deficiency of BChE would affect the metabolism of all of these drugs. However it is the interference with succinylcholine metabolism that is of most concern to doctors, especially anaesthesiologists. The enzyme succinylcholine is hydrolyzed by BChE to succinylmonocholine and then to succinic acid.

BuChE shows significant genetic polymorphism in humans, with 24% of the population having at least one genetic variant allele. Most variants have a decreased enzyme activity, which is clinically important because individuals with low activity are highly sensitive to succinylcholine.

This condition is recognized most often when respiratory paralysis unexpectedly persists for a prolonged period of time following administration of standard doses of succinylcholine. The mainstay of treatment in these cases is ventilatory support until diffusion of succinylcholine from the myoneural junction permits return of neuromuscular function of skeletal muscle. The diagnosis is confirmed by a laboratory assay demonstrating decreased plasma cholinesterase enzyme activity.

Pseudocholinesterase deficiency is most common in people of European descent; it is rare in Asians.

36 Metallic Irritants

GENERAL

1. **Sankhya or Somalkhar is the vernacular name of which of the following poisons?**
   A. Copper sulphate
   B. Lead tetroxide
   C. Mercuric chloride
   D. Arsenic trioxide

2. **Acrodynia is seen in poisoning with:**
   A. Arsenic
   B. Mercury
   C. Lead
   D. Copper

3. **Plumbism is the name given to chronic poisoning with:**
   A. Mercury
   B. Lead
   C. Copper
   D. Either mercury or lead

4. **Aldrich-Mees' lines are seen on .... in poisoning due to ....**
   A. Sclera, arsenic
   B. Gums, lead
   C. Fingernails, arsenic
   D. Fingernails, mercury

5. **Hyperpigmentation of palm and soles is seen in poisoning with:**
   A. Arsenic
   B. Mercury
   C. Lead
   D. Copper

6. **Saturnism is the name given to chronic poisoning with:**
   A. Mercury
   B. Copper
   C. Thallium
   D. Lead

7. **Glass blowers' shakes are seen in chronic poisoning with:**
   A. Arsenic
   B. Mercury
   C. Silica poisoning
   D. Lead

8. **Which of the following facts regarding metal fume fever are correct?**
   A. It is characterized by an influenza like syndrome, with sudden onset of chills, fever, thirst, myalgias and headache within 4-8 hours of inhalation of freshly oxidized metallic fumes
   B. The metals responsible are mainly zinc, brass, copper, tin, magnesium, iron, nickel, manganese, cadmium, chromium and cobalt
   C. The course of metal fume fever is generally benign with symptoms resolving completely within 24-48 hours without any sequelae
   D. All of the above

9. **Reinsch's test is used for:**
   A. Morphine
   B. Dhatura
   C. Arsenic
   D. Nux vomica
10. **Marsh test is used for the detection of:**
   A. Arsenic
   B. Lead
   C. Strychnine
   D. Opium
11. **Gutzeit test is done mainly for:**
   A. Lead
   B. Arsenic
   C. Mercury
   D. Copper
12. **Quicksilver is the common name of:**
   A. Artificial silver
   B. Mercury fulminate
   C. Arsenious oxide
   D. Mercury
13. **Which of the following poisonings can mimic the disease cholera?**
   A. Arsenic trioxide
   B. Copper sulphate
   C. Zinc chloride
   D. Barium Chloride
14. **Sodium formaldehyde sulphoxylate was once recommended in which of the following poisonings?**
   A. Arsenic trioxide
   B. Mercuric chloride
   C. Lead tetroxide
   D. Manganese dioxide
15. **Which of the following is Scheele's green?**
   A. Copper aceto-arsenite
   B. Copper carbonate
   C. Lead sulphate
   D. Copper arsenite
16. **Hydrargyrism is chronic poisoning with:**
   A. Lead
   B. Mercury
   C. Copper
   D. Arsenic
17. **Which of the following is Malachite green?**
   A. Copper aceto-arsenite
   B. Copper carbonate
   C. Lead sulphate
   D. Mercuric iodide
18. **Which of the following poisons is most likely to cause ulceration of the large bowel, especially caecum?**
   A. Morphine
   B. Mercury
   C. Methyl alcohol
   D. Datura
19. **Which of the following is Emerald green?**
   A. Copper aceto-arsenite
   B. Lead Carbonate
   C. Lead sulphate
   D. Mercuric iodide
20. **Paris Green is a:**
   A. Stomach poison
   B. Contact poison
   C. Fumigant
   D. rodenticide
21. **Which of the following poisons is present in Donovan's solution?**
   A. Lead
   B. Copper
   C. Arsenic
   D. All of the above
22. **Danbury tremors are seen in poisoning with:**
   A. Copper
   B. Mercury
   C. Lead
   D. Arsenic
23. **Which of the following poisons is present in Fowler's solution?**
   A. Arsenic
   B. Mercury
   C. Thallium
   D. Osmium

24. Amenorrhoea and Infertility are the possible complications of chronic poisoning with:
A. Arsenic
B. Lead
C. Mercury
D. Organophosphorus

25. Shaking palsy is associated with which of the following poisons:
A. Arsenic
B. Mercury
C. Copper
D. Dhatura

26. Which of the following is the most toxic metal?
A. Cadmium
B. Lead
C. Thallium
D. Aluminum

27. Which of the following is the white vitriol?
A. Copper sulphate
B. Ferrous sulphate
C. Zinc sulphate
D. None of the above

ARSENIC

28. Which of the following are non-poisonous salts of arsenic?
A. Arsenic disulphide
B. Arsenious oxide
C. Arsenic trisulphide
D. Both (A) and (C)

29. The fatal dose of arsenic trioxide is:
A. 200-300 micrograms
B. 2-3 mg
C. 200-300 mg
D. 2-3 g

30. In acute arsenic poisoning, maximum arsenic concentration is found in .... followed by ....
A. Liver, kidney
B. Liver, brain
C. Brain, liver
D. Liver, spinal cord

31. Once a person is poisoned with arsenic, it may remain for years in:
A. Bone
B. Hair
C. Liver
D. Kidney

LEAD

32. Sugar of lead is the name given to which of the following poisons?
A. Lead acetate
B. Lead carbonate
C. Lead chromate
D. Lead tetroxide

33. The earliest and most consistent manifestation of chronic lead poisoning is:
A. Facial pallor
B. Anemia
C. Lead colic
D. Lead line

34. Feature most commonly encountered in chronic lead poisoning is:
A. Lead line
B. Lead palsy
C. Dry belly aches
D. Encephalopathy

35. One of the classical signs of chronic lead poisoning is basophilic stippling. In which of the following cells is this seen?
A. Basophils
B. Red blood cells
C. Lymphocytes
D. All White blood cells

36. Basophilic stippling is seen in:
A. Thalassemia
B. Sideroblastic anaemia
C. Chronic lead poisoning
D. All of the above

37. Lead is absorbed through:
A. Skin
B. GIT
C. Lungs
D. All of the above

38. *Sindur* used by ladies is:
A. Lead acetate
B. Lead tetroxide
C. Lead chromate
D. Lead carbonate

39. Anti-knocking agent used in petrol is:
A. Lead chromate
B. Lead sulfide
C. Lead tetraethyl
D. Any compound of lead

40. Acute lead poisoning in children presents as:
A. Status epilepticus
B. Ataxia
C. Focal deficit
D. Papilloedema

MERCURY

41. The usual fatal dose of mercuric chloride in a 70 kg human being is:
A. 0.5-1.0 microgram
B. 0.5-1.0 mg
C. 0.5-1.0 g
D. 5-10 g

42. Calomel is:
A. Mercurous chloride
B. Mercuric chloride
C. Mercuric sulfide
D. Mercuric oxide

COPPER

43. Usual fatal dose of copper sulfate is:
A. 10-20 micrograms
B. 10-20 milligrams
C. 1-2 g
D. 10-20 g

44. Bluish green vomitus in copper sulfate poisoning can be differentiated from that due to bile by the addition of:
A. Ammonium hydroxide
B. Potassium permanganate
C. Nitric acid
D. Egg albumen

MISCELLANEOUS

45. The best antidote for thallium is:
A. BAL
B. EDTA
C. Potassium ferric hexacyanoferrate
D. Sodium thiosulfate

46. The French General Napoléon Bonaparte (1769-1821) was supposed to have been poisoned with:
A. Copper
B. Lead
C. Mercury
D. Arsenic

47. Clapton's line is seen in:
A. Acute iron poisoning
B. Chronic zinc poisoning
C. Chronic copper poisoning
D. Chronic mercury poisoning

48. Antidote for acute iron poisoning is:
A. Deferoxamine
B. Sodium EDTA
C. BAL
D. Penicillamine

49. A patient is brought to casualty with poisoning. Stomach wash lavage fluid produces a black precipitate on heating. Which is the most likely poisoning?
A. Tik-20
B. Silver nitrate
C. Morphine
D. Hydrogen cyanide

50. "Lunar caustic" is also known as:
A. Iron sulphate
B. Mercury nitrate

C. Cadmium nitrate
D. Silver nitrate

51. Chronic exposure to which of the following poisons produces "argyria" or "argyriosis"?
A. Lead
B. Arsenic
C. Silver
D. Mercury

52. Bluish grey pigmentation of conjunctivae, mucus membranes and nails are most frequently associated with chronic poisoning by salts of:
A. Arsenic
B. Mercury
C. Copper
D. Silver

53. Butter of antimony is:
A. Antimony potassium tartarate
B. Antimony trichloride
C. Antimony sulphide
D. Antimony hydride

54. Cuprimine is:
A. Desferroxamine
B. Penicillamine
C. EDTA
D. Copper sulphate

MULTIPLE ANSWER TYPE (PGI, CHANDIGARH PATTERN)

55. Which of the following facts are correct about Burtonian line?
A. It may be seen in silver poisoning
B. It is not seen in edentulous patients
C. It is normally seen in gum margins, but is also seen radiologically near the epiphysis of long bones
D. It is more commonly seen in females
E. If the gums are infected, then the pigmentation may be more extensive

56. Following are features of chronic lead poisoning?
A. Encephalopathy
B. Palsy
C. Bronchitis
D. Colic and constipation
E. Cataract formation

57. The following statements are true about lead palsy:
A. It is seen both in acute and chronic lead poisoning
B. It is more common in adults than in children
C. It is more common in men than in women
D. The arm is more commonly affected than the leg
E. It occurs in about 90% of patients with chronic lead poisoning

58. Following salts may be used as *sindur*:
A. Lead tetroxide
B. Lead tetraethyl
C. Mercuric chloride
D. Mercuric sulfide
E. Mercurous chloride

59. Which of the following statements about mercuria lentis are correct?
A. It is seen in acute mercury poisoning
B. It is observed usually with a slit lamp
C. Visual blurring is often present, and sometimes there is concentric constriction of visual fields
D. It is characterized by a brown reflex of the anterior lens capsule of the eye
E. Frequently punctate hemorrhages can be seen on the sclera

ANSWERS

GENERAL

1. D.
2. B. ***Related facts:*** The term comes from "*acro*" meaning extremities (this term is seen in such words as acromegaly – or enlargement of extremities), plus the Greek word "*odyne*" or pain (as in anodyne or a pain killer). The term literally means pain in the extremities. It is seen in chronic mercury poisoning. Other names for this disease are Swift's disease, Feer's disease, Selter's disease, erythredema, Pink disease and dermato-polyneuritis.

   It is frequently seen in infants which are chronically exposed to mercury as in teething powders, lotions, ointments or napkin rinses (mercurous chloride or calomel is bactericidal and germicidal and was once used for napkin rinses). The child is restless, irritable and feverish. There is tachycardia, generalized erythema, hyperhidrosis (excessive sweating), stomatitis and dystrophy of hair and nails. Hands and feet are red and swollen, although cold and painful. Mortality is about 10%.
3. B. ***Related fact:*** The word comes from Latin *plumbum*, meaning lead. This Latin root also gives us the word "plumber", a person who works with lead. **P**lumbism is common in people who work with lead, e.g. **p**otters, **p**ewters, **p**ainters, **p**rinters and **p**lumbers. Lead often gets administered slowly through food or water and in such situations too plumbism can occur. Plumbism was common in days when water was supplied to homes through lead pipes or copper pipes with lead-soldered joints.
4. C. ***Related fact:*** Sometimes these lines are known just as Mees' lines (technically they are known as *transverse striate leukonychia*). Mees' lines are transverse, 1-2 mm white striations in the fingernails, which may be deformed or fall out within 2-3 weeks of exposure. They occur both in acute as well as chronic arsenic poisoning.

   Although Mees' lines reflect a transient disruption of nail plate growth, some physicians believe these lines are actual arsenic deposits.

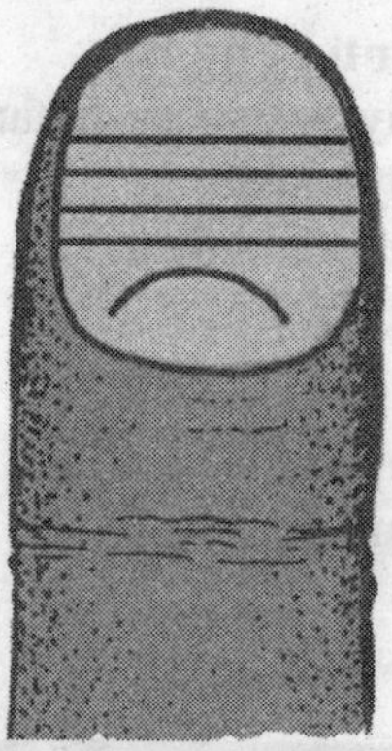

Fig. 36.1: Aldrich-Mees' lines on fingernails seen in arsenic poisoning

Mees' lines are rather uncommonly seen; they are thought to occur in just about 5% of the patients of arsenic poisoning.

The lines are named after **C.J. Aldrich** (American physician, early 20th century) and **R.A. Mees** (Dutch scientist, 20th century), who first described them.

A variation of this question is often asked like this→A middle aged man presents with paraesthesia of hands and feet. Examination reveals presence of Mees' lines in the nails and rain drop pigmentation in the hands. The most likely causative toxin for the above mentioned symptoms is (a) Lead (b) Arsenic (c) Thallium (d) Mercury. The answer is (b) Arsenic.

Additional info: Although Mees' lines are *classically* associated with arsenic poisoning, they are also seen in several other systemic insults such as Hodgkin's disease, CHF, leprosy, malaria, chemotherapy abd carbon monoxide poisoning. They have even been described in a patient with helminthic and amebic infections.[1]

It is important to appreciate that these lines represent a transient problem relating to the growth disturbance of the nails. Several other similar lines in nails have been described, most common being Muehrcke's lines (specific for hypoalbuminemia), and Beau's lines (seen in any severe systemic illness that disrupts nail growth, Raynaud's disease, pemphigus and trauma). A detailed discussion of these lines is beyond the scope of this book.

5. A.

6. D. ***Related fact:*** In ancient times, each major heavenly body were supposed to be composed of one major metal. Thus sun was supposed to be composed of gold, and moon of silver. The planet Saturn was supposed to be composed of lead. Thus chronic poisoning with lead came to be known as saturnism.

7. B. ***Additional info:*** These are also known as **Hatter's shakes**, because they were once very common in workers involved in hat industry. Watch out for this synonym too.

   Variant: Hatter's shake are seen in chronic poisoning with (a) arsenic (b) mercury (c) phosphorus (d) lead. The answer is (b) Mercury.

8. D. ***Additional Notes:*** Other facts to remember about Metal fume fever are:
   - Recognized for centuries, but first characterized by Potissier in 1822.
   - Caused by freshly oxidized metallic fumes having a particle size smaller than 0.5 to 1.0 microns.
   - Usually caused by welding or melting of metals (tasks involving oxidation of metals) mentioned above. Other occupations involved are soldering, forging and casting of metal.
   - Quite common. More than 1000 cases annually are reported.
   - Most commonly seen in Zinc, iron and copper.
   - Cadmium and tin produce a more severe illness.
   - Also known as MFF, Monday morning fever (workers complain of illness developing at the beginning of the week. It resolves completely during the weekend. It recurs the next work week again), the smothers, brass founder's ague, brazier's disease, foundry fever, galvanizer's poisoning, smelter's chills, zinc chills, zinc fume fever, brass chills and copper fever.
   - Repeated episodes are frequent, especially after a patient has been free from exposure for several days.
   - The syndrome is toxic in origin. Not dependent on prior sensitization.
   - The course of the fever is generally benign. Fever can be as high as 104°C. Chest examination and radiographs show no changes.
   - Theories about causation (i) Release of endogenous pyrogens (ii) Production of antigenic metal proteinates (iii) Delayed hypersensitivity pneumonitis (iv) Direct toxic effect on alveolar cells.

---

[1] Hepburn MJ, English JC 3rd, Meffert JJ. Mees' lines in a patient with multiple parasitic infections. Cutis. 1997 Jun;59(6):321-3

9. C. *Additional Notes:* Developed by German Hugo Reinsch, this test is done in this way. 20 ml of stomach contents or vomitus is taken. Same amount of urine can also be taken or even dissolved suspect powder. It is placed in a conical flask along with 4 ml Hydrochloric acid. A small strip or coil of copper is added. The flask is gently heated for an hour. Copper strip (or coil) is removed and examined. The interpretation is as follows:

If there is a silvery deposit→**mercury.**

If there is black deposit→**arsenic, antimony** or **bismuth** (any of these three could be there).

To Differentiate between the last three, place copper in 2 ml of 10% potassium cyanide.

Deposit dissolves→**Arsenic.**

Deposit does not dissolve→**Antimony** or **bismuth.**

So Reinsch's test is basically done for four poisons (i) **arsenic** (ii) **mercury** (iii) **antimony** and (iv) **bismuth.**

10. A. *Additional facts:* This test was developed by the British chemist **James Marsh** (1794-1846) in 1836. Later Berzelius modified the test and the test became known as the Marsh-Berzelius test.

The origin of the test is interesting. In 1832, Marsh was asked to testify in a supposed case of arsenic poisoning. A person known as John Bodle was supposed to have poisoned his grandfather by putting arsenic in his coffee. Marsh who was working at the Royal Arsenal in Woolwich at that time, was called by the prosecution to try to prove that arsenic was present in the coffee. At that time, the standard test for arsenic was to pass hydrogen sulfide through the suspected sample. If arsenic was present, it would from a yellow precipitate of arsenic sulfide (As_2S_3). Marsh performed the test successfully, but alas, the yellow precipitate did not keep very well, and by the time it was presented to the jury it deteriorated. The jury was not convinced, and John Bodle was acquitted. To make matters more frustrating for Marsh, the accused John Bodle confessed later that he had indeed killed his grandfather. Stung by this, Marsh decided to devise a better test to demonstrate the presence of arsenic. The result of his work culminated in the celebrated Marsh test (Fig. 36.2).

To perform this test, first of all, a hydrogen generator is taken (A). Hydrogen is generated in this generator by zinc and dilute H_2SO_4. For obvious reasons, zinc itself should be free of traces of arsenic. The suspected

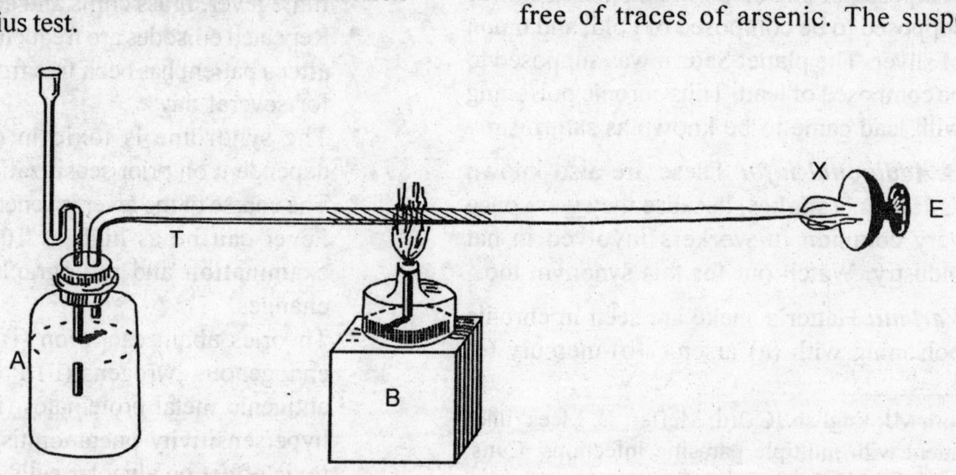

Fig. 36.2: Marsh test. Please refer to text for details

sample containing arsenic is introduced into a hydrogen generator. If arsenic is present in the suspected sample, this would produce arseniuretted hydrogen or arsine (AsH_3) by the following reaction:

$$2As + 3H_2 \rightarrow 2AsH_3$$

This gas is made to eject through a narrow tube (T) which is heated (B). As it comes out in a jet it is ignited (X), the flame being cooled by placing a piece of cold porcelain in the flame (E). Arsine is decomposed back to arsenic and hydrogen, forming a brownish-black film of arsenic in a cold zone.

$$2AsH_3 \rightarrow 2As + 3H_2$$

The beauty of this test (over the earlier tests) was that this film of arsenic could *actually* be shown to the lay jury to make the test appear more convincing! This was the first accurate test to be developed for arsenic, which could also be demonstrated convincingly to a lay jury. Later it underwent several useful modifications.

11. **B.** ***Related facts:*** This test was developed by the German chemist Max Adolf Gutzeit (1847–1915). Like the Marsh test, this test too is based on the formation of arsine and is basically just a modification of the Marsh test. The suspected sample is added to the hydrogen generator (containing zinc and sulfuric acid). If arsenic is present in the sample, AsH_3 will form. A filter paper moistened with an acidulated silver nitrate solution is held over the resulting fumes. The formation of a yellow spot on the paper indicates the presence of inorganic arsenic compounds. In some variations of the test, the filter paper may be treated with mercuric chloride or mercuric bromide. Formation of a yellow spot over the filter paper indicates the presence of arsenic.
12. **D.**
13. **A.**
14. **B.** The use of sodium formaldehyde sulfoxylate was first advocated by S. M. Rosenthal in 1935, but its use never caught up. It was a controversial treatment from the very beginning. The recommended procedure was to perform a gastric lavage with 5% solution of sodium formaldehyde sulfoxylate, followed by 2% $NaHCO_3$, and finally leave 250 cc of the sodium formaldehyde sulfoxylate in the stomach.

    Sodium formaldehyde sulfoxylate is a powerful reducing agent and is thought to convert poisonous mercury salts to elemental mercury, limiting its absorption. Another recommended treatment was gastric lavage with egg white; it formed mercury albuminate, limiting the absorption of mercury. Other protein containing solutions such as milk have also been tried in an effort to bind mercury.
15. **D.** ***Related fact:*** It was used as a weedkiller. Mnemonic: CAS→Copper Arsenite= Scheele's green.
16. **B.**
17. **B.** Mnemonic: MCC→**M**alachite Green = **C**opper **C**arbonate.
18. **B.** ***Related fact:*** This ulceration is seen if the victim survives for a few days. It is as a consequence of excretion of mercury into the gut. The superficial ulceration may resemble that of bacillary dysentery.
19. **A.** Copper aceto arsenite is known by two other names—Paris Green and Schweinfurt Green. Mnemonic: CAAPES—**C**opper **A**ceto **A**rsenite = **P**aris Green, **E**merald Green, **S**chweinfurt Green.
20. **A.** Insecticides can be classified in a number of ways – on the basis of their chemistry, their toxicological action, or their mode of penetration. In the latter scheme, they are classified according to whether they take effect upon ingestion (*stomach poisons*), inhalation (*fumigants*), or upon penetration

of the body covering (*contact poisons*). Since most synthetic organic insecticides penetrate by all three of these pathways, they should better be distinguished from each other by their basic chemistry. However since this question has been asked time and again, a brief introduction to the three types of poisons is given below:

Stomach poisons: Stomach poisons are toxic only if ingested through the mouth and are most useful against those insects that have biting or chewing mouth parts, such as caterpillars, beetles, and grasshoppers. The chief stomach poisons are the arsenicals — e.g., Paris Green (copper acetoarsenite), lead arsenate, and calcium arsenate; and the fluorine compounds, among them sodium fluoride and cryolite. They are applied as sprays or dusts onto the leaves and stems of plants eaten by the target insects. Stomach poisons have now mostly been replaced by synthetic organic insecticides, which are less dangerous to humans and other mammals.

Fumigants: These are toxic compounds that enter the respiratory system of the insect through its spiracles, or breathing openings. They include such chemicals as hydrogen cyanide, naphthalene, nicotine, and methyl bromide and are used mainly for killing insect pests of stored products (e.g. wheat grains) or for fumigating nursery stock.

Contact poisons: These poisons penetrate the skin of the pest and are used against those arthropods, such as aphids, that pierce the surface of a plant and suck out the juices. Nicotine, pyrethrum and rotenone are examples of contact poisons.

Paris Green was first used as an insecticide in 1867. It has never been used as a rodenticide.

21. C. Donovan's Solution was prepared by Michael Donovan (b. 1760), a Dublin apothecary. It is an aqueous solution of iodides of mercury and arsenic and was used to treat veneral diseases.

22. B. ***Additional info:*** Danbury in Connecticut, USA was known as the hat making capital of the world in the 19th century. During the industry boom of the 1880s, over five million hats a year were produced there in 56 different factories.

The production process involved using a mercury compound, mercury nitrate, to remove fur from pelts and turn it into felt more easily. Abraham Lincoln's famous beaver stovepipe hats were made in this fashion.

Hat makers, exposed to large amounts of vaporized mercury, began to experience its effects on their nervous systems. Doctors even recorded seeing "holes the size of quarters" inside some hatters' brains. These workers displayed classical symptoms of chronic mercury poisoning, one of which is tremors. This is why, these tremors came to be called Danbury tremors. These are also known as *Hatter's shakes*. Watch out for this fact.

The state of Connecticut outlawed the use of mercury in hat making in the early 1940s. But there are signs that mercury remains in soil and river sediment not far from where factories once stood.

23. A. Fowler's solution, also known as *Liquor arsenicalis*, was prepared by Stafford physician Thomas Fowler (b. 1736). It is a solution of potassium arsenite containing the equivalent of 1% As_2O_3. It was used in the treatment of blood disorders and intermittent fever. It was used as a tonic also.

24. B.

25. B.

26. C.

27. C. ***Related facts:*** The word vitriol comes from Latin *vitrum* meaning glass. Sulphates of several metals such as copper, iron, zinc and cobalt are known as vitriols on account of their glassy appearance or luster. Remember the following:

- Blue vitriol—Copper sulphate.
- Green vitriol—Ferrous sulphate.
- Red vitriol—Cobalt sulphate.
- White vitriol—zinc sulphate (Formerly called vitriol of zinc).
- Oil of vitriol—sulphuric or vitriolic acid; popularly so called because it has the consistency of oil.
- Vitriol of Mars—ferric sulphate, a white crystalline substance which dissolves in water, forming a red solution.

ARSENIC

28. D.

29. C. ***Related fact:*** In older books, frequently the fatal dose was mentioned as 3 grains (1 grain being equal to 60 mg). Students may often find this choice (as the correct intended choice), so watch out for this too.

Arsenic is available in two forms—a trivalent form (arsenite) and a pentavalent form (arsenate). Pentavalent form is less toxic than the trivalent form because it is less water soluble.

30. A. ***Related facts:*** Arsenic concentrations in fatal cases (mg/L or mg/kg) are as follows (in decreasing concentrations) (See table 36.1).

31. A. Both Arsenic and phosphorus belong to group 7 of period table. Arsenic thus mimics phosphorus and replaces it in the bone. There it remains for years.

Hair keep growing and after the poisoning has stopped, new hair that forms at the root would be devoid of arsenic. Hair at the tips that contained arsenic would be trimmed off during regular hair cuts. Thus after a few months, arsenic would not be found in the hair. But if hair were not trimmed off, arsenic would indeed be found in those portions of the hair that grew during the time of arsenic poisoning. Arsenic in soft tissues such as liver and kidney does not remain for any appreciable period after poisoning has stopped.

Arsenic gets deposited in hair and bones for entirely different chemical reasons. In bones, it replaces phosphorus as we have seen above. In hair it attaches to the sulfydryl groups of keratin. It is useful to remember that in exhumations, bones and hair are almost routinely examined, if arsenic poisoning was suspected during life.

LEAD

32. A. ***Related fact:*** Lead carbonate is known as **White lead** and Lead oxide as **litharge.** Lead acetate used to be called 'sugar of lead' because of its sweet taste; it was added to wines as a sweetener! Romans used to sweeten their wines with sugar of lead. It is hypothesized that they got chronic lead poisoning as a result. They became lethargic (because of chronic lead poisoning), and the great Roman Empire fell.

33. A. This is a dubious fact. The only justification of inclusion of this question is the

Table 36.1: Arsenic concentrations in various organs in fatal arsenic poisoning (mg/L or mg/kg)

Rank	1	2	3	4	5
Organ	Liver	Kidney	Spleen	Blood	Brain
Average	29	15	8.8	3.3	1.7
(Range)	(2.0-120.0)	(0.2-70.0)	(0.5-62.0)	(0.6-9.3)	(0.2-4.0)

regular frequency with which this question is asked in the examinations.

34. **C.** This is another dubious fact, touted most often in MCQ books. Once again the only justification of its inclusion is the frequency with which this question has been asked in various examinations.

35. **B.** ***Related fact:*** Lead increases hemolysis (besides decreasing haem synthesis as well), as a result of which immature red cells are released in circulation. These are reticulocytes and red cells with basophilic stippling. Lead inhibits the enzyme **pyrimidine 5′ – nucleotidase,** which normally eliminates degraded RNA. This leads to clumping of ribosomal RNA, which is seen as stippling.

36. **D.** ***Additional info:*** Basophilic stippling is a nonspecific finding noted in the blood of patients with thalassemia and sideroblastic anaemia. Though this finding is also seen in chronic lead poisoning, it is not noted always. Nor is the amount of RBCs showing basophilic stippling any indication of the degree of lead intoxication.

37. **D.** ***Related fact:*** Lead is absorbed through all portals of entry. Occupational exposure results mainly from inhalation, while in most other situations the mode of intake is ingestion. Tetraethyl lead can be absorbed readily through skin.

38. **B.** Nowadays a number of other synthetic materials are used in *sindur*, but there was a time when lead tetroxide was used as *sindur*. This could cause chronic lead poisoning in ladies.

39. **C.** ***Related information:*** Petrol is a mixture of several hydrocarbons, some of which have a tendency to burn prematurely when the gaseous mixture is compressed in the engine mechanism. Lead tetraethyl is added to petrol to prevent this premature burning. However this lead is released in the environment causing chronic lead poisoning.

40. **A.** ***Related facts:*** Lead causes injury to several organs, including the kidney (renal failure, hypertension), bone marrow (anemia) and, especially, the CNS. Lead poisoning is difficult to diagnose unless the physician has a high index of suspicion. The symptoms and signs of lead poisoning reflect the blood lead levels (BLL). Gastrointestinal symptoms including abdominal cramps, constipation and vomiting are associated with BLL in excess of 20 micrograms/dL. Lead encephalopathy is more common in children than adults and is characterized by lethargy, headache, seizures and other signs of cerebral edema, including status epilepticus and coma. BLL found in children with encephalopathy range from 100 micrograms/dL to 300 micrograms/dL.

Status epilepticus (and convulsions) are treated in a conventional manner with benzodiazepines and other anticonvulsants, including phenobarbital and phenytoin. Patients with lead encephalopathy may require high doses of anticonvulsants for seizure control. Persistent status epilepticus may require neuromuscular blockade with EEG monitoring.

In the past, many of the children presenting with acute lead poisoning died due either to poor diagnosis or lack of proper treatment. Those that survived had a high incidence of epilepsy, cognitive impairment, poor memory and learning problems. Radiographs of the long bones often showed ‘lead lines’ in the metaphysis, and basophilic stippling of red blood cells. Most of these children were investigated for seizure disorders or brain tumours until the correct diagnosis was contemplated and established.

Lead poisoning in children can easily be diagnosed by completing a urine coproporphyrin test at the bedside. Glacial acetic acid is added to a sample of urine, followed by the addition of ether and 1.5 N hydrochloric acid. An orange fluorescence of the urine sample by illumination with a Wood's light indicates a positive test.

Note that physical findings of chronic lead toxicity includes papilloedema. Other physical findings are gingival lead lines (purple-blue lines consisting of lead sulfide precipitates within the gingival tissue), buccal stains and macular gray stains. However (d) may not be a correct choice as it is a physical finding rather than a symptom.

MERCURY

41. C. ***Additional fact:*** The usual fatal dose of mercurous chloride in a 70 kg human being is 1.5-2.0 g.

42. A. ***Related fact:*** Mercuric chloride is corrosive sublimate. Mercuric sulfide is vermillion or *sindur*. In fact any blood red colored salt may be used as *sindur*. Mercuric sulfide is one; lead tetroxide is another. Watch out for this fact, as it lends itself for a very good MCQ.

COPPER

43. D.

44. A. ***Related fact:*** When ammonium hydroxide is added to the vomitus of a copper sulfate poisoned patient, it turns deep blue in color. In bile the color remains unchanged.

MISCELLANEOUS

45. C. ***Additional info*****:** In acute poisoning, a stomach wash is done with potassium ferric hexacyanoferrate, ($KFe_{(III)}[Fe_{(II)}(CN)_6]$) – sometimes termed as Prussian blue. After the stomach wash, the same drug is instilled through a duodenal tube directly into the duodenum since thallium may diminish gastric and intestinal motility. The dose is 125 mg/kg twice a day, with 50 ml of 15% mannitol. Mannitol is given as a laxative, since one of the most commonly reported side effects of this drug is constipation.

Administration should be continued until urinary thallium excretion is less than 0.5 mg/24 hours.

True Prussian blue [or Ferric Ferrocyanide ($Fe_4[Fe(CN)_6]_3$) or ferric hexacyanoferrate] is also advocated as an antidote for thallium poisoning, although this is said to be less effective than Potassium ferric hexacyanoferrate. However both antidotes are believed to be more effective than activated charcoal in binding thallium and preventing its absorption from the GI tract. Ferric Ferrocyanide is available as Radiogardase™ (500 mg capsules). Structure given below:

In the gut, Prussian Blue traps thallium by

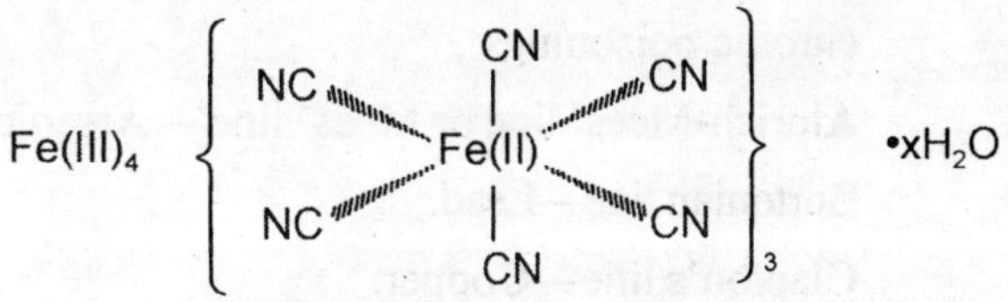

Fig. 36.3: Ferric ferrocyanide (Radiogardase™)

exchanging thallium for potassium in the molecule's lattice. Thallium is thus passed out of the body in the stool rather than be reabsorbed.

Because thallium has an entero-enteric cycle, thallium excreted into the intestine is trapped and redistribution of the poison slowed.

Since Prussian blue (in its both forms as mentioned above) contains CN ions, there was some concern about CN poisoning occurring in patients receiving this drug. However in vitro experiments have demonstrated that release of cyanide does not occur in human conditions. Long-term administration of Prussian Blue to animals also does not produce any toxic effects.

Without treatment, the half-life of thallium is about 8 days. With colloidally soluble potassium ferric hexacyanoferrate therapy the half-life is reduced to 3 days. When this therapy is combined with forced diuresis the half-life of thallium is reduced to 2 days.

46. **D.** ***Related fact:*** Napoleon died a mysterious death after six years in exile. It is widely believed that after Napoleon lost the legendary battle of Waterloo in 1815, and the English exiled him to the remote island of St. Helena, they slowly poisoned him to death with arsenic.

47. **C.** It is a greenish line seen on the dental margin of gums in chronic copper poisoning. Allegedly due to the formation of copper sulfide. First described by the London physician and surgeon Edward Clapton (1830-1909).

Remember all three lines seen in different chronic poisonings:

Aldrich-Mees' line or Mees' line— Arsenic.

Burtonian line—Lead.

Clapton's line—Copper.

48. **A.**

49. **B.** ***Related facts:*** Silver nitrate, on exposure to light or on contact with organic matter such as skin may turn to finely divided silver which is blackish in color. The vomiting in such cases is also blackish for the same reason.

50. **D.** ***Related facts***: "Lunar caustic" is silver nitrate in the form of sticks used in cauterization.

51. **C.**

52. **D.**

53. **B.** ***Related facts:*** Called so because of its waxy quality.

54. **B.** ***Related info:*** Cuprimine and Depen are the most popular brand names of Penicillamine.

MULTIPLE ANSWER TYPE (PGI, CHANDIGARH PATTERN)

55. **A,B,E.** It is true that Burtonian line is seen normally in chronic lead poisoning, but it is also seen in several other chronic metal poisonings such as silver, copper and mercury. This line is about 1 mm wide and is due to the deposition of lead (or other metal, such as silver, copper or mercury) sulfide in the gum margin.

56. **A,B,D.**

57. **B,C,D.** Lead palsy is seen in only about 10% of patients with chronic lead poisoning. Facts mentioned in b,c and d are correct. Among the arms, the right arm is more commonly affected than the left. If a patient uses a particular group of muscles excessively in his occupation, then these are the muscles likely to be affected by weakness.

58. **A,B.** While the common teaching in this country is that lead tetroxide is vermillion or *sindur*, any blood red colored salt may be used as *sindur*. Both lead tetroxide and mercuric sulfide are red in color.

59. **B,C,D.** ***Related facts***: Mercuria lentis is a classical symptom of chronic mercury poisoning or "hydrargyrism". "Tunnel vision" or concentric constriction of visual fields is often associated with mercuria lentis.

37 Vegetable Poisons

1. **Which of the following statements about toxalbumin is not true?**
   - **A.** It is also known as phytotoxin
   - **B.** It is a toxic protein
   - **C.** It is a degradation product of the albumin of hens' eggs and generates as a result of egg's decay
   - **D.** It resembles a bacterial toxin in action
2. **Which of the follwing statements about castor oil is true?**
   - **A.** It contains the poison ricin
   - **B.** It contains the poison crotin
   - **C.** It contains the poison abrin
   - **D.** It does not contain any poison
3. **Which of the following plants is also known as "marking nut"?**
   - **A.** *Semecarpus anacardium*
   - **B.** *Claviceps purpurea*
   - **C.** *Ricinus communis*
   - **D.** *Croton tiglium*
4. **Which of the following plants has a black, roughly cone shaped nut having a thick pericarp?**
   - **A.** Abrus precatorius
   - **B.** Semecarpus anacardium
   - **C.** Calotropis gigantea
   - **D.** Plumbago rosea
5. ***Claviceps purpurea* contains which of the following poisons?**
   - **A.** Bhilawanol
   - **B.** Calotropin
   - **C.** Ergotamine
   - **D.** Capsaicin
6. **Which of the following poisons produces changes which simulate contusions?**
   - **A.** Ricinus communis
   - **B.** Semecarpus anacardium
   - **C.** Capsicum annum
   - **D.** Abrus precatorius
7. **All of the following are vegetable poisons *except*:**
   - **A.** Madar
   - **B.** Cantharides
   - **C.** Croton
   - **D.** Castor
8. **'Hunan hand' is seen in toxicity due to:**
   - **A.** Chilli powder
   - **B.** Marking nut
   - **C.** Castor oil
   - **D.** Poppy seeds
9. ***"Suis"* are classically made from which of the following plants?**
   - **A.** *Capsicum annum*
   - **B.** *Abrus precatorius*

C. *Calotropis gigantea*
D. *Plumbago rosea*

10. Uscharin is an active ingredient of:
A. Semecarpus anacardium
B. Calotropis procera
C. Colocynth
D. Datura alba

11. The juice from which of the following plants is used by tanners for removing hair from the hides and for deodourising them?
A. Calotropis procera
B. Semecarpus anacardium
C. Abrus precatorius
D. Plumbago rosea

MULTIPLE ANSWER TYPE (PGI, CHANDIGARH PATTERN)

12. Which of the following are names of *Abrus precatorius*?
A. *Indian liquorice*
B. Lal chitra
C. *Gunchi*
D. Red pepper
E. *Ratti*

13. Which of the following are NOT toxalbumins?
A. Abric acid
B. Abrin
C. Bhilawanol
D. Ricin
E. Crotin

14. Which of the following are genuinely useful treatment steps in *Ratti* poisoning?
A. Gastric lavage if poisoning is oral
B. Digitalis IV
C. Supportive measures, with emphasis on rehydration
D. Dissect out *suis* if the poisoning is through *sui*
E. Give antiabrin IV

15. Which of the following are NOT the toxic principles of *Ratti*?
A. Glycyrrhizin
B. Semecarpol
C. N-methyl tryptophan
D. Curare
E. Abric acid

16. *Suis* are mostly used for:
A. Homicide
B. Suicide
C. Cattle poisoning
D. Parasuicide
E. Enhancing aroma of foods

ANSWERS

1. C.
2. D.
3. A. ***Related facts:*** *Claviceps purpurea* is known as ergot; *Ricinus communis* as *arandi* and *Croton tiglium* as *jamalgota* or *naepala.* Remember these names also as they can also be asked in MCQs. For instance, this question has often been asked in examinations→ Jamalgota is (a) *Ricinus communis* (b) *Croton tiglium* (c) *Abrus precatorius* (d) *Colocynth.* The answer is (b) *Croton tiglium.*
4. B.
5. C.
6. B. ***Related fact:*** These are known as false bruises or false contusions.
7. B.
8. A. ***Related fact:*** "Hunan hand" is a contact dermatitis resulting from the direct handling of chili peppers containing capsaicin. The condition has been termed so because cooks working in Chinese restaurants often experience it (Hunan is the name of a province in China). Capsaicin is not water soluble, so it is difficult to wash it off one's hands after handling hot peppers.
9. B. The *suis* (needles) are made in this way→The seeds are decorticated and ground. Then they are mixed with datura, opium and onion and then made into a paste with the help of spirit and water. The paste is then drawn in the form of long needles about 15 mm long and dried in the sun. Each needle weighs about 90-120 mg.

   These needles are mounted on a handle (two needles on one handle), and the handle is struck on the back or belly of the animal. The animal dies in about 3-5 days. This method is used either for revenge (killing the cattle of an enemy) or for obtaining hides.

   The advantage of this method (from the perspective of the criminal) is that the punctures made by *suis* give the appearance of a viper bite, and no one suspects the killer. This fact has often been asked in the form of an MCQ as below:

   Qu. Puncture marks made by a *sui* made from *Ratti* resemble:

   (a) Cobra bite (b) Viper bite (c) Hydrophid bite (d) None of the above. The intended answer is (b) Viper bite.
10. B. ***Related facts:*** This plant is known in Hindi as *Madar*, *Akdo*, *Akda*, or simply as *Ak*. Besides uscharin, the plant contains several other active chemicals, main ones being calotropin, calactin and calotoxin.
11. A. ***Related facts:*** The juice (which is milky in nature) is used by people to remove their own unwanted hair too! It is also used as a vesicant and for treatment of chronic skin conditions.

MULTIPLE ANSWER TYPE (PGI, CHANDIGARH PATTERN)

12. A,C,E. *Abrus precatorius* is also known as **Jequirity** or **Jequirity bean.** The seeds are hard, red and black and look quite attractive (Fig. 37.1). Though the seeds are highly poisonous, they are often strung into necklaces and rosaries in India and other tropical areas. For this reason this seed is also known

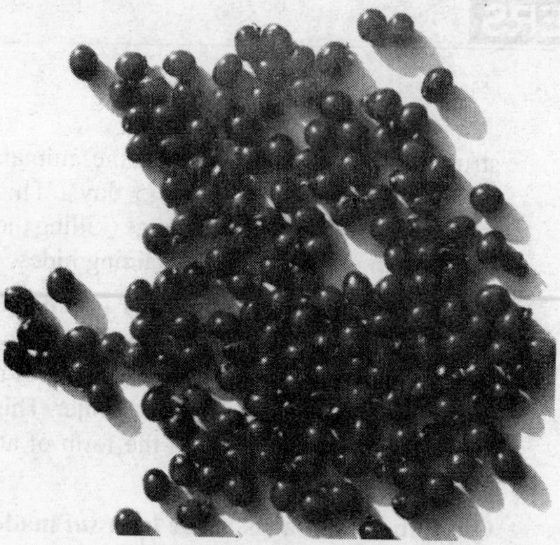

Fig. 37.1: *Ratti* seeds ***(See also Colour Plate 2)***

as **rosary bead, Buddhist rosary bead** or **Prayer bead.**

13. A,C.

14. A,C,D. Gastric lavage and dissection of *suis* are genuine treatment protocols. Supportive measures with a special emphasis on rehydration is also important, since vomiting and diarrhoea are major symptoms in *ratti* poisoning. Digitalis has no known beneficial value in *ratti* poisoning. It is a common myth among students that antiabrin is given for *ratti* poisoning. An anti-serum indeed used to be supplied (by Merck and Co.) under the name of "anti-abrin" or "jequiritol" but was found to be useless and is no longer available.

15. B,D. The active principles of *Ratti* are (i) Abrin (ii) Abric acid (iii) Glycyrrhizin and (iv) N-methyl tryptophan.

Semecarpol is the active principle of *Semecarpus anacardium* (marking nut). Curare is the active principle that comes from *Strychnos toxifera, Strychnos curare* and *Chondrodendron tomentosum.*

16. A,C.

38 Animal Poisons

1. **Intravascular hemolysis and depression of the coagulation mechnism is seen after the bite of:**
   A. Viper
   B. Cobra
   C. Common Krait
   D. Banded Krait

2. **Which of the following statements about snakes is WRONG?**
   A. In general belly scales on a poisonous snake are large and cover the entire breadth of the belly
   B. Head scales in true vipers are large
   C. Fangs in a poisonous snake may be canalized
   D. Poisonous snakes are generally nocturnal in nature

3. **Ophitoxaemia means:**
   A. Metallic poisoning
   B. Poisoning with Spanish Fly
   C. Snake bite
   D. Poisoning caused by eating poisonous fishes

4. **Third supralabial is large and touches both the eye and the nasal shield in:**
   A. Cobra
   B. Coral snake
   C. Krait
   D. Both A and B

5. ***Bungarus caeruleus* is the zoological name of which of the following poisonous snakes?**
   A. Common krait
   B. Common cobra
   C. Saw-scaled viper
   D. Russel's Viper

6. **Which of the following is true in a Krait?**
   A. Scales in the middle of the back are enlarged and hexagonal
   B. Fourth infralabial is the largest of all the infralabials
   C. Fourth infralabial is the smallest of all the infralabials
   D. Both A and B

7. **The predominant toxin present in cobra venom is:**
   A. Hemolysin
   B. Neurotoxin
   C. Lecithinase
   D. Phosphatidase

8. **Venom of sea snake is mostly:**
   A. Neruotoxic
   B. Hemolytic
   C. Myotoxic
   D. Hepatotoxic

9. **The fatal dose of dried cobra venom is:**
   A. 15 microgram
   B. 15 mg

C. 15 g
D. 150 g

10. **Blister beetle is also known as:**
A. Honey bee
B. Lice
C. Tse-Tse fly
D. Spanish Fly

11. **Cantharidin is the active principle of:**
A. Honey bee
B. Spanish fly
C. Wasp
D. Scorpion

12. **Priapism means:**
A. Excessive tearing from the eyes, especially red tears
B. Primary impotence
C. Painful erection of penis
D. Excessive itching as if bugs were running underneath the skin

13. **Priapism is a feature of:**
A. Poisoning by Spanish Fly
B. Cobra bite
C. Viper bite
D. Scorpion bite

14. **The fatal dose of cantharidin is:**
A. 15-50 micrograms
B. 15-50 milligrams
C. 1-2 g
D. 10 g

15. **"Irukandji syndrome" is seen in bite by:**
A. Saw scaled viper
B. A peculiar type of jellyfish
C. Spanish Fly
D. Scorpion

MULTIPLE ANSWER TYPE (PGI, CHANDIGARH PATTERN)

16. **Following are symptoms of Spanish Fly poisoning:**
A. Pin-point pupil
B. Hematuria
C. Nausea and vomiting of bloody mucus
D. Dry and hot skin
E. Priapism

17. **Treatment of Spanish Fly poisoning involves:**
A. Stomach wash
B. Hot bath
C. Pressure on the eye balls
D. Inhalation of camphor
E. Administration of amphetamines

18. **Postmortem appearances in Spanish Fly poisoning are:**
A. Inflammation and vesication around mouth
B. Ulceration of oesophageal mucosa
C. Marked congestion of stomach mucosa with petechial hemorrhages
D. Shiny greenish particles of insect sticking to stomach mucosa
E. Inflammation of bladder mucosa

19. **Which of the following is NOT seen with bite of a pit viper?**
A. CVS collapse
B. Absence of local signs
C. Convulsions
D. DIC
E. Paralysis

ANSWERS

1. A.
2. B. ***Related fact:*** A very tricky question indeed, and the student must keep in his mind ALL the features of a poisonous and non-poisonous snake.

   Fangs are present ONLY in poisonous snakes. These are modified teeth. They may be grooved (as in elapids, such as cobras, kraits, and coral snakes), or they may be canalized (as in vipers).

   Remember that in a POISONOUS SNAKE, belly scales are LARGE. Head scales are SMALL in true vipers. In pit vipers, cobra, king cobra, coral and kraits (all poisonous snakes), head scales are LARGE. In a NON-POISONOUS SNAKE belly scales are small and do not cover the entire width of the belly, and head scales are large.

Table 38.1: Comparison of head and belly scales in poisonous and non-poisonous snakes

Scales	*Poisonous*	*Non-poisonous*
Head	Small in true vipers – Larger in Cobra, king cobra, coral and Kraits	Large
Belly	Large (cover the entire breadth of the belly)	Small (do not cover the entire breadth of the belly)

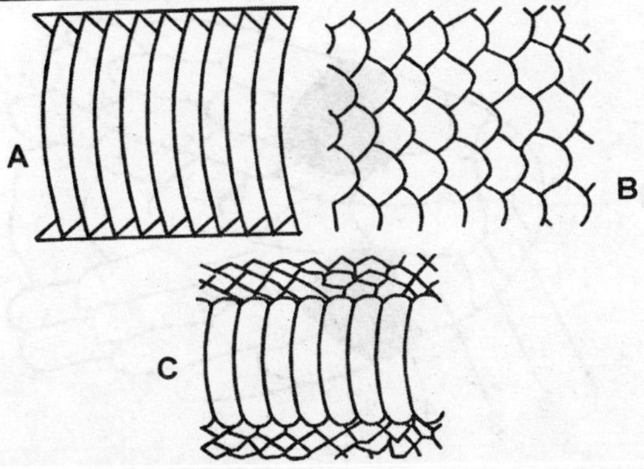

Fig. 38.1: Belly scales in poisonous snakes cover the entire belly (A). Belly scales in non-poisonous snakes do not cover the entire belly (B) and (C)

In Figure 38.1, belly scales are shown. In (A) belly scales are big enough to cover the entire width of the belly. This is a poisonous snake. In (B), the belly scales are small, and in (C) belly scales are larger but do not cover the entire width of the belly. They are both examples of non-poisonous snakes.

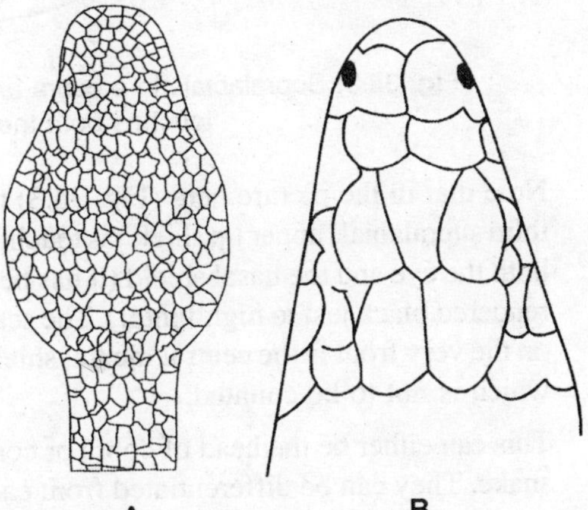

Fig. 38.2: (A) Head scales are small in true viper (poisonous). (B) Head scales are larger in a non-poisonous snake

Figure 38.2 shows heads of two snakes. The first head contains several small scales. This is the head of a true viper. On the right side, there is a head which contains large scales. This is the head of a non-poisonous snake (do remember though that cobra, king cobra, coral and kraits – though poisonous – also have large head scales).

3. C.
4. D. A note about counting the scales in snakes may be in order here. The central scale (just over the snout) is called the mental shield. Behind this shield, scales are counted by numerals (1st, 2nd, 3rd and so on). The same numbering system is applied both in upper (supralabials) and lower jaw (infralabials).

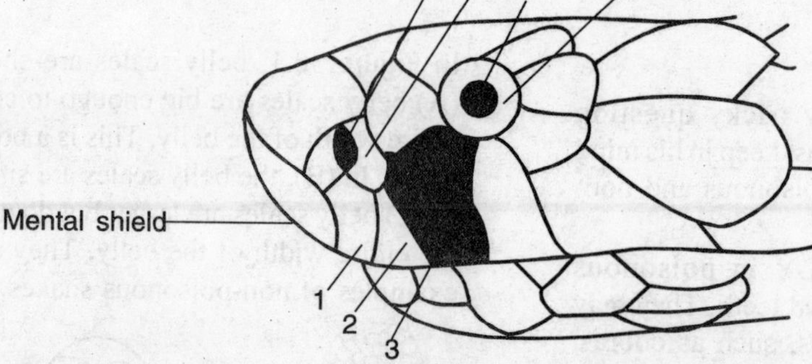

Fig. 38.3: Supralabials in a cobra and coral snake. Note that the third supralabial touches both the nasal and the eye shield

Note that in the picture here (Fig. 38.3) the third supralabial (upper lip shield) is touching both the eye and the nasal shield (it has been rendered black just to highlight it). The scale on the very front is the central mental shield, which is not to be counted.

This can either be the head of cobra or coral snake. They can be differentiated from each other by the fact that coral snakes have "coral spots" on their belly.

5. **A *Related fact:*** Names of others:
Common Cobra→*Naja naja.*
Saw scaled viper→*Echis carinatus.*
Russel's viper→*Vipera russelli.*

Together all the four snakes (given in the choices) are collectively referred to as the "Big Four". These four are most commonly found poisonous snakes in India.

6. **D.** The first picture below (Fig. 38.4) shows central hexagonal scales on the middle of the back of Krait.

The second picture (Fig. 38.5) is a view of the lower jaw of the krait from below. Note the central mental shield just below the snout, which is not to be counted. Behind this, on either side, the infralabials (lower lip shields) are counted by numerals. Note that here are only four infralabials, of which fourth is the largest (it has been rendered black just to highlight it).

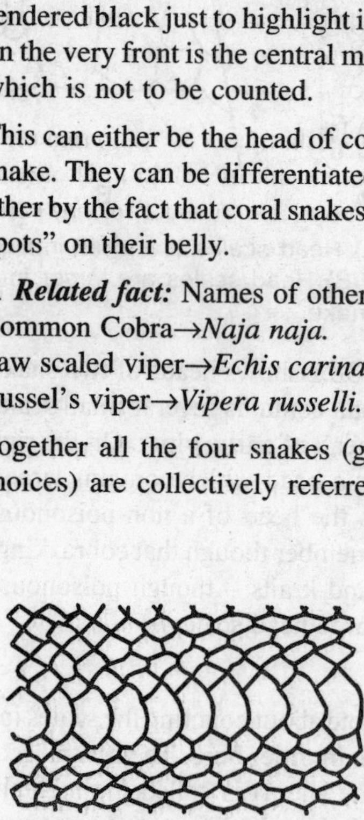

Fig. 38.4: Central hexagonal scales on the middle of the back of krait

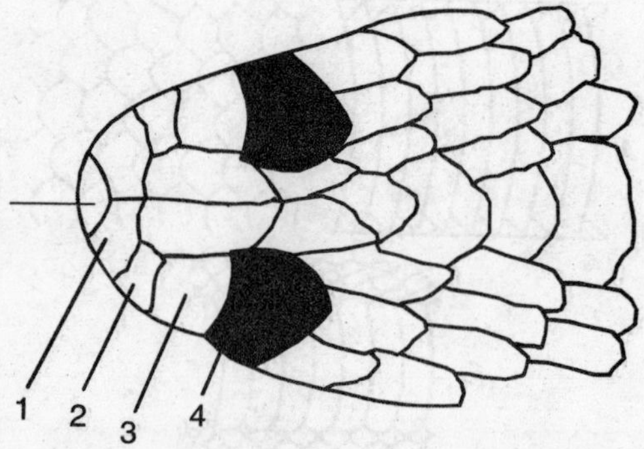

Fig. 38.5: Fourth infralabial in krait is the largest (View is from below)

7. B. ***Related fact:*** Dominant feature of elapid bites (Cobra, kraits and coral snakes) is neurotoxicity, while the principal feature of viperid bites (saw scaled and Russel's viper) are haemostatic abnormalities such as bleeding from the bite site, incoagulability of blood etc.

8. C. ***Related facts:*** The venom of colubrine snakes is mainly neurotoxic, that of viperine snakes mainly hemolytic and that of sea snakes mainly myotoxic.

Table 38.2: Nature of poison and main symptoms produced by various classes of snakes

Class of snakes	*Examples*	*Nature of poison*	*Main symptoms*
Colubridae	Cobra, Krait, coral snake	Neurotoxic	Convulsions, weakness of muscles, paralysis
Viperidae	Saw scaled viper, Russel's viper	Hemotoxic	Disseminated intravascular coagulation (DIC), haemorrhage, localized swelling
Hydrophidae	Sea snakes	Myotoxic	Generalized muscular pain followed by myoglobinuria

9. B. ***Related facts:*** Following table must be remembered by students to solve this type of question:

Table 38.3: Fatal dose and total yield of venom (in one bite) in various snakes

Snake	*Fatal dose in terms of dried venom*	*Total yield in one bite in terms of dried venom*
Krait	6 mg	20 mg
Saw scaled viper	8 mg	25 mg
Cobra	15 mg	200-350 mg
Russel's viper	20 mg	150-200 mg

10. D.

11. B.

12. C.

13. A.

14. B. ***Related fact:*** The fatal dose of powdered beetle (powdered cantharides) is 1.5-3.0 g.

15. B. ***Related fact:*** Irukandji (*Carukia barnesi*) is a small transparent jellyfish found in northern Australia, especially north Queensland around the Cairns region. Its bell is up to 2.5 cm across, but the tentacles may be up to one metre long.

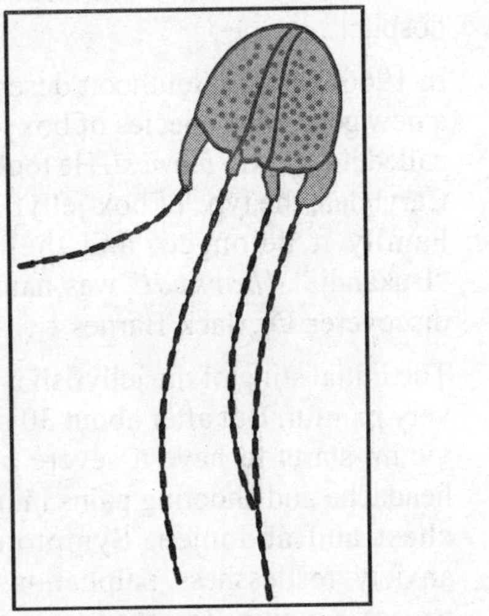

Fig. 38.6: *Carukia barnesi* or irukandji. The body is only about 1.5 cm in diameter (about the size of a thumbnail), and can be identified by the 'string of pearls' nematocysts on its tentacles

There are several small and large species of Irukandji. All species belong to a family of box jellyfish (carybdeids) with 4 tentacles – one in each corner. Out of these, the only one PROVEN to cause the Irukandji syndrome is *Carukia barnesi*. "Box jellyfish", are commonly known as *stinger* or *sea wasp*. They can be found from around November to April along the north Queensland coast. Visitors to the north Queensland coast are routinely warned about "Box jellyfish".

This jellyfish was first named by Dr Hugo Flecker in 1952, after an Aboriginal tribe (Irukandji) that lived in that region. However, it was a doctor - Jack Barnes - who, in 1964, was finally able to identify the jellyfish and demonstrate that it produced the Irukandji syndrome. He spent several hours in a wet-suit lying in the water near Cairns searching for this jellyfish. To Dr Barnes' delight, a thumbnail-sized jellyfish swam past his mask. He stung himself, his son Nick, and a lifesaver friend to check that the jellyfish he had caught was indeed responsible for 'irukandji syndrome'. All three ended up in hospital.

In 1966, Dr Ron Southcott described this as a new genus and species of box jellyfish. He called it *Carukia barnesi*. He took '*car*' from Carybdea, the type of box-jellyfish in whose Family it belonged, and the '*ruk*' from "Irukandji". '*barnesi*' was named after its discoverer Dr. Jack Barnes.

The initial sting of the jellyfish is usually not very painful. But after about 30 minutes, the victim starts to have a severe backache or headache and shooting pains in his muscles, chest and abdomen. Symptoms include anxiety, restlessness, palpitations, sweating, nausea, vomiting, marked tremors and high blood pressure. In rare cases, the victim suffers pulmonary oedema which could be fatal if not treated. This array of systemic symptoms is known as the Irukandji syndrome.

The symptoms are similar to those seen in phaeochromocytoma (adrenal medullary tumour), with excessive release of catecholamines into the bloodstream. Recent work has shown that the venom contains a potent neuronal sodium channel agonist and that *C. barnesi* venom powerfully stimulates noradrenaline (very similar to adrenaline) release explaining, at least in part, the clinical features of the "Irukandji syndrome".

No antivenom exists. First aid includes application of vinegar-soaked pad to the stung area and pain killers. Treatment is mainly symptomatic.

MULTIPLE ANSWER TYPE (PGI, CHANDIGARH PATTERN)

16. B,C,E.

17. A.

18. A,B,C,D,E.

19. B,C,E. ***Related facts:*** Viper venom is mainly hemotoxic. CVS collapse, DIC, Intravascular hemolysis with hemoglobinuria etc. are common with viper bites. Local signs such as local pain, swelling, ecchymosis etc are marked.

39 Food Poisoning and Poisonous Foods

1. **The term "food poisoning" includes:**
   A. Poisoning due to bacteria, their toxins, viruses and protozoa
   B. Poisoning due to poisons of vegetable origin such as *Lathyrus sativus*
   C. Poisoning due to foods of animal origin such as poisonous fish
   D. All of the above
2. **Which one of the following type of food poisoning is often fatal?**
   A. Salmonella
   B. Staphylococcal
   C. Botulism
   D. Clostridium
3. ***Lathyrus sativus* or *kesari dal* contains a:**
   A. Neurotoxin
   B. Cardiotoxin
   C. Hemolytic toxin
   D. Myotoxin
4. ***Salmonella* typically produces:**
   A. Infective type of food poisoning
   B. Toxic type of food poisoning
   C. Both infective and toxic type of food poisoning
   D. Botulism
5. **Which of the following statements about infective type of food poisonings is not true?**
   A. The organisms belong mainly to Salmonella group
   B. It is caused by eating canned or preserved foods
   C. It follows the multiplication within the body of pathogenic organisms contained in the food
   D. It causes diarrhoea after about 24 to 48 hours of eating food
6. **People eating raw or undercooked eggs are likely to have food poisoning by:**
   A. *Listeria monocytogenes*
   B. *Staphylococcus aureus*
   C. *Salmonella* spp
   D. *Clostridium botulinum*
7. **Beta-N-oxalylamino-L-alanine (BOAA) is the toxic principle of:**
   A. Cassava
   B. Mexican poppy
   C. Fava beans
   D. *Lathyrus sativus*
8. **Persons who consume *kesari dal* for long periods may show:**
   A. Status asthmaticus
   B. Complete paraplegia
   C. Myocardial infarction
   D. Kidney failure

9. **Lathyrism is caused by:**
   A. Clostridium perfringens
   B. *Kesari dal*
   C. Monosodium glutamate
   D. Flavoring agents.

10. **'Chinese restaurant syndrome' is due to:**
   A. Arsenic
   B. Monosodium glutamate
   C. Chinese tea
   D. Excess chilly

MULTIPLE ANSWER TYPE (PGI, CHANDIGARH PATTERN)

11. **Which of the following facts about *Campylobacter jejuni* are correct?**
   A. It is a straight gram positive rod
   B. The organism is most commonly isolated in children younger than five years
   C. *Campylobacter* food poisoning is more common in winter months
   D. Most frequent sources of Campylobacter in food are unpasteurized milk and raw or undercooked poultry products
   E. Birds are a common reservoir, and small outbreaks have been associated with contamination of milk by birds pecking milk container tops

12. **Which of the following facts about *Kesari dal* are CORRECT?**
   A. It grows under extreme conditions of drought
   B. It contains twice as much protein as wheat
   C. It causes a syndrome similar to myocardial infarction
   D. It is also known as sweet pea, grasspea or chickling pea
   E. Steeping the pulse in hot water and parboiling removes 90% of the toxin

ANSWERS

1. **D.** Food poisoning is a very loosely defined term. Technically it must encompass all kinds of illnesses which can occur as a result of ingestion of food. This would include the three choices above, as well as poisoning due to chemicals added to the food such as coloring agents, preservatives etc.

   However the term food poisoning as most typically used by lay people refers to a situation where there is simultaneous attack of many persons at the same time, who partook of the same food and who display the same typical signs and symptoms. This usually happens in marriages and banquets and represents *only* the bacterial type of food poisoning. For the purposes of this question however, choice (D) must be taken as correct.

2. **C.**

3. **A.**

4. **A.** ***Additional info***: Bacterial food poisoning is mainly of three types (i) infective type (ii) toxic type and (iii) botulism.

   In the infective type of food poisoning, the bacteria multiply within the body and cause typical symptoms like diarrhoea and vomiting. Important features which immediately distinguish it from toxic type are (i) fever (due to infection) (ii) a delayed onset of symptoms – typically about 24-48 hours (time taken by bacteria to multiply). Bacteria typically causing infective type of food poisoning are (i) *Salmonella* spp (ii) *Shigella* spp (iii) *Campylobacter* spp (iii) Invasive *Escherichia coli* (iv) *Vibrio parahaemolyticus* (v) *Yersinia* spp.

   In the toxic type of food poisoning, bacteria have already produced toxins in the food, and the patient ingests preformed toxins. These toxins are exotoxins. Important features of this type of food poisoning is (i) absence of fever (because there is no actual infection by bacteria) (ii) a short period of onset of symptoms – typically less than six hours (because the toxin is already preformed). Bacteria typically causing toxic type of food poisoning are (i) *Staphylococcus aureus* (ii) *Bacillus cereus* (iii) *Clostridium perfringens* (synonym *Clostridium welchii*) (iv) Enterotoxigenic *Escherichia coli*. In both infective and toxic type of food poisoning, the major feature is diarrhoea and vomiting.

   The third type is botulism. Though it is caused by preformed bacterial exotoxins produced by *clostridium botulinum*, it is not clubbed with toxic type of food poisoning, because unlike it, its major feature is *not* diarrhoea and vomiting but muscle paralysis. It is the *most* dangerous type of food poisoning.

5. **B.** Eating canned or preserved foods usually causes toxic type of food poisoning.

6. **C.** ***Additional info***: Infection of the egg with *Salmonella* is supposed to occur from the chicken's gastrointestinal tract through cracks in the shell. However lately outbreaks have occurred through consumption of non-cracked, nonsoiled eggs. These eggs have presumably been infected *before* the formation of the shell.

7. **D.** ***Additional info:*** Beta-N-oxalylamino-L-alanine (BOAA), is also referred to as Beta-

N-oxalyl-L-alpha-beta-diamino-propionic acid (ODAP). It is a neurotoxin which mimics glutamate. This mimicry causes excessive triggering of the fast excitatory signals running through the brain and nervous system resulting in exhaustion and death of neurons. When consumed in large quantities, kesari dal causes a spastic disorder called lathyrism (sometimes called neurolathyrism).

8. **B.**

9. **B.**

10. **B.** ***Related facts:*** Chinese restaurant syndrome [Synonyms: Hot dog headache; Glutamate-induced asthma; MSG (monosodium glutamate) syndrome] was first described in 1968, when reports of a series of reactions to Chinese food were described.[1]. It was supposed to be caused by monosodium glutamate.

Monosodium glutamate, or MSG (sold in India mostly as *Ajinomoto*) is the sodium salt of glutamic acid and is used to enhance the flavor of foods, especially Chinese foods, such as noodles. The typical history given by the patient is that he took a large amount of Chinese food in a restaurant. Sometime after the ingestion he develops typical symptoms typically comprising a burning sensation and numbness of face which quickly spreads to neck, shoulders, upper limbs, back, abdomen and occasionally the thighs. Two other typical symptoms are (i) bronchospasm, which could even be life-threatening, and (ii) Angioedema.

Other symptoms are rather non-specific and comprise nausea, vomiting, headache and chest pain.

In children, MSG typically causes a seizure like syndrome. This has been termed "shudder attacks". Watch out for this question too.

Typically the MCQ would be like this:

"Shudder attacks" in children are due to:

(a) Sulfites (b) Erythrosine (c) Karaya gum (d) MSG.

The correct answer is (d). Note that the examiner has cleverly concealed the full name of the chemical.

The actual pathophysiology of Chinese restaurant syndrome has not been worked out, but it is believed that arterial receptors such as aortic chemoreceptors are involved, with glutamate (an important constituent of MSG), an excitatory neurotransmitter in the CNS, playing a major role.

There is another illness which occurs after eating in a "Chinese restaurant". This too goes by the name of "Chinese restaurant syndrome", although it has nothing to do with MSG.

It is typically associated with eating reheated fried rice (note that fried rice is a typical food served in Chinese restaurants). The causative agent is *Bacillus cereus*, an aerobic, spore-forming gram-positive, rod shaped bacteria. Its spores survive the initial boiling of rice that is then allowed to cool in bulk. During the slow cooling, spores germinate and vegetative bacteria multiply, then sporulate again. Sporulation is also associated with toxin production. Portions of unused boiled rice are usually kept for preparation of fried rice on the next day. If the batch was contaminated with *Bacillus cereus*, overnight storage in a refrigerator is sufficient to allow toxin production. The toxin is heat-stable, and can easily withstand the brief high temperatures used to cook fried rice. Within 16 hours of eating contaminated fried rice, patients suffer a bout of vomiting that generally lasts for less than a day. This syndrome is largely of historical importance now.

---

[1]Schaumburg H. Chinese-restaurant syndrome. N Engl J Med. 1968 May 16;278(20):1122

MULTIPLE ANSWER TYPE (PGI, CHANDIGARH PATTERN)

11. **B,D,E.** ***Additional info*****:** *Campylobacter* is a curved Gram-negative rod. Its infection is more common in summer months. *Campylobacter* species responsible for food poisoning are *C.jejuni, C. coli* and *C.lari*.

12. **A,B,D,E.** ***Additional facts:*** Till 1980's in central India wages of landless labourers were given in the form *Kesari Dal* which was cheaper than cereals or coarse grains. Consumption of staple diet of *Kesari Dal* led to crippling disease of neuro lathyrism. Over the last few years the rising cost of pulses has made *Kesari Dal* more expensive than wheat or rice and hence it is no longer given to labourers as wages for work done; as a result the disease has virtually disappeared from central India.

11 POISONS ACTING ON THE BRAIN AND SPINAL CORD

40 *Somniferous Poisons*

OPIUM

1. Opium is the dried juice of which of the following plants?
A. *Capsicum annum*
B. *Datura fastuosa*
C. Papaver somniferum
D. *Cannabis sativa*

2. Which of the following terms best describes the somniferous group of poisons?
A. Psychotropic substances
B. Analeptics
C. Narcotics
D. Neuroleptics

3. The usual fatal dose of opium is:
A. 2 micrograms
B. 2 milligrams
C. 20 milligrams
D. 2 grams

4. Which of the following antidotes are no more used in opium poisoning today?
A. Naloxone
B. Naltrexone
C. Nalorphine
D. Nalmefene

5. Which of the following antidotes to morphine can be administered orally?
A. Naloxone
B. Naltrexone
C. Nalmefene
D. All of the above

6. "Opioids" differ from "Opiates" in which sense?
A. Opioids are derived directly from opium but opiates are not
B. Opioids include natural, semisynthetic and synthetic derivatives of morphine
C. Opioids are less potent than opiates
D. Opioids are longer acting than opiates

BARBITURATES

7. The most effective treatment in barbiturate poisoning is:
A. Hemodialyis
B. Analeptics
C. Intravenous fluids
D. Artificial respiration

8. In barbiturate poisoning, the urine may be scanty and contain the following, *except*:
A. Albumen
B. Sugar
C. Haematoporphyrin
D. Acetone

9. Approximate duration of action in hours of long acting barbiturates is:
A. 1-2 hours

B. 3-6 hours
C. 6-12 hours
D. 16-24 hours

10. Phenobarbitone is:
A. Long acting
B. Intermediate acting
C. Short acting
D. Ultra short acting

MULTIPLE ANSWER TYPE (PGI, CHANDIGARH PATTERN)

11. The following drugs belong to the phenanthrene group:
A. Morphine
B. Codeine
C. Papaverine
D. Noscapine
E. Thebaine

12. Which of the following are synthetic drugs related to opium?
A. Diphenoxylate
B. Fentanyl
C. Loperamide
D. Methadone
E. Meperidine

13. Which of the following is the same as pethidine?
A. Meperidine
B. Tramadol
C. Pentazocine
D. Demerol
E. Nalbuphine

14. The following alkaloids are present in opium *except*:
A. Hyoscyamine
B. Morphine
C. Papaverine
D. Nicotine
E. Propoxyphene

15. Which of the following are tests for morphine?
A. Marquis' test
B. Meixner test
C. Deniges' test
D. Melzer's test
E. Husemann's test

ANSWERS

OPIUM

1. C.
2. C. ***Related fact:*** It is very important to appreciate that the term "narcotic" refers to the somniferous group of poisons ONLY in a medical sense. In a legal sense, the term "narcotic" acquires entirely a different meaning. A narcotic drug is defined LEGALLY in section 2(xiv) of *The Narcotic Drugs and Psychotropic Substances Act, 1985.* According to this section:

   "Narcotic drug" means coca leaf, cannabis (hemp), opium, poppy straw and includes all manufactured goods;

   > (manufactured goods refer to drugs which are produced by refining, alteration or transformation of any narcotic or psychotropic substance).

   Thus narcotic drug has distinct meanings medically and legally (this may remind one of the term "abortion", which too has a different medical and legal meaning). Medically narcotic may refer only to a somniferous drug, but legally it may actually refer even to a stimulant (like cocaine) or deliriant (like cannabis).
3. D. ***Related facts:*** It is useful to remember the fatal doses of some other important related drugs which may be asked as MCQs. It is easier (and more meaningful) to remember them against a backdrop of their usual therapeutic doses. The students may find the following list useful:

Table 40.1: Fatal doses of some common opioids (in comparison with their therapeutic doses)

Opiate	*Usual therapeutic dose*	*Usual fatal dose*
Heroin	-	50 mg
Morphine	10-15 mg	200 mg
Codeine	10-60 mg	800 mg
Pethidine	50-150 mg	1 g

4. C. ***Related facts:***
   - The first opiate antagonist to be introduced in practice was→N-allylnorcodeine (in 1915).
   - Nalorphine developed in 1954, Naloxone in 1960 and naltrexone in 1963. Nalmefene is the **MOST RECENT** entrant for the treatment of opium poisoning.
   - Antidotes not used today are→Nalorphine and Levallorphan→Why? →Because they are (i) weak competitive antagonists and (ii) have undesirable Kappa receptor agonist properties (producing dysphoria).
5. B. ***Related facts:*** Routes of administration for various morphine antidotes are:
   - Naloxone→IV most preferred. Otherwise also give sublingually, intramuscularly, or even instilled down an endotracheal tube. Since repeated doses may be required, naloxone infusion may be better.
   - Dose of naloxone→1.2 mg for adult and 0.4 mg for child. Repeated again. A total of 75 mg in 24 hours can be given.
   - Naltrexone→Orally. Dose 50 mg / day. May also be used to treat opiate addiction.
   - Nalmefene→Naltrexone derivative. Pure opiate antagonistic effects. IV most commonly. But can also be given intra-

muscularly or subcutaneously. Dose →Begin with 0.1 mg, and if withdrawal reaction does not occur, administer 0.5 mg, followed by 1 mg in 2-5 minutes if necessary.

6. B. ***Related facts:*** Opiates are drugs *derived from opium*, and include natural products morphine, codeine, thebaine and many semisynthetic congeners derived from them. Opioid – on the other hand – is a much broader term which refers to *any* agent that binds to opioid receptors. It is a more inclusive term applying to all agonists and antagonists with morphine-like activity. The term Opioid would thus include completely synthetic products such as methadone, pethidine (meperidine) and propoxyphene, which are not included under opiates.

The term opioid derives from the Greek suffix "eidos" which means "similar to" or "like". Thus Opioids are Opium like, and refer broadly to all compounds related to opium. Drugs like diphenoxylate, fentanyl, loperamide, and methadone are synthetic derivatives of opium, and are thus referred to as opioids.

Opioids have a depressant action on the CNS of humans and dogs, but they have an excitatory effect on the CNS of cats and horses.

Interestingly the Greek suffix "*eidos*" appears in a number of other medical terms (the medical student may find it easier to remember the terms this way – this is known as etymological learning and is very close to this author's heart). It is seen in adenoid (gland like), arachnoid (spider's web like), arytaenoid (cup or ladle like), choroid (leather or parchment like), cirsoid (varix like), clinoid (bed like), colloid (glue like), coracoid (like the beak of a crow), coronoid (like the beak of a crow again), cricoid (ring like), deltoid (like the Greek letter delta), ethmoid (sieve like), fibroid (thread like), glenoid (like a shallow socket), hyoid (like the Greek letter upsilon – it looks rather like U), lambdoid (like the Greek letter lambda), mastoid (like the female breast), odontoid (like a tooth), pterygoid (like a wing), scaphoid (like a boat), sesamoid (like a seed), sigmoid (like the Greek letter Sigma), sphenoid (wedge like), styloid (pillar like), thyroid (like a shield), trapezoid (like a small table), typhoid (like a smoke or mist) and xiphoid (sword like). It is interesting to see that as many as four Greek letters - delta, upsilon, lambda and sigma – appear in these terms, signifying medical personnel's interests in classical literature and learning.

BARBITURATES

7. A.

8. D.

9. C. For this question and its variants, please remember the following Table 40.2.

10. A.

Table 40.2: Onset and duration of action of some common barbiturates

Class of barbiturates	*Onset of action within*	*Duration of action*	*Major examples*
Long acting	2 hours	6-12 hours	Barbitone, phenobarbitone
Intermediate acting	0.5-1 hour	3-6 hours	Amobarbitone, Butobarbitone
Short acting	—	<3 hours	Cyclobarbital, pentobarbital, seconal
Ultra-short acting	Immediate	5-10 minutes	Pentothal sodium, hexobarbital sodium, kemithal sodium

MULTIPLE ANSWER TYPE (PGI, CHANDIGARH PATTERN)

11. **A,B,E.** ***Related facts***: Papaverine and noscapine (narcotine) belong to the other major group of drugs found in poppy, the benzylisoquinolines.
12. **A,B,C,D,E.** ***Related facts***: Three terms are normally used in relation to drugs related to opium —natural, semisynthetic and synthetic. Natural drugs are those which are normally found in poppy capsules (morphine, codeine, thebaine etc). If a natural drug molecule is taken and is altered chemically to produce another molecule which retains morphine like activity, it is known as semisynthetic derivative. Examples are heroin (produced by acetylating morphine), hydrocodone, naloxone and naltrexone. Synthetic drugs are completely synthesized in the laboratory without using any natural drug as a starting molecule. All five drugs mentioned above are purely synthetic drugs. Diphenoxylate is used as an antidiarrhoeal, Fentanyl as an adjunct to anaesthesia, Loperamide and Meperidine as anlagesics and Methadone for opiate abstinence syndrome.
13. **A,D.** ***Related facts***: Pethidine is the International Nonproprietary Name (INN) while meperidine is the United States Approved Name (USAN) of the same drug. Demerol is one of the several proprietary names of pethidine.

    An International Nonproprietary Name (INN) is the official non-proprietary or generic name given to a pharmaceutical substance, as designated by the World Health Organization. The plethora of named proprietary preparations containing a given substance can lead to confusion about the identity of the active ingredient. INNs facilitate communication by providing a standard name for each substance. WHO issues INN names in English, Latin, French, Russian, and Spanish. Arabic and Chinese versions, although not included in the original scheme, are now also being issued.

    A United States Approved Name (USAN) is the official non-proprietary or generic name given to a pharmaceutical substance, as defined in the United States Pharmacopeia (USP).
14. **A,D,E.** ***Related facts:*** Propoxyphene is a synthetic opium derivative and is not a natural alkaloid of opium.
15. **A,C,E.** ***Additional information***: These are old tests for morphine, but may still be asked in examinations. For **Marquis' test** the reagent is 3 cc of pure concentrated sulphuric acid to which 2 drops of 40% formaldehyde solution has been added. Morphine gives a fine purple-red color with this reagent, changing to violet and then to blue.

    Deniges' test→The test solution (presumably containing morphine) is made slightly acidic. A drop of hydrogen peroxide is added and made alkaline with ammonia. The solution is stirred with a bright piece of copper wire. A brisk effervescence ensues, and a wine-red color develops if morphine is present.

    Husemann's test→A fragment of the residue (presumably containing morphine) is warmed on a water bath with few drops of concentrated sulphuric acid in a watch glass for about half an hour. Morphine if present is converted to apomorphine, which appears as brownish or almost black. Cool and add one drop of concentrated nitric acid. A red-violet or blue color is produced, changing rapidly to dark blood red and then to yellowish red.

    Meixner test and Melzer's test arc both for poisonous mushrooms.

41 *Inebriant Poisons*

GENERAL

1. **Absolute alcohol is:**
   A. 90% alcohol
   B. 95-99% alcohol
   C. 99-100% alcohol
   D. 100% alcohol

ETHYL ALCOHOL

2. **Specific gravity of ethyl alcohol is:**
   A. 0.59
   B. 0.79
   C. 0.99
   D. 1.09
3. **Caloric content of ethyl alcohol is:**
   A. 4 Kcal/g
   B. 4 Kcal/cc
   C. 7 Kcal/g
   D. 7 Kcal/cc
4. **The alcohol content of whisky (v/v) is around:**
   A. 15%
   B. 30%
   C. 45%
   D. 90%
5. **Metabolism of ethyl alcohol follows:**
   A. Zero order kinetics
   B. First order kinetics
   C. Second order kinetics
   D. Third order kinetics
6. **The fatal dose of ethyl alcohol in an average adult is:**
   A. 100-150 cc
   B. 5-6 g/kg of body weight
   C. 1500 cc
   D. 50-60 g/kg of body weight
7. **The fatal blood level of ethyl alcohol is:**
   A. 30 mg%
   B. 80 mg%
   C. 500 mg%
   D. 1000 mg%
8. **At equilibrium, the ratio of concentration of ethyl alcohol between whole blood and CSF (whole blood:CSF) is:**
   A. 2:1
   B. 1.2:1
   C. 1:1.2
   D. 1:2
9. **The legally permissible blood alcohol level in India for driving is:**
   A. 0 mg %
   B. 30 mg %
   C. 80 mg %
   D. 100 mg %
10. **McEwan's sign is seen in:**
    A. Dhatura poisoning

B. Drowning
C. Putrefaction
D. Ethyl alcohol poisoning

11. If "C" is the concentration of alcohol in the blood in decigrams%, "p" the weight of the body in kg, "a" the alcohol ingested in gm and "r" the Widmark constant, then according to the Widmark's formula:
A. p=acr/100
B. p=acr
C. c=apr
D. a=cpr

12. In chronic alcoholism which of the following is seen?
A. Delirium tremens
B. Wernicke's encephalopathy
C. Korsakoff's psychosis
D. All of the above

13. Absorption of ethyl alcohol occurs in the following manner:
A. 20% from stomach, 50% from small intestines and the rest from large intestines
B. 10% from oral mucosa, 20% from stomach, 40% from small intestines and the rest is excreted in feces unchanged
C. 80% from stomach and 20% from small intestines
D. 20% from stomach and 80% from small intestines

14. Beer-drinkers' cardiomyopathy first reported in mid 1960s was due to:
A. Cobalt
B. Ethyl alcohol
C. Methyl alcohol
D. Yeast

15. The term "alpha alcoholism" refers to:
A. Physical dependence on alcohol
B. Only psychological dependence on alcohol
C. Alcoholism resulting in disease states like cirrhosis of liver
D. Profound craving for alcohol

16. Which of the following neurological disease of slow onset, seen in chronic alcohol abusers, is due to demyelination of the corpus callosum?
A. Wernicke's disease
B. Jamaica Ginger paralysis
C. Marchiafava-Bignami syndrome
D. Punch-drunk syndrome

17. Jamaica-ginger paralysis is due to:
A. Chronic intake of alcohol
B. Methanol
C. Tri-ortho-cresyl phosphate
D. Castor oil

18. Which of the following is the MOST RELIABLE method for determination of blood alcohol concentration?
A. Cavett's test
B. Breath alcohol analyser
C. Gas liquid chromatography
D. Kozelka and Hine test

19. In India, if a motor vehicle is involved in an accident, a breathalyzer test on the driver is:
A. Permissible under section 185 of *Motor Vehicles Act 1988*
B. Permissible under section 203 of *Motor Vehicles Act 1988*
C. Permissible under section 204 of *Motor Vehicles Act 1988*, but only when conducted by a medical personnel
D. Not legally permissible

20. Misconduct in public by a drunken person is liable to be prosecuted under section:
A. 85 I.P.C.
B. 86 I.P.C.
C. 510 I.P.C.
D. 510 Cr.P.C.

21. If someone was forced to drink alcohol or alcohol was given to him without his knowledge and under its influence he did some criminal act, what punishment will he get?

A. He will get the benefit of section 84 IPC and not get any punishment
B. He will get the benefit of section 85 IPC and not get any punishment
C. He will get the benefit of section 86 IPC and get only one fifth of punishment normally prescribed for that particular crime
D. He will be punished normally as it is everyone's duty to see that he is not given alcohol by force or fraud

METHYL ALCOHOL

22. Methyl alcohol is excreted mainly through:
A. Feces
B. Urine
C. Sweat
D. Breath

23. Methyl alcohol poisoning leads to:
A. Respiratory acidosis
B. Metabolic acidosis
C. Respiratory alkalosis
D. Both metabolic and respiratory acidosis

24. The best antidote for methyl alcohol poisoning is:
A. Alkaline diuretics
B. Acid diuretics
C. I.V. Fructose
D. Ethyl alcohol

25. Rate of oxidation of methanol is:
A. $1/50^{th}$ of that of ethanol
B. $1/5^{th}$ of that of ethanol
C. 5 times that of ethanol
D. 50 times that of ethanol

26. Fatal dose of methanol is:
A. 6-20 ml
B. 60-200 ml
C. 500-750 ml
D. 1000-1500 ml

27. Toxic effects of methyl alcohol poisoning is due to:
A. Acetaldehyde formation
B. Formation of urate crystals in retina causing its damage
C. Formaldehyde formation
D. Metabolic alkalosis

28. The visual disturbances of methyl alcohol poisoning include all of the following *except*:
A. Blurred vision
B. Concentric diminution of visual fields for color and form
C. Photophobia
D. Pinpoint pupils

29. The dangerous concentration of methyl alcohol in blood is:
A. 0.8 mg%
B. 8 mg%
C. 80 mg%
D. 800 mg%

30. Hemodialysis reduces the half life of methyl alcohol from 40 hours to about:
A. 40 seconds
B. 1 hour
C. 4 hours
D. 20 hours

KEROSENE

31. Most important and common complication of acute kerosene poisoning is:
A. Acute hepatic failure
B. Bronchopneumonia
C. Acute renal failure
D. Kerosene encephalopathy

MISCELLANEOUS

32. Mickey Finn refers to:
A. Methyl alcohol
B. Amphetamines

C. Hallucinogenic mushrooms
D. Chloral hydrate

MULTIPLE ANSWER TYPE (PGI, CHANDIGARH PATTERN)

33. Which of the following is a valid antidote against methyl alcohol?
A. Ethyl alcohol
B. Activated charcoal
C. 4-methyl pyrazole
D. Folinic acid
E. Potassium ferrocyanide

34. Methyl alcohol is absorbed from:
A. Intestines
B. Stomach
C. Hair
D. Lungs
E. Skin

35. Which of the followings are dihydroxy alcohols?
A. Isopropanol
B. Ethylene glycol
C. Methanol
D. Glycerine
E. Propylene glycol

36. Which of the following facts will demonstrate that the alcohol detected in the blood may have been produced as a result of postmortem decomposition?
A. *n*-Propanol and n-butanol are simultaneously detected in blood
B. Blood level of ethanol is less than 70 mg%
C. Absence of ethylglucuronide in the blood
D. Bone shows a very high concentration of ethyl alcohol as well as methyl alcohol
E. Urine and vitreous humor would not show alcohol

37. Which of the following are true about methyl alcohol poisoning?
A. Blindness is produced due to the formation of formic acid
B. Fomepizole is very helpful
C. Ethanol is very useful
D. Gastric lavage is not helpful
E. Activated charcoal is highly effective

38. Proof spirit can be defined as:
A. A mixture of alcohol in water corresponding to 57.1% by volume
B. A mixture of two or more different liquors
C. Spirit which at a temperature of 51°F, weighs exactly twelve-thirteenths of an equal volume of distilled water
D. Spirit which has been "proved" to be spurious by chemical testing
E. Spirit which is sold in "tamper-proof" cans

39. In India, if a motor vehicle is involved in an accident, a police officer can legally ask a medical practitioner to take blood samples of the driver for a laboratory test under which of the following conditions?
A. Blood samples may be taken straightaway without first conducting a breath test
B. If breath tests have been done and presence of alcohol in breath has been established by these tests
C. If the person has refused to give breath samples
D. When the driver is a female above 18 years of age
E. When the driver is a child below 12 years of age

40. Alcohol is rapidly absorbed in which of the following situations?
A. When the person has had a gastrectomy
B. When alcohol is taken with food high in fat
C. When alcohol is taken with carbonated soda
D. When alcohol is taken with ice
E. When the person has ingested parasympathomimetic drugs such as prostigmine

ANSWERS

GENERAL

1. **C.** ***Additional info:*** Absolute alcohol (also known as dehydrated alcohol) is ethyl alcohol containing no more than one percent water. Different manufacturers have different standards, but most manufacturers prepare it at 99.5% concentration.

   It is not possible to obtain absolute alcohol by simple fractional distillation, because a mixture containing at least 95.4% alcohol and 5.6% water becomes a constant boiling mixture or an azeotropic mixture.

   > An azeotrope (from the Greek "*a*" without, "*zein*" to boil, and "*trope*", turning, change; literally, "boiling without change".) is a liquid mixture of two or more components which has a unique constant boiling point. This azeotrope may boil at a higher, lower, or intermediate temperature, relative to the boiling points of its constituent liquids, and the liquid retains the same composition as it is boiled. As a consequence, the vapor has the same composition as the liquid and simple distillation will not separate the constituents as it would with most liquid mixtures. To get a higher concentration it is necessary to use a special kind of distillation known as azeotropic distillation.

   To obtain 100% pure alcohol a small quantity of benzene is added to rectified spirit and the mixture is then distilled. Absolute alcohol is obtained in third fraction that distills over at 78.2°C.

   Because a small amount of the benzene used remains in the solution, the product of this process will cause extensive liver damage if consumed.

   There is also an absolute alcohol production process by dehydration using glycerine.

ETHYL ALCOHOL

2. **B.**
3. **C.** ***Related facts***: Some other interesting facts and figures about ethyl alcohol which can be asked as MCQs are:
   - The numeral 7 comes twice in relation of alcohol. Another fact with numeral 7 is →A man of average size can metabolize about 7 g alcohol/hr (range 5-13 g/hr). This is equivalent to about 9 cc of absolute alcohol.
   - One average peg of whiskey contains 30 cc of liquor. Taking whiskey to be around 45% of alcohol, this equals 13.5 cc (or about 10.5 g) of absolute alcohol. This means, an average man can metabolize an average peg of whiskey in about 1.5 hours.
   - Using the Widmark formula (*See answer to question 10 below*), it can easily be calculated that an average peg of whiskey raises the blook alcohol level of an average 70 mg man by about 22 mg%.
   - Similarly it can be shown that if a drunk man stops taking alcohol, his blood alcohol levels will fall at a rate of about 15 mg %/hour.
4. **C.** An alcoholic beverage may be defined as any drinkable liquid containing from 0.5% to 95% ethyl alcohol. The student may find an odd question sometimes on the alcohol content of various drinks. Table 41.1 gives the alcohol contents of most common drinks.

Table 41.1: Some common alcoholic beverages and their alcoholic content

Alcoholic beverage	*Alcohol content in % (v/v)*
Beers (lager)	3.2-4.0%
Malt liquor	3.2-7.0%
Ales	4.5%
Porter	6.0%
Stout	6.0-8.0%
Table wines	7.1-14.0%
Sparkling wines	8.0-14.0%
Fortified wines	14.0-24.0%
Aromatized wines	15.5-20.0%
Sake	14.0-16.0%
Aquavit	35.0-45.0%
Okolehao	40.0%
Brandies	40.0-43.0%
Whiskies	40.0-75.0%
Vodkas	40.0-50.0%
Gins	40.0-48.5%
Rum	40.0-95.0%
Tequila	45.0-50.5%

5. A. There are no such terms as second order kinetics and third order kinetics. Most drugs follow first order kinetics, i.e. a *constant fraction* of the drug is metabolized in a unit time. Ethyl alcohol differs from most drugs in the sense that it follows zero order kinetics, i.e. a *constant amount* of ethyl alcohol is metabolized in a unit time (this constant amount is given in the answer to one of the previous questions – 9 cc of absolute alcohol per hour).

Many students find the concept of zero order kinetics and first order kinetics difficult to understand, perhaps because most books give it in complex mathematical forms. It can be understood in a simple way as below:

- Suppose there are fifty molecules of a given enzyme in the body. Each molecule metabolizes one molecule of the drug in one hour. If a person ingests two molecules of drug, these two occupy two molecules of enzyme and are metabolized in one hour. Rest 48 molecules (of enzyme) do nothing during this period.
- Suppose now the person ingests four molecules of the drug. It is quite simple to understand that now four molecules of the enzymes would be occupied for next one hour, and the drug would still be metabolized in the same amount of time, i.e. one hour. If the person ingests eight molecules, or for that matter any amount upto 50 molecules, the drug would still be metabolized in the same amount of time. This is first order kinetics, i.e. increasing quantities of drug gets metabolized (in the same amount of time) as the ingested quantity (of the drug) increases. In other words a *constant fraction* rather than a *constant amount* of drug is metabolized in a unit time. Note that in the above case, if the person ingests two molecules, it would be mathematically correct to say that 50% of the drug (or one molecule) was metabolized in half an hour. Similarly if the person ingested eight molecules, 50% of the molecules (or 4 molecules) would still be metabolized in half an hour. In other words, a *constant fraction* of the drug gets metabolized in a given time. 100% of the drug gets metabolized in one hour in all cases (as long as the person ingests less than 50 molecules).
- Now let us suppose that there is a different drug metabolized by a different enzyme. The number of these molecules of enzyme in the body is just one. This molecule too metabolizes its substrate in one hour. If a person ingests one molecule of the drug, it would be metabolized in one hour. But if this person ingests two molecules of drug, the second molecule will have to wait till the first molecule gets metabolized. Two molecules will be metabolized in two hours, four in four hours and so on. In other words, a *constant amount* (i.e. one molecule) of the drug gets metabolized in a given time. This is zero order kinetics.

Alcohol follows this pathway (since the molecules responsible for alcohol degradation are very less in the body to start with).

- Note that in the very first example, if the person ingests more than 50 molecules of drug (say 100 molecules), only 50 molecules can get metabolized in the first hour and the next 50 molecules will be metabolized in the next hour. The complete amount of drug will now take two hours to metabolize. This as we know is zero order kinetics. In other words, after a certain limit, even first order kinetics changes to zero order kinetics. This happens when the enzymes get saturated.

6. B. ***Additional facts:*** It is difficult to relate fatal dose of ethyl alcohol with those of other poisons as human body has a unique ability to metabolize this poison effectively. Thus the same fatal dose taken over an extended period of time say, 2-3 days, may not be fatal. Indeed many heavy drinkers do take this amount within 2-3 days. The fatal dose mentioned above must be taken within a very short time.

In an average 70 kg man, the total fatal dose works out to about 400 g, which is about 500 cc of absolute alcohol (specific gravity of ethyl alcohol = 0.79). Thus if the question offers fatal doses in cc, the correct answer is 500 cc of absolute alcohol (taken within a short time).

7. C. ***Related fact:*** It is useful to remember the figure 500.

- Fatal dose of absolute alcohol is 500 cc.
- Fatal blood levels of ethyl alcohol are 500 mg%.

8. C. This is a tricky question. Remember that plasma, serum, saliva, urine and CSF contain more water than whole blood (on account of blood containing solid matter in the form of RBCs), and therefore all these fluids are expected to contain *more* alcohol at equilibrium. Body organs such as liver and brain are expected to contain less alcohol than whole blood, as their water content is lesser. Alveolar air also contains lesser alcohol than whole blood.

The commonly recognized ratios of concentration between whole blood and various body samples are as follows (Table 41.2).

Table 41.2: Ratio of alcohol concentration in blood and various body organs/fluids at equilibrium (shaded rows indicate where organ/sample concentration is *lesser* than that of blood)

S.No.	*Body organ/ fluid/sample*	*Blood:sample concentration*
1.	Urine	1:1.3
2.	Saliva (pure, as obtained by special cannulae in the parotids)	1:1.21
3.	CSF	1:1.2
4.	Sweat	1:1.2
5.	Vitreous	1:1.2
6.	Tears	1:1.14 (range 1.08 to 1.20)
7.	Plasma or serum	1:1.12 to 1:1.2
8.	Saliva (mixed with mucous secretions from the mouth, as is likely to be obtained in ordinary laboratory conditions)	1:1.02 to 1:1.08
9.	Mother's milk	1:1
10.	Brain	1:0.85
11.	Liver	1:0.85
12.	Alveolar air	1:1/2100

Note that body organs/samples have been arranged in decreasing concentrations, with urine having the maximum concentration at equilibrium and alveolar air the least. Only the last three organs/samples (shaded) actually show lesser concentration of alcohol than blood at equilibrium.

9. B. *Related fact:* This is according to section 185 of *Motor Vehicles Act 1988.* On first offence, the punishment is imprisonment of 6 months and/or fine of Rs. 2000 If the second offence is committed within three years, the punishment is 2 years and/or fine of Rs. 3000.

The clause of 30 mg/100 ml was added by an amendment in 1994. It came into effect from 14 November 1994.

> **The legal limit in (mg%) in other countries is as follows:**
>
> Australia 50, Bulgaria 0, Denmark 80, France 50, Hungary 0, Netherlands 50, Romania 0, Spain 80, Yugoslavia 50, Austria 80, Canada 80, Ireland 80, Germany and Italy 80, Norway 50, Russia 0, Turkey 0, Belgium 80, Czechoslovakia 80, Finland 50, Greece 50, Luxembourg 80, Poland 20, Sweden 20, USA 100 (in several states. Some states in the US have reduced the legal level to 80 mg).

10. D. *Related fact:* Ethanol is a mydriatic, but towards the terminal states, i.e. the stages of stupor and coma, the pupils may become constricted. They dilate once again at about the time of death.

McEwan's sign involves pinching the skin of the face or neck, or light slapping. It dilates the constricted pupils momentarily, after which they constrict again. This can be remembered as C→D→C. It is intended to be a diagnostic sign of alcoholic coma (differentiating from other causes of coma, such as diabetic coma etc.). It is however a highly unreliable sign and must not be depended upon.

11. D. *Examples to consolidate the fact in mind:* (i) Let us assume that we want to find out the amount of alcohol which a 70 kg robust adult male must consume in order to raise his blood level to 30 mg% (the legal driving limit in India). We will go like this:

a=cpr

a=0.3 x 70 x 0.68

a= 14.28 g

To convert it into c.c., we must divide this by 0.79 (the sp gr of alcohol). We get 18 cc.

This is 100% alcohol. Considering that on an average, whisky is 45% alcohol, it comes to 18x100/45, or 40 cc.

30 cc makes one standard peg. So it means one must consume a little more than one standard peg of whisky (about one plus one-third of a peg) to raise his blood concentration of alcohol to that of legal driving limit in India.

(ii) Let us now solve this question: How much blood alcohol level will be obtained in an average 70 kg man, if he consumes an average peg of whiskey?

a=cpr

Weight of alcohol in an average peg of whiskey (a) = 10.5 g (*See answer to question 3 above*)

10.5 = c x 70 x 0.68

c = 0.22 decigram % or 22 mg %

(iii) If a drunk person stops taking alcohol, by what rate his blood alcohol level will fall?

We know that an average person metabolizes about 7 g of absolute alcohol every hour.

7 = c x 70 x 0.68

This gives c = 0.15 decigram % or 15 mg %

A question can be asked on the Widmark factor or "r". Remember it is LESS for women. For men it is 0.68; for women it is 0.55. Sometimes only a single digit is given. In that case, take 0.6 for men and 0.5 for women. Actually it represents the Volume of Distribution V_d, which is less for women, who have more fat compared to men.

The units of "c" are most often confused. In most books one would find the unit of "c" written as "g/L", which is another way of representing "decigrams%".

Additional info: This formula was developed by the Swedish toxicologist Erik Matteo Prochet Widmark (1889-1945).

12. D.

13. D.

14. A. ***Additional Notes:*** A cobalt salt (usually cobalt sulphate or cobal chloride) is usually added to illegally produced beer as a foam stabilizer. This would improve the "head" of the beer. In August 1965, an alarming outbreak of cardiac failure occurred among the heavy beer-drinkers of Quebec City. Similar outbreaks had previously occurred in Omaha, Nebraska, and in Louvain, Belgium. The onset was fairly sudden, with severe abdominal pain, vomiting, hemetemesis, ascites, pericardial effusion, and a peculiar dusky, diffuse cyanosis. The mortality was 42%. At postmortem examination, the heart was found to be heavier than normal and the walls of all chambers were hypertrophied. There was watery and fatty vacuolation of the myofibres, and complete absence of inflammatory cell exudates. The disease remained a mystery till it was recognized that changes in the thyroid were similar to those produced by cobalt salts. Inquiry showed that cobalt sulphate had been added to improve the "head" of the beer, and that cobalt, NOT ALCOHOL, was responsible for the outbreak. Some heavy drinkers of the bad beer however escaped injury. Why they escaped? This problem has remained unsolved.

15. B. ***Additional info:*** American physiologist Elvin Morton Jellinek (1890-1963) has defined alcoholism as "any use of alcoholic beverages that causes any damage to the individual or society or both". He then went on to list five subtypes of alcoholism which are widely used by clinical psychologists and psychiatrists today.

The first subtype is *alpha alcoholism.* It is defined as psychological reliance on alcohol "to relieve bodily or emotional pain." The second subtype, *beta alcoholism* is a form of heavy drinking that results in physical disease states (ulcers, cirrhosis of the liver, damage to the nerves, and kidney problems) in the absence of either physical dependence or psychological dependence on alcohol.

The third subtype – *gamma alcoholism*— is a severe form of alcoholism. It involves demonstrable tolerance to alcohol, withdrawal symptoms and craving (indicative of physical dependence), and loss of control of drinking. Gamma alcoholics crave the need for alcohol, yet can live without alcohol for a short period of time.

In the fourth subtype—the *delta alcoholism* – the drinker cannot stay away from liquor for even a day or two without suffering from withdrawal symptoms.

Finally, Jellinek noted a fifth subtype, *epsilon alcoholism*, or "periodic alcoholism". These are individuals that engage in periodic binges, with long periods of abstaining in between.

16. C. ***Related facts:*** Also known as Marchiafava's syndrome or Marchiafava's disease, this progressive neurological disease is most frequently seen in middle-aged or elderly alcoholic males but rarely encountered in some nonalcoholic subjects too. The main symptoms are gait problems, fits and seizures, stupor, coma and dementia. It is mainly due to demyelination of the corpus callosum. In some cases, the damage extends to nearby subcortical white matter and/or the anterior commissure.

This condition was first described in 1903 by two Italian pathologists Ettore Marchiafava (1847-1935) and Amico Bignami (1862-1919). Since the condition was first described in Italy, and since the victims consumed red Italian wines, it was for long thought that the condition in some way was related to Italian wines. But now it is known that this is not true. Death usually occurs 4 to 6 years after onset.

17. **C.** ***Related facts:*** Jamaica-ginger paralysis was seen in the USA during the time of Prohibition (This was the period between 1920-33, when alcohol had been made illegal throughout USA. This was done by 18th amendment to the United States Constitution). People desiring to drink alcohol resorted to alternate ways to get alcohol. Since some medical remedies naturally contain alcohol, many people began taking these medical remedies. One such remedy was the fluid extract of Jamaica ginger, which was a popular folk remedy in the United States since 1860s for headache and indigestion. It was also used as a promoter of menstrual flow and for mild upper respiratory infections. Better known as Jake, it was a covert way of drinking alcohol; it was especially suited for this purpose since it was easily obtainable from pharmacies and its alcohol content was a minimum of 70%! Official medicinal extracts of ginger had to contain five grams of ginger as powder or resin to each milliliter of alcohol. Sold as such, it was opaque, thick and irritating to drink, so unscrupulous dealers added more alcohol to it making it not only more palatable, but more "potent" too! It was often highly adulterated with other ingredients such as molasses, glycerin, herbs or castor oil. In 1930, as the prices of castor oil rose, the alternative adulterant TOCP was used.

TOCP was an industrial chemical sold as a plasticizer (a substance added to plastics or other materials to make or keep them soft or pliable. PVC is flexible and durable because of such plasticizers). It was used in the manufacture of products such as lacquer, leather and airplane finishes. TOCP binds to cells in the spinal cord, producing serious toxicity and neuronal death. Victims would develop numbness and pain in their legs, followed by muscle weakness and finally paralysis with foot drop. Within one week, the same symptoms would occur in the upper extremities, resulting in wrist drop. Although fatalities were unusual, recovery was slow and many cases would result in permanent neurological damage and long-term disability. It also caused impotence. The victims who exhibited resultant gait disorders were said to have the "Jake Leg" or "Jake Walk". Between 1930-31, the number of cases spread from New York to California and reached epidemic proportions with at least 50,000 individuals affected.

The tragedy recurred again in 1959 in Morocco, when about 10,000 people were similarly poisoned with TOCP. The victims had eaten food cooked in olive oil adulterated with lubricating oil; and the latter happened to be contaminated with TOCP! It was thus a unique case, where an adulterant was itself adulterated! It is useful to remember that in our own country, argemone oil is frequently used to adulterate cooking oils, especially mustard oil.

18. **C.** ***Additional facts*****:** F.L. Kozelka and C.H. Hine of the University of Wisconsin described their method for determination of

alcohol in 1941. It is a color or spot test, and like all color or spot tests has a high rate of false-positive and false negative results. It is a macro method, implying that the test requires fairly large volumes of blood such as 1 mL.

Cavett's test is a micro method (i.e. it works well with smaller volume such as 0.1 mL), which utilizes the principle that alcohol is easily oxidised to acetic acid by oxidising agents such as potassium dichromate and sulphuric acid. If N/20 dichromate solution is used to oxidise alcohol, one ml of such a solution would oxidise about 0.575 mg of alcohol. This fact is utilized for determination of alcohol levels in the blood.

Both these methods suffer from several problems (i) both are chemical oxidation methods and as such not specific for ethanol, which could be a serious problem if a dead body has undergone decomposition or a living subject suffers from diabetes and keto-acidosis (ii) neither method can be automated, which is a big limitation when one has many samples to analyze (iii) finally one needs to work with corrosive reagents - sulphuric acid and potassium dichromate in both these methods.

With breath alcohol analyser (commonly known as breathalyser), one can detect alcohol in breath, and there are even instruments which aim to calculate the exact concentration of alcohol in blood. All of these are based on the tacit assumption that at equilibrium, the ratio of alcohol between blood and breath is 1:2100 (i.e. 1 ml of blood would contain exactly the same amount of alcohol as 2100 ml of exhaled breath). However for venous blood, this ratio is not a constant but changes as a function of ethanol metabolism. If one wants to determine blood-alcohol one needs to analyse blood by a more reliable method.

The most reliable method of all these methods is gas liquid chromatography.

19. B. Section 203 of *Motor Vehicle Act 1988* gives detailed instructions on who can conduct breathalyzer tests and under which circumstances. Following is a summary:

- A police officer in uniform or an officer of the Motor Vehicles Department (duly authorised by that Department) can ask *any* person suspected of drunken driving to provide one or more specimens of breath for breath test either at the spot or nearby. Note that such a driver may not actually be involved in an accident. The sample can be requested simply if the police officer suspects him of drunken driving.
- If the vehicle is *actually* involved in an accident, the police officer is authorized to collect such breath samples even if the drunken driver was himself injured and was admitted in a hospital for treatment. In the latter case however, the physician incharge of the patient has to be informed, and breath samples can only be taken if he (the physician incharge) thinks that this would not interfere with the proper care or treatment of the patient.
- If breath tests reveal the presence of alcohol, the police officer can arrest the driver without warrant (except when the person is at a hospital as an indoor patient).
- The police office can also arrest the driver without warrant, if he refuses or fails to provide breath samples (except when the person is at a hospital as an indoor patient).
- A person arrested in consequence of failure to provide breath samples shall be given another opportunity to provide a specimen of breath for a breath test while at a police station.

- The results of a breath test made under section 203 are admissible in evidence in a court of law.

20. C. Section 510 IPC states that "Whoever, in a state of intoxication, appears in any public place, or in any place which it is a trespass in him to enter, and there conducts himself in such a manner as to cause annoyance to any person, shall be punished with simple imprisonment for a term which may extend to twenty-four hours, or with fine which may extend to ten rupees, or with both".

21. B. Such a person will get the benefit of section 85 IPC and not get any punishment whatsoever. Section 85 of IPC relates to act of a person incapable of judgment by reason of intoxication caused against his will. It states:

Nothing is an offence which is done by a person who, at the time of doing it, is, by reason of intoxication, incapable of knowing the nature of the act, or that he is doing what is either wrong, or contrary to law; provided that the thing which intoxicated him was administered to him without his knowledge or a against his will.

Note that section 84 IPC is meant for mentally unsound people only.

METHYL ALCOHOL

22. D. About 80% of methyl alcohol is excreted unchanged from lungs. About 3-5% is excreted unchanged in the urine.

23. D. ***Related fact:*** The metabolic acidosis is due to the formation of formic acid. Respiratory acidosis occurs due to depression of the central respiratory center by methanol.

24. D.

25. B.

26. B.

27. C.

28. D.

29. C.

30. B.

KEROSENE

31. B. ***Related fact:*** Kerosene has a very low surface tension, because of which it rapidly spreads over the surfaces it comes in contact with, such as respiratory parenchyma. Hepatic and renal failure are unknown in kerosene poisoning. CNS may be depressed, but encephalopathy is unknown.

Remember other important pointers in relation to kerosene poisoning:

- Double bubble sign is seen in→ Kerosene poisoning (if kerosene is not there in the choice, look for hydrocarbons, which should be the correct choice) . Things to remember about this sign:
  - o It is a radiological sign.
  - o Upright X-ray.
  - o Two liquid densities in the stomach. Air-hydrocarbon interface and hydrocarbon-fluid interface.
- Most important line of treatment in kerosene poisoning is→Prevention of aspiration, and respiratory support.
  - o Endotracheal intubation.
  - o Oxygen.
  - o Continuous positive airway pressure.
  - o High frequency Jet Ventilation (HFJV) using high respiratory rates (220-260) with small tidal volumes.
  - o Extracorporeal membrane oxygenation (ECMO) when all other measures have failed.
- Induction of vomiting is→**NOT** recommended in Kerosene, because of the risk of aspiration.

- Stomach wash→Doubtful value. If done, do only after endotracheal intubation.
- Corticosteroids→**NOT** recommended in Kerosene, because of the increased chances of bacterial superinfection.
- Following measures are **contraindicated** in Hydrocarbon/kerosene poisoning:
  - o Emetics.
  - o Activated charcoal.
  - o Olive oil/mineral oil.
  - o Cathartics.
  - o Catecholamines (dopamine, adrenaline etc).
- Fatal dose (Kerosene)→10-30 ml.
- Fatal period (Kerosene)→less than 24 hours.

MISCELLANEOUS

32. D. ***Related facts:*** Chloral hydrate when mixed with alcohol is given the name "Mickey Finn" or "knockout drops". Its hypnotic action is very rapid in such cases. Used for daylight robberies, railway robberies etc. At one time, it was used to Shanghaii sailors (*Shanghaii is an interesting toponym, and means "to render unconscious by means of drugs". The term came into general use around 1870. Shanghaii was a seaport on the Hang Pu river in the Yangtze delta. It was opened up to international trade under the Treaty of Nanking in 1842. Since American sailors were unwilling to go there, unconventional methods had to be used to get them to the ship. Shanghaiing them with chloral hydrate was one such method. Shanghaii, apparently meant "to take to Shanghaii"*). Also used to seduce women and knock out private detectives in movies. However it takes a lot longer to put people to sleep with this drug, than the movies would imply.

Other pointers about Chloral Hydrate:

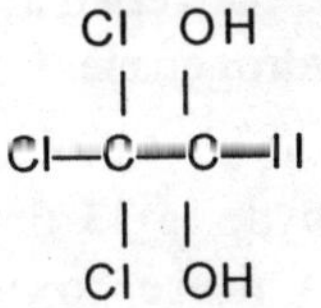

Fig. 41.1: Chloral hydrate

- Structure very similar to ethyl alcohol.
- Rapidly metabolized in the liver to **trichloroethanol**, which is also hypnotic. (Which of the following poisons gets metabolized in the liver to Trichloroethanol→Chloral Hydrate).
- Peculiar pungent odour, pungent bitter taste. Because of peculiar pungent odour and taste, can not be administered homicidally to a victim, except in alcohol.
- Which of the following poisons is most commonly mixed in country made liquor to enhance its potency→Chloral Hydrate.
- Fatal dose→5-10 g.
- Fatal period→8-12 hours.

MULTIPLE ANSWER TYPE (PGI, CHANDIGARH PATTERN)

33. A,C,D. To understand why these three act as antidotes against methyl alcohol poisoning, let us recapitulate the metabolism of methyl alcohol (Fig. 41.2).

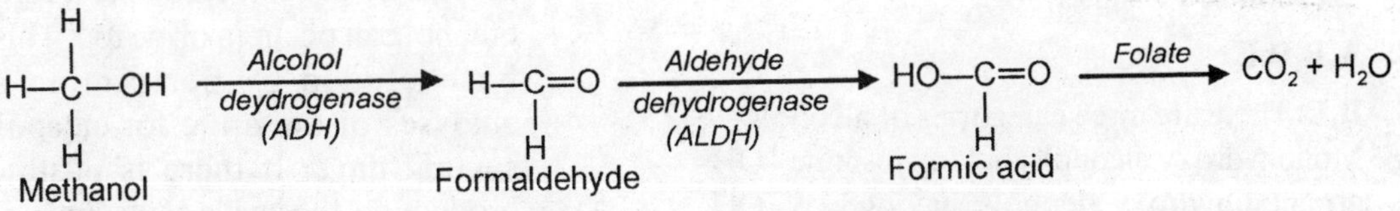

Fig. 41.2: Metabolism of methanol

We can see that methanol is converted to harmless carbon dioxide and water in three steps.

Step 1: Methanol is converted by Alcohol Dehydrogenase (ADH) to formaldehyde.

Step 2: Formaldehyde is converted to Formic acid by Aldehyde dehydrogenase.

Formaldehyde and formic acid are very toxic compounds (formaldehyde is 33 times and formic acid 6 times more toxic than methanol,). If their formation can be stopped, much of the toxicity of methanol can be avoided.

Its formation is stopped in two ways:

i. By giving oral ethyl alcohol. Ethyl alcohol is a preferential substrate for ADH. So most molecules of ADH get engaged in metabolizing ethyl alcohol. Methanol does not get converted to formaldehyde and is excreted as such.
ii. By giving 4-Methyl pyrazole (Fomepizole), which is a competitive inhibitor of ADH.

Step 3: Formic acid is converted to carbon dioxide and water which is a folate dependent pathway.

If despite giving ethyl alcohol and/or 4-methyl pyrazole, some methanol has been converted to formaldehyde (and then to formic acid), our main aim is to complete the metabolism of formic acid as soon as possible. This is done by giving folic acid, as this facilitates the conversion of formic acid to harmless carbon dioxide and water as shown above.

Remember that the trade name of 4-methyl pyrazole is FOMEPIZOLE. For a related question see Chapter 50.

34. A,B,D,E.

35. B,E. There are three categories of alcohols—Monohydroxy alcohols, having just one –OH group; dihydroxy alcohols, having two –OH groups and trihydroxy alcohols, having three –OH groups. Dihyroxy alcohols are referred to also as glycols. Methanol, ethanol and isopropanol are examples of monohydroxy alcohols, ethylene glycol and propylene glycol are examples of dihyroxy alcohols and glycerine is an example of trihydroxy alcohols.

36. A,B,C,E. ***Related facts*:** Postmortem production of alcohol is a known phenomenon. Bacteria, yeast and mold can produce alcohol in the body after death. Following facts must be considered by the forensic pathologist to differentiate genuine antemortem intake of alcohol from postmortem production.

i. There are witnesses having seen the victim drinking. This goes in favor of antemortem ingestion.
ii. There is putrefaction of body. In this condition, one must consider postmortem production of alcohol.
iii. Postmortem production of alcohol is generally never more than 70 mg %. There are rare reports of postmortem production upto 200 mg%, but never more than that. Postmortem levels above 200 mg% suggest that the alcohol was ingested before death.
iv. Urine and vitreous humor are generally immune to the postmortem production of alcohol. Presence of alcohol in blood in a putrefying body with concomitant absence from urine and vitreous is highly suggestive of postmortem production of ethanol.
v. Rarely if the deceased was diabetic and had an urinary infection with *Candida albicans*, postmortem production of ethanol can occur in urine too. This must be excluded by performing serial analyses of the urine for ethanol over several days. If there is postmortem production, the levels of alcohol will rise.

vi. Microorganisms produce – besides ethanol – a number of other by products, which are never seen in true antemortem ingestion. These products are used as "markers" for postmortem ethanol production. Most useful markers are *n*-propanol and *n*-butanol. Other markers that can be used are acetone, isopropanol, *t*-butanol, isoamylalcohol, and *n*-amylalcohol.

vii. Ethylglucuronide, a phase II metabolite of ethanol is never produced by microorganisms. It is seen only in true antemortem ingestion.

37. A,B,C. ***Related facts*:** Gastric lavage is quite useful in methyl alcohol poisoning. Activated charcoal is not helpful in methyl alcohol poisoning. For all other poisons in which it is not effective, please see Chapter 31 (General Principles of Treatment).

38. A, C. The origin of the term "proof spirit" lies in the antiquities of history. In olden times (as it is now) it was usual for suppliers and traders to adulterate ethyl alcohol with water and it needed to be "proved" that it was indeed ethyl alcohol at the right concentration. To do this, the sample (of alcohol to be tested) was mixed with gunpowder and ignited. If the sample had a very low alcohol content (say 30% v/v), ignition did not take place. As the concentration of alcohol in this weaker solution was increased, a point came, when the gunpowder could just be ignited. This concentration came to be called as proof spirit, as the presence of spirit in such a mixture had been "proved"! This concentration was found to be equal to 57.1% by volume (i.e. 100 cc of mixture contained 57.1 cc of ethyl alcohol).

Since it was impractical to use gunpowder every time one wanted to test the strength of alcohol, a simpler method – hydrometer – began to be used (it works on the specific gravity of the mixture). In the 1740s, the Customs and Excise and the London distillers began to use Clark's hydrometer to measure spirit strength. By the Hydrometer Act, 1818, a more accurate version (of hydrometer) by Bartholomew Sikes was universally adopted. Measurement of proof strength of alcohol by this method came to be known as Sikes system (or sometimes Sykes system). This system remained unchallenged for over 160 years – until 1980 (see below).

In 1952, Britain passed *The Customs and Excise Act* which defined spirits of proof strength as follows:

'Spirits shall be deemed to be at proof if the volume of the ethyl alcohol contained therein made up to the volume of the spirits with distilled water has a weight equal to that of twelve-thirteenths of a volume of distilled water equal to the volume of the spirits, the volume of each liquid being computed as at fifty-one degrees Fahrenheit'.

In other words, proof spirit (100 proof) meant that the spirit at a temperature of 51°F (11° C), weighed exactly twelve-thirteenths of an equal volume of distilled water.

It is worth noting that the US adopts a much simpler method of defining proof. The percentage of alcohol in the mixture is measured at 60°F (approximately 15.6°C). The percentage is then doubled to get the proof strength. Thus 40% alcohol is 80 proof, 50% alcohol is 100 proof and so on. Students may find it a bit confusing that British and American proof systems do not overlap exactly. For instance, 70 proof alcohol (British) is 80 proof (American). For a quick conversion of British proof to American, one can divide the British proof by 7, then multiply by 8.

Mainly to avoid such confusions, on 1st January, 1980, in common with other EC countries, Britain adopted the system of measurement recommended by the International Organization of Legal Metrology (*Organization Internationale de Métrologie Légale* or OIML), a body with most major nations among its members. The OIML system measures alcoholic strength simply as a percentage of alcohol by volume at a temperature of 20°C. Thus if a sample contains, say, 43.5% alcohol (at 20°C), it would simply be labelled as 43.5% alcohol v/v. This system replaces the older Sikes system of measuring the strength of spirits. However it is not uncommon still to find bottles of liquor depicting the concentration of alcohol in both modern (percentage by volume) and older Sikes (proof) system.

39. B,C. It is important to realize that under section 204 of *Motor Vehicles Act 1988*, the police officer is *not* authorized to take blood sample of the offending driver straightaway, without first giving an opportunity to him for a breath test. Provisions under section 204 of *Motor Vehicles Act 1988* are important for a medical practitioner to appreciate. These are:

- Blood samples can be taken at the police station by a medical practitioner called there by the police officer under the following circumstances:
  - o If the offending driver has refused to give breath samples and has been arrested in consequence.
  - o If the driver did give breath samples and alcohol was found in them.
  - o If the offending driver is a female and the medical practitioner a male, blood samples can be taken only in the presence of a female, whether a medical practitioner or not.
- If the offending driver himself was injured and was undergoing treatment, blood samples can still be taken at the hospital under similar circumstances. The only important rider here is that the physician incharge must certify that such collection of samples would not hamper the treatment in any way. The requirement of a female attendant in case of a female driver is also not applicable here.
- All laboratory tests conducted under section 204 are admissible in evidence.
- All laboratory tests under this section must be done at a laboratory established, maintained or recognised by the Central Government or a State Government.

40. A,C,E. Remember that almost 80% alcohol is absorbed from the intestine. Thus any situation which "sends" alcohol quickly to intestines is likely to "quicken" absorption. Gastrectomy is one such situation. Drugs which increase gastric motility such as parasympathomimetic drugs (prostigmine) hasten absorption for the same reason. Carbonated drinks hasten absorption, presumably because the bubbles greatly increase the alcohol carrying surface area.

Warm drinks dilate gastric mucosal capillaries, hastening absorption; the converse happens with cold iced drinks. Food, especially that which is high in fats and proteins delays absorption; about 10-20% of the ingested alcohol may not even be absorbed in this situation.

The optimum concentration at which alcohol is absorbed best is 10-20%. One would imagine that absorption would be quicker at higher concentrations, but this is not so. The factors which reduce alcohol absorption at higher concentrations are (i) pyloric spasm

(ii) secretion of gastric mucus due to irritation (iii) reduced gastric motility, thus delaying passage of alcohol in duodenum.

Alcohol is absorbed more rapidly in habituated drinkers than novices, presumably because habituated drinkers have a rapid gastric emptying time.

The Table 41.3 gives situations where the absorption of alcohol is increased and decreased.

Table 41.3: Various conditions when absorption of alcohol is increased or decreased

S.No	*Absorption of alcohol increased*	*Absorption of alcohol decreased*
1.	When the concentration of alcohol is between 10%-20%	When the concentration of alcohol is below 10% or above 20%
2.	When alcohol is swallowed rapidly	When alcohol is slowly gulped
3.	When alcohol is taken on empty stomach	When alcohol is taken with food, especially that rich in fat and proteins
4.	When alcohol is taken with carbonated soda	—
5.	When drink is warm	When drink is ice cold
6.	In habitual drinkers	In novices
7.	In patients of gastrectomy	
8.	With simultaneous ingestion of parasympathomimetic drugs (e.g. prostigmine)	With simultaneous ingestion of parasympatholytic drugs (e.g. atropine), or with sympathomimetic drugs (e.g. adrenaline and benzedrine)
9.	Drugs which increase gastric motility (e.g. insulin)	
10.	—	Achlorhydria and chronic gastritis

42 Deliriant Poisons

1. **The alkaloid found in *Datura* seeds is:**
   A. Pilocarpine
   B. Physostigmine
   C. Atropine
   D. Prostigmine
2. **Imaginary threads are pulled from the tips of fingers in poisoning from:**
   A. Datura poisoning
   B. Cocaine poisoning
   C. Hashish poisoning
   D. Opium poisoning
3. **The usual fatal dose of datura seeds is:**
   A. 10 to 20
   B. About 50
   C. 100 to 125
   D. 200 to 300
4. **Which of the following plants is colloquially known as deadly nightshade?**
   A. *Hyoscyamus niger*
   B. *Atropa belladona*
   C. *Datura stramonium*
   D. *Datura atrox*
5. **Which of the following plants is colloquially known as Jimson weed?**
   A. *Hyoscyamus niger*
   B. *Atropa belladona*
   C. *Datura atrox*
   D. *Datura stramonium*
6. **Which of the following plants is colloquially known as Henbane?**
   A. *Hyoscyamus niger*
   B. *Atropa belladona*
   C. *Datura atrox*
   D. *Datura stramonium*
7. **Which one of the following is NOT a cannabis preparation?**
   A. Brown sugar
   B. Ganja
   C. Bhang
   D. Sinsemilla
8. **Which of the following is a highly potent form of marijuana obtained from unpollinated female plants?**
   A. Sinsemilla
   B. Bhang
   C. Charas
   D. *Afim*
9. **Active principle of cannabis is:**
   A. Pilocarpine
   B. Atropine
   C. Morphine
   D. THC

10. **World's most commonly used illicit drug is:**
   A. Brown sugar
   B. LSD
   C. Cannabis
   D. Cocaine

MULTIPLE ANSWER TYPE (PGI, CHANDIGARH PATTERN)

11. **Which of the following parts/products are related to cannabis?**
   A. *Afim*
   B. *Bhang*
   C. *Post ka doda*
   D. Sinsemilla
   E. *Charas*

ANSWERS

1. **C.**
2. **A.**
3. **C.**
4. **B.** *Nightshade* is the name given to any plant of the genus Solanum (family Solanaceae), which has about 2,300 species, and certain other plants of the same family and other families. The species usually called nightshade in North America and England is *Solanum dulcamara* (it is also known as bittersweet and *woody nightshade)*. Its foliage and egg-shaped red berries are poisonous, the active principle being solanine, which can cause convulsions and death if taken in large doses. The *black nightshade* (*S. nigrum*) is also generally considered poisonous, but its fully ripened fruit and foliage are cooked and eaten in some areas.

   The aptly named *deadly nightshade* is the belladonna (*Atropa belladonna*), a tall, bushy herb of the same family and the source of several alkaloid drugs. *Enchanter's nightshade* is a name applied to plants of the genus Circaea (family Onagraceae). *Malabar nightshade* refers to twining herbaceous vines of the genus Basella (family Basellaceae).
5. **D.** ***Related fact:*** *Datura stramonium* is also known colloquially by another name —*thorn apple*. This fact can also be asked in an MCQ.

   Please note that *Datura fastuosa* is also known as Thorn apple, making the whole issue somewhat confusing.
6. **A.** ***Related fact:*** Remember table 42.1 for common names:

Table 42.1: Botanical and common names of some common deliriant plants

S.No.	Botanical name	Common name
1.	*Atropa belladona*	Deadly nightshade
2.	*Datura stramonium*	Jimson weed, Thorn apple
3.	*Hyoscyamus niger*	Henbane, *Khorasani ajwayan*
4.	*Datura fastuosa*	Thorn apple
5.	*Datura alba*	Safed Dhatura
6.	*Datura niger*	Kala Dhatura

   Note that both *Datura stramonium* as well as *Datura fastuosa* are known as Thorn apple. *Datura fastuosa* are found in plains, while *Datura stramonium* grows at high altitudes in Himalayas.
   Datura alba and *Datura niger* are two different varieties of *Datura fastuosa*.
7. **A.**
8. **A.** Sinsemilla is a very popular form of cannabis in the USA. The female plants are specially tended and kept seedless by preventing pollination in order to induce a high resin content.

   The word comes from American Spanish, *sin* without + *semilla* seed (*semilla* is also related to semen).

   Cannabis is a dioecious plant, which means that the male and female flowers develop on separate plants (although monoecious examples do exist with both sexes on one plant). Plants with male flowers are called "staminate", and those with female flowers "pistillate". Sinsemilla is produced by eliminating "staminate" plants from the field. In lieu of setting seed in the earliest flowers, the "pistillate" plants continue to produce additional flowers, which are covered by resin glands, thus increasing the amount of THC obtainable from a single plant.

Since 1975, sinsemilla has been the primary style of North American and European marijuana production.

9. **D.** THC stands for delta-9 **T**etra**H**ydro**C**annabinol. It is a cannabinoid found both in male and female plants. As THC is known to stimulate appetite and soothe nausea, it has found medical uses. Dronabinol (sold under the trade name Marinol) is a synthetic version of THC. Dronabinol was approved by the Food and Drug Administration (FDA) in 1985 for treating the nausea produced by chemotherapy in cancer patients (especially those who do not respond to the more commonly used anti-emetics). In 1992 it was approved for prescription to people with AIDS to stimulate appetite and combat weight loss.

   Dronabinol is sold in 2.5 mg, 5 mg and 10 mg capsules. Dose ranges from 2.5 - 20 mg a day. The most common side effect is feeling euphoric or high. Other side effects include dizziness, drowsiness and abnormal thinking. Nabilone is an analog of dronabinol used for the same purpose. It is manufactured by Lilly and is available commercially in the US under the trade name Cesamet.

   Another THC based drug is Sativex, which has been developed by a British company, GW Pharmaceuticals. While Dronabinol contains just THC, Sativex contains THC as well as other cannabinoids found in the marijuana plant. It is used as a mouth spray for multiple sclerosis to alleviate pain. In April 2005, Canadian authorities approved the marketing of Sativex, but it has not been approved elsewhere including the US.

10. **C.**

MULTIPLE ANSWER TYPE (PGI, CHANDIGARH PATTERN)

11. **B,D,E.** Bhang consists of dried mature leaves and flower stems of cannabis, which are ground with water and mixed with fruit juice or milk. Sinsemilla is a popular form of cannabis in USA. *Charas* refers to the dried resin of cannabis.

    Afim is raw opium, which comes from *Papaver somniferum. Post ka doda* refers to the capsule of *Papaver somniferum* after opium has been extracted from it.

43

Spinal Poisons

1. **How many uncrushed seeds of *Strychnos Nux vomica* when taken as such can cause death?**
   A. 1-2 seeds
   B. 5 seeds
   C. 10 seeds
   D. They can not cause death
2. **Strychnine poisoning can be confused with which of the following disease?**
   A. Migraine
   B. Tetanus
   C. Cholera
   D. Lower nephron nephrosis
3. **Strychnine mainly acts at:**
   A. Kidneys
   B. Posterior horn cells of the spinal cord
   C. Anterior horn cells of the spinal cord
   D. Heart
4. **Strychnine poisoning may resemble all of the following medical conditions/ poisonings *except*:**
   A. Tetanus
   B. Meningitis
   C. Intracerebral bleeding
   D. Dhatura poisoning
5. **In India, the plant *Strychnos Nux vomica* is known as**
   A. *Kuchila*
   B. Marking nut
   C. Ratti
   D. Jamalgota
6. **Lateral bending of the victim – seen in many cases of strychnine poisoning – is known as:**
   A. Opisthotonus
   B. Emprosthotonus
   C. Pleurosthotonus
   D. Risus sardonicus
7. **Opisthotonus is seen in:**
   A. Strychnine poisoning
   B. Severe cerebral palsy
   C. Traumatic brain injury
   D. All of the above
8. **What is the effect of external stimuli, such as touching the patient, a slight current of air, light and sound, on convulsions in a patient poisoned with strychnine?**
   A. The convulsions disappear till the external stimuli is there, only to return when the stimuli is taken off
   B. The convulsions increase in intensity
   C. The convulsions decrease in intensity
   D. The lower limbs go in convulsions but upper limbs relax immediately
9. **In strychnine poisoning, the symptoms usually start:**
   A. Within 15 minutes to an hour

B. After 12-18 hours
C. After 2-3 days
D. After 2 weeks

10. **The usual fatal period in strychnine poisoning is:**
A. 1-2 minutes
B. 1-2 hours
C. 24 hours
D. 3-5 days

11. **The usual cause of death in strychnine poisoning is:**
A. Asphyxia
B. Cardiac failure
C. Renal failure
D. Hepatic failure

12. **The taste of strychnine is:**
A. Tasteless
B. Intensely bitter
C. Sweetish pungent
D. Sour

13. **Which of the following organs of the deceased is not of much use for the detection of strychnine?**
A. Bone
B. Liver
C. Kidneys
D. Brain

MULTIPLE ANSWER TYPE (PGI, CHANDIGARH PATTERN)

14. **Which of the following facts about *Strychnos Nux vomica* are CORRECT?**
A. The plant belongs to the family Ranunculaceae
B. The plant is found in *jungles* of India
C. The seeds are hexagonal in shape
D. The seeds contain brucine
E. The outer surface of the seeds is very smooth and satin-like due to the presence of innumerable fine, silky hairs

15. **The main signs and symptoms of strychnine poisoning are:**
A. Flaccid paralysis of lower limbs
B. Trismus
C. Alternate contraction and dilation of pupils
D. Risus sardonicus
E. Delirium

16. **Which of the following types of spams are seen in Strychnine poisoning?**
A. Emprosthotonos
B. Trismus
C. Pleurosthotonus
D. Risus sardonicus
E. Opisthotonus

17. **Which of the following facts are CORRECT about convulsions in strychnine poisoning?**
A. They are first tonic and then become clonic
B. Convulsions can usually be controlled by benzodiazepines and barbiturates
C. The convulsions are continuous and end only at death
D. There is spasm of diaphragm too
E. There is chattering of teeth which is known as the "death chatter"

18. **Which of the following measures are USEFUL in the treatment of strychnine poisoning?**
A. Induction of vomiting
B. Administration of activated charcoal
C. Forced alkaline diuresis
D. Intubation and mechanical ventilation
E. Amphetamine

19. **The classical autopsy features of strychnine poisoning are:**
A. Absence of rigor mortis
B. Postmortem caloricity
C. Green blue post mortem staining
D. Frothing at the mouth
E. Signs of asphyxia

20. Which of the following facts about strychnine poisoning are CORRECT?
A. Suicidal poisoning is very common with strychnine
B. The seeds are sometimes taken as an aphrodisiac
C. It is the leading cause of homicide in the world today
D. The seeds are sometimes used as a cattle poison and also as an arrow poison
E. Strychnine was one used as a medicine, mainly as a tonic

ANSWERS

1. **D.** ***Related fact:*** Uncrushed seeds of *Strychnos Nux vomica* do not cause death, as they have a hard coating which is not dissolved by stomach or intestinal juices. If the question refers to crushed seeds, then the correct answer is 1 seed (in the given question 1-2 seeds would be the correct answer). *So do look out for what the question is referring to* – **crushed** or **uncrushed** seeds! If the question asks the dose in terms of weight of strychnine, the correct answer is 30-50 mg. If the question asks for weight of strychnos seeds, the answer is 1-3 gm of strychnos seeds.
2. **B.**
3. **C.** ***Related fact:*** Glycine is a major post-synaptic inhibitory neurotransmitter in mammalian spinal cord and brain stem. Strychnine and glycine act at two separate binding sites on the glycine receptor in an allosteric manner; i.e. the binding of one compound at its site lowers the affinity of the glycine receptor for the other compound at its site. Strychnine acts mainly on the inhibitory synapses in ventral horns
4. **D.** ***Related fact:*** Since strychnine causes seizures, all medical conditions causing seizures need to be excluded. These include (i) tetanus (ii) idiopathic seizure disorders (iii) drug withdrawal (iv) meningitis (v) intracerebral bleeding. Other poisonings that may cause myoclonus or seizures are (i) cyclic antidepressants (ii) theophylline (iii) chlorinated hydrocarbon insecticides (DDT) (iv) amphetamines (v) cocaine.
5. **A.** ***Related facts:*** Other common names of *Strychnos Nux vomica* are Dog button (because it is sometimes used to kill stray dogs), Quaker Buttons[1] and poison nut. Watch out for these choices as well.

   Names in other languages: French - *Noix vomique*; German – Brecknusz, Krahenaugen; Italian – *Noce vomica*; Spanish - *Nuez vomica.*
6. **C.**
7. **D.** ***Additional info:*** Opisthotonus is the backward bending of individuals. It is classically seen in strychnine poisoning, but is also seen in individuals with severe cerebral palsy or traumatic brain injury. In infants and children opisthotonos is exhibited more often and is also more exaggerated than in adults. Opisthotonus in infants may be apparent in the first hours of life.
8. **B.** ***Related facts:*** The convulsions increase in intensity with the application of external stimuli. That is why (i) gastric lavage is not done in strychnine (because it is a very strong physical stimulus) (ii) the room of the patient has to be noise free (sound stimulus is minimized) and darkened (light stimulus is minimized).
9. **A.**
10. **B.**

---

[1]Quakers was a religious sect founded by George Fox, of Leicestershire, England, about 1650, the members of which call themselves Friends. Fox's teaching was primarily a preaching of repentance.

Men and women listening to the preachings sometimes fell down and lay struggling as if for life. For this reason, they were called Quakers, in derision.

Seeds of Nux vomica are called Quaker buttons, presumably because they cause similar trembling!

11. **A.** This asphyxia is due to the spasm of respiratory muscles.

12. **B.** ***Additional info:*** Strychnine has been described as the MOST bitter substance in the world. It can be detected in dilutions as high as 1/700,000. More recent reports however suggest that the maximum detectable dilution is about 1/100,000, but it is still quite high to rate it as the most bitter substance in the world.

13. **A.** ***Related fact:*** The highest concentrations of strychnine are found in liver, stomach, kidneys and blood. The following data taken from the analytical results seen in 15 fatal cases is illustrative[1]:

Table 43.1: Strychnine concentrations in Fatalities (mg/L or mg/kg)

Organ	*Average*	*Range*
Liver	116	2-257
Stomach	113	7.5-282
Kidney	42	3.2-106
Blood	20	0.5-61
Brain	14	2.4-26
Urine	8.3	1-33

This table (Table 43.1) clearly illustrates that the best organs to analyse in Strychnine poisoning are liver, stomach and kidneys, and to some extent blood. Strychnine is not found in any appreciable quantities in brain and spinal cord. It is a myth that brain and spinal cord MUST be preserved in strychnine poisoning. There is no scientific basis for believing so.

A variant of this question is often asked like this: **In *Nux vomica* poisoning, which one of the following is also required to be preserved?**

(a) Long bone (b) Brain (c) Muscles (d) Skin

For this question the correct answer should be (b), because the other three tissues contain even lesser quantities of strychnine than brain (or none at all).

This is however not a correctly framed question, because there is no protocol saying that brain MUST be preserved in strychnine poisoning. The choice (B) appears correct simply because it is the best choice available.

MULTIPLE ANSWER TYPE (PGI, CHANDIGARH PATTERN)

14. **B,D,E.** *Strychnos nux vomica* belongs to the family *Loganiaceae* (order *Gentianales*) and not to *Ranunculaceae*. The tree is a native of India, growing in Bengal, Malabar, on the Coromandel Coast, in Ceylon, in many islands of the Indian Archipelago, in Cochin China, and in northern Australia.

The seeds are not hexagonal, but circular. They are flat disc shaped, much like a coat button. The seeds contain strychnine which is the main alkaloid, but they also contain a less poisonous alkaloid brucine, which is about 10-20 times less toxic than strychnine. The seeds also contain a glucoside *loganin* (mnemonic—Remember the family *Loganiaceae*). Loganin is inert.

15. **B,D.** In strychnine poisoning the main symptom is rigidity of the whole body and NOT flaccid paralysis. Trismus is also known as lockjaw. Alternate contraction and dilation of pupil is classically seen in aconite and NOT in strychnine poisoning. Risus sardonicus or "sardonic smile" is due to contraction of facial muscles, which produce a kind of grimacing. Delirium is NOT seen in strychnine poisoning. On the contrary the mind is completely clear in this poisoning (remember strychnine acts mainly on the spinal cord and NOT on the brain).

[1] Baselt R.C. (2004) Disposition of Toxic Drugs and Chemicals in Man, 7th Edition. Biomedical Publications, Foster City, California (pages 1039-40).

16. A,B,C,D,E. Emprosthotonus is the forward bending of the victim, pleurothotonus (sometimes spelled with an "s" as in pleurosthotonus), lateral bending and opisthotonus, backward bending. All these three kinds of bendings are seen in strychnine poisoning.

The terms are derived from Greek *emprosthen*, "forward"; *opistho*, "behind"; *pleurothen*, "from the side" and *tonos*, "tension".

17. B,D. Convulsions in strychnine poisoning are clonic first and then become tonic. The convulsions are NOT continuous. Each convulsion lasts for only half to two minutes to be followed by a relaxation period of about 10-15 minutes after which another bout of convulsion starts and so on. No chattering of teeth has been described in strychnine poisoning.

18. B,D. Induction of vomiting is contraindicated, because it can initiate severe convulsions. Forced alkaline diuresis is of no value. Amphetamine is a stimulant and can actually worsen the condition. Activated charcoal is very beneficial in strychnine poisoning as it can adsorb a good amount of poison. Intubation is necessary because respiration is compromised.

19. B,D,E. Rigor mortis actually starts early in strychnine poisoning. The color of the postmortem staining in strychnine is normal. Postmortem caloricity, or rise in temperature of the body after death, is classically described as a feature of strychnine poisoning.

20. B,D,E. Suicidal poisoning is very rare with strychnine, because the death is very agonizing. Homicide with strychnine is possible, but is very difficult because of its intensely bitter taste. That's why homicide with strychnine is very rare.

44 Peripheral Nerve Poisons

1. **Which of the following is the mode of action of curare?**
   A. It inhibits the peripheral enzymes
   B. It blocks the receptors at the myoneural junction
   C. It blocks impulses in the spinal cord
   D. It first depresses and then stimulates the cerebral cortex

2. **Which of the following acts as a peripheral nerve poison?**
   A. Curare
   B. Strychnos Nux vomica
   C. Opium
   D. Bhang

3. **Which one of the following statements regarding curare is NOT true?**
   A. Causes flaccid paralysis of skeletal muscles
   B. It is found in various species of *Strychnos*
   C. It is not poisonous when swallowed
   D. It causes hypertension

4. **Death by curare is due to:**
   A. Cardiac failure
   B. Coma
   C. Asphyxia
   D. Cardiac failure followed by coma

5. **Which poison was given to the Greek philosopher Socrates to execute him?**
   A. Curare
   B. Strychnos nux vomica
   C. *Conium maculatum*
   D. Datura

6. **Cases of human poisoning with poison hemlock occur because:**
   A. The hemlock roots are mistaken for parsnips
   B. The hemlock leaves are mistaken for parsley
   C. The hemlock seeds are mistaken for anise
   D. All of the above

7. **Death in poison hemlock occurs is due to:**
   A. Kidney failure
   B. Respiratory failure
   C. Fulminant hepatitis
   D. Hemolysis

8. **Fatal dose of coniine is:**
   A. 60 picograms
   B. 60 micrograms
   C. 60 mg
   D. 60 g

9. **Which is the best antidote for *Conium maculatum* poisoning?**
   A. Atropine
   B. Physostigmine

C. Amphetamine
D. No specific antidote exists

MULTIPLE ANSWER TYPE (PGI, CHANDIGARH PATTERN)

10. Which of the following facts about Poison Hemlock are correct?

A. Its botanincal name is *Conium maculatum*
B. Only root is toxic
C. Its toxic principle is similar to nicotine
D. Its leaves when crushed, emit the odor of bitter almonds
E. Its main symptoms are tremors, diaphoresis, sweating, mydriasis and convulsions

11. Which of the following are active principles of *Conium maculatum*?

A. Coniine
B. Ergometrine
C. Ricin
D. Gamma-coniceine
E. Abrin

12. Which of the following measures are most helpful in *Conium maculatum* poisoning?

A. Gastric lavage
B. Administration of general anaesthesia
C. Activated charcoal
D. Hemodialysis
E. Benzodiazepines

ANSWERS

1. **B.**
2. **A.**
3. **D.** Curare is not a single chemical, but a generic term for many different types of preparations, which includes many components but most frequently the deadly poisons of the bark of *Strychnos toxifera* or *Strychnos guianensis* (Family Loganiaceae). Among the many alkaloids present in curare preparations, the most common ones are curarine and tubocurarine.

   From some other species of Strychnos (*Strychnos nux vomica*), we get strychnine – a completely different chemical – with which curare should not be confused.

   Sir Walter Raleigh and several other early explorers to South America reported on curare and its effect, but apparently it was the noted geographer Alexander von Humboldt (1805) who was the first reliable eyewitness of curare preparation.

   Curare is not poisonous by mouth. Animals, which have been killed by curare can be eaten with no harmful effects. Indeed curare is used as an arrow poison to kill animals for eating.

   Curare causes hypotension due to released histamine. Thus choice (D) is the intended choice.
4. **C.** Death from curare is caused by asphyxia, because the skeletal muscles (including muscles of respiration) become relaxed and then paralyzed. Autopsy findings are also those of asphyxia for the same reason.
5. **C.** ***Related facts:*** *Conium maculatum* is the botanical name of Poison Hemlock. Poison hemlock (*Conium maculatum*) is different from water hemlock (*Cicuta maculata*). The latter is also a poisonous plant, and its active principle is cicutoxin. Socrates was given poison hemlock in 399 B.C. The Greeks in fact used it routinely for inflicting capital punishments. The Old Testament describes rhabdomyolysis in Israelites who consumed quail fed on hemlock. *Conium maculatum* is a recognized medicine under Unani system, where it is known by the name *Shokran*.
6. **D.**
7. **B.** ***Related facts:*** It is useful to remember that poison hemlock contains several piperidine alkaloid toxins (e.g. coniine) that are structurally similar to nicotine. Nicotine activation at autonomic ganglia initially can cause tachycardia, salivation, mydriasis, and diaphoresis. In severe cases, acetylcholine (nicotinic) receptor antagonism develops leading to bradycardia, ascending paralysis, and CNS depression (coma). Death is typically from respiratory failure.
8. **C.**
9. **D.**

MULTIPLE ANSWER TYPE (PGI, CHANDIGARH PATTERN)

10. **A,C,E.** ***Related facts***: All parts of this plant are toxic. The crushed leaves emit an unpleasant "mousy" odor. Odor of bitter almonds is typically associated with cyanide.

Note that its typical symptoms are similar to those produced by nicotine, because its active principles are structurally similar to nicotine.

11. **A,D.** ***Related facts***: The complete list of active principles of *Conium maculatum* is gamma-coniceine, coniine, N-methyl coniine, conhydrine, and pseudoconhydrine.

12. **A,C,E.** Aggressive GI decontamination is the best measure that can be undertaken in this poisoning. Benzodiazepines are useful in controlling convulsions.

12 POISONS ACTING ON OTHER PARTS OF THE BODY

45 Cardiac Poisons

CYANIDE

1. **The oral fatal dose of liquid hydrocyanic acid is:**
   A. Just a drop
   B. 2 mg
   C. 20 mg
   D. 50 mg
2. **The oral fatal dose of potassium cyanide is:**
   A. Just a speck of powder
   B. 1-2 mg
   C. 5-10 mg
   D. 200-300 mg
3. **The odor of cyanide is same as that of:**
   A. Aromatic oil
   B. Sewer gas
   C. Bitter almonds
   D. Rotten fish
4. **The average fatal period for hydrocyanic acid poisoning is:**
   A. Instantaneous
   B. 2 to 10 minutes
   C. 30 to 60 minutes
   D. 1 to 2 hours
5. **In cyanide poisoning, which of the following is not useful?**
   A. Oxygen
   B. BAL
   C. Amyl nitrite
   D. Activated charcoal
6. **Which of the following statements about methemoglobin are correct?**
   A. In the methemoglobin molecule, the normal ferrous (Fe^{2+}) iron of the heme moiety has been oxidized to ferric (Fe^{3+}) iron
   B. Methemoglobin is unable to act as a carrier of oxygen
   C. It can be produced by oxidizing agents
   D. All of the above
7. **Normal levels of methemoglobin in the body are:**
   A. Zero percent
   B. Less than one percent
   C. 5-6 percent
   D. About 10 percent
8. **Nitrites are used in cyanide poisoning because they:**
   A. Chemically neutralize cyanide
   B. Cause chelation of cyanide
   C. Energize the heart
   D. Form methemoglobin
9. **Maximum tolerated concentration of methemoglobin without adverse symptoms from methemoglobin is:**
   A. 5%

B. 10-12%
C. 20-30%
D. 40%

10. What is the usual dose of sodium nitrite, which is administered in cyanide poisoning?
A. 2 ml of 100% solution
B. 10 ml of 3% solution
C. 50 ml of 25% solution
D. 100 ml of 50% solution

11. The enzyme rhodanese:
A. Is a mitochondrial enzyme
B. Binds cyanide to itself and thus sequesters It away from the system
C. Should be administered immediately in cyanide poisoning
D. Is common in Rhodesians, making them virtually immune to cyanide

12. Amyl nitrite in cyanide poisoning is administered:
A. Orally
B. By inhalation
C. Intravenously
D. Sublingually

13. Which of the following facts about sodium nitrite – as used in cyanide poisoning - is correct?
A. It must be given very fast, preferably within 2-4 seconds to be effective
B. The best way to administer sodium nitrite is sublingually
C. It must be administered very slowly, preferably over 2-4 minutes
D. It is preferably given in a concentration of 50%

14. Cyanide antidote kit does NOT contain:
A. Sodium thiosulfate
B. Sodium nitrite
C. Sodium bicarbonate
D. Amyl nitrite

ACONITE

15. Which one of the following drugs is useful in the treatment of aconite poisoning?
A. Atropine
B. Physostigmine
C. Sodium thiosulphate
D. Antiaconitine

16. Which of the following poisons is colloquially known as sweet poison, *Meetha Zehar* or *Meetha Bish*?
A. Hydrogen cyanide
B. Yellow *kaner*
C. Aconite
D. *Digitalis purpurea*

17. What is the state of pupil in aconite poisoning?
A. Contracted
B. Dilated
C. Alternately contracting and dilating
D. No effect

OLEANDER

18. Thevetin, thevetoxin and cerberin are found in:
A. Yellow oleander
B. White oleander
C. *Cerbera odollam*
D. Aconite

NICOTINE

19. Which of the following actions most correctly describes action of nicotine on the human body:
A. It depresses the respiratory effort
B. It first stimulates and then depresses the cells of the peripheral autonomic ganglia
C. It first depresses and then stimulates the cells of the midbrain
D. It acts as a hepatotoxic poison

MISCELLANEOUS

20. *Jaborandi* is:
A. *Digitalis purpurea*
B. Areca or betel nut
C. *Nerium odorum*
D. *Pilocarpus microphyllus*

21. The usual adult fatal dose of pilocarpine is:
A. 100 microgram
B. 1 mg
C. 100 mg
D. 10 g

22. Which of the following is the correct antidote for *Jaborandi* poisoning?
A. BAL
B. Atropine
C. Physostigmine
D. Amyl nitrite

MULTIPLE ANSWER TYPE (PGI, CHANDIGARH PATTERN)

23. Which of the following is a valid cyanide antidote?
A. Sodium nitrite
B. Sodium thiosulfate
C. Vitamin B_{12a}
D. Alpha-ketoglutaric acid
E. Stroma free methemoglobin

24. Which of the following enzymes are inhibited by cyanide?
A. Succinic dehydrogenase
B. Superoxide dismutase
C. Carbonic anhydrase
D. Acetylcholinesterase
E. Cytochrome oxidase

25. Which of the following nitrites are used for treatment in cyanide poisoning?
A. Potassium nitrite
B. Cobalt nitrite
C. Sodium nitrite
D. Ammonium nitrite
E. Amyl nitrite

26. Main symptoms of *jaborandi* poisoning are
A. Salivation
B. Dilated pupils
C. Dry skin
D. Lachrymation
E. Slow irregular pulse

ANSWERS

CYANIDE

1. **D.**
2. **D.** ***Related fact:*** Compare it with the fatal dose of phosphorus which is just 120 mg!
3. **C.** ***Additional info:*** This odor can not be preceived by everybody. Approximately half of the human population (figures in various studies vary between 20% and 60%) do not possess this ability. The ability to smell HCN is inherited as a sex-linked recessive trait. Among the people who can not smell HCN, males far outnumber females.
4. **B.**
5. **B.** ***Related facts:*** Cyanide is adsorbed very well by activated charcoal, and its use is recommended. For poisons not adsorbed well by cyanide, please see chapter 31 (General Principles of Treatment).
6. **D.** ***Related fact:*** In normal reduced hemoglobin, all four iron atoms are ferrous. In methemoglobin, one or more of the iron atoms are in the ferric state. It cannot carry oxygen and it is produced by oxidising agents such as amyl and sodium nitrite.
7. **B.** ***Related fact:*** Under normal conditions, small amounts of methemoglobin are constantly being formed. The levels of methemoglobin are kept in check by NADH (reaction catalysed by methemoglobin reductase), which acts to reduce it back to hemoglobin. Normal levels are not zero percent, but very low – mostly below 1 percent.
8. **D.** ***Related fact:*** Cyanides have an intense affinity for ferric (Fe^{3+}) iron. Cytochrome oxidase molecules have the ferric (Fe^{3+}) iron, to which cyanide attaches, rendering them ineffective. The physician's goal in cyanide poisoning is therefore to produce an alternate source of ferric (Fe^{3+}) iron which can compete with cytochrome oxidase for the cyanide ion. This is done by administering nitrites to the patient, which oxidize normal hemoglobin to methemoglobin.
9. **C.** ***Related fact:*** Remember that the physician administers nitrites (amyl nitrite and sodium nitrite) in cyanide poisoning in order to produce methemoglobinemia. He must remember that the levels achieved must not exceed 20-30%, because then the oxygen carrying capacity of blood is severely compromised, especially in patients who are already anaemic. In fact there are cases, where the physician induced methemoglobinemia caused death rather than the cyanide poisoning for which nitrites were administered.

   Because of this, recently physicians have tried administering stroma free methemoglobin[1] which provides exogenous methemoglobin for combination with cyanide, without the need to produce it endogenously.

   Methemoglobin levels peak about 30 minutes after administration of sodium nitrite.

---

[1] Stroma-free methemoglobin is produced by lysing the RBCs and removing the membranes. This brings hemoglobin out in solution (stroma-free hemoglobin solution or SFHS). The iron groups in the Hb molecule are then oxidized to the +3 state (to produce methemoglobin) and used as an antidote for lethal CN poisoning. This treatment was pioneered (in 1985) by Raymond P. Ten Eyck, M.D. of the Boonshoft school of medicine, Wright state university. However this is still at an experimental stage.

10. B. ***Related fact:*** Do not confuse it with choice (C). This would have been the correct choice if the dose of sodium thiosulfate were asked.

11. A. ***Related facts:*** Rhodanese is a mitochondrial enzyme. Amyl nitrite and sodium nitrite administered in CN poisonings make methemoglobin, which captures cyanide ion away from cytochrome oxidase. Cyanmethemoglobin is thus formed. Cyanmethemoglobin keeps releasing cyanide ions back in the system (albeit at a very slow pace), which must be taken care of. This is done by sodium thiosulphate which is administered along with amyl nitrite and sodium nitrite.

 The reaction can be written as follows:

$$CN^- + S_2O_3^{2-} \xrightarrow{\textit{Rhodanese}} SCN^- + SO_3^{2-}$$

 This reaction is catalysed by Rhodanese present within mitochondria.

 Addition of sulfur to the cyanide molecule (formation of thiocyanate) is irreversible. Thus cyanide can not diffuse back in the system. Thiocyanate (though it contains cyanide) is harmless and is excreted in the urine.

 Since Rhodanese transfers a sulfur atom from thiosulfate to cyanide, it is also known as *Thiosulfate cyanide sulfurtransferase*.

 The role of sulfur donors thus is very important in the treatment of cyanide poisoning. There are natural sulfur donors in the body too in the form of cysteine. It can take care of small amounts of cyanide (as in ingestion of some cyanogenetic plant products), but not the massive amounts encountered in frank poisonings.

12. B. ***Related fact:*** Amyl nitrite pearls are broken in a gauze sponge and the patient is asked to inhale the gauze for about 30 seconds each minute. If the patient is intubated the gauze is held between the oxygen source and the endotracheal tube. Please note that it is only an emergency measure. It does not raise the methemoglobin level anywhere near the desired 20-30% level; it merely does so to about 5%. When the IV line is started (through which sodium nitrite is administered), inhalation can be stopped.

13. C. ***Related fact:*** Sodium nitrite has its own adverse effects, the most important being the production of excessive methemoglobin and hypotension (because of its potent vasodilator action). These adverse effects are avoided by a slow infusion, preferably over 2-4 minutes.

14. C. ***Related fact:*** This was once known as Lilly antidote kit or Lilly Cyanide kit, as it was manufactured by Eli Lilly and Company. This company no longer manufactures this kit now. It is now available from Taylor pharmaceuticals, a Division of Akorn, Inc. Each package contains 12 amyl nitrite pearls, two 10-mL vials of 3% sodium nitrite for injection, and two 50mL vials of 25% sodium thiosulfate for injection. This kit is the mainstay of cyanide antidotal therapy in the United States. For a related question, see Chapter 50.

ACONITE

15. A. In aconite poisoning, heart beat is accelerated at first, but as poisoning deepens, it becomes slow (braydcardia), feeble and irregular. If bradycardia develops, atropine 1 mg subcutaneously is useful.

16. C. ***Additional facts:*** The idea of sweet poison sounds rather paradoxical, as poisons are commonly understood to be bitter or repulsive in taste. However some poisons have been described which have a somewhat sweetish taste. These are (i) Aconite (ii) Lead acetate (iii) Glycols (iv) Beryllium compounds (v) Methyl salicylate and (vi) Bromoform

($CHBr_3$). There is even one gaseous poison (N_2O) that is supposed to be sweetish in smell and taste. It is commonly known as laughing gas. Some people think that carbolic acid also has a sweetish tinge. Of these only Aconite is called *Meetha Zehar* or *Meetha Bish* in vernacular language (it literally translates in English as "sweet poison"). Lead Acetate is also called sugar of lead. There is evidence that it was used to sweeten wine in the Roman Empire! Akee – a poisonous fruit – has a somewhat "nutty" taste, which is not bad either.

The medicolegal significance of sweet poisons is that they are easier to administer with a homicidal intent.

17. **C.** Alternately contracting and dilating pupils are the classical finding in aconite poisoning. This feature, also known as hippus, is not seen in any other poisoning.

OLEANDER

18. **A.**

NICOTINE

19. **B.**

MISCELLANEOUS

20. **D.** ***Additional info:*** *Jaborandi* refers to a three to seven-metre-high shrubby tree with smooth grey bark, large leathery leaves and thick, small, reddish-purple flowers. The leaves contain an essential oil which gives off an aromatic balsam smell when they are crushed. *Jaborandi* is native to South and Central America and to the West Indies. Several Pilocarpus species are called *jaborandi* and used interchangeably in commerce and herbal medicine, including the main Brazilian species of commerce: *P. jaborandi*, and *P. microphyllus*, and the Paraguay species *P. pennatifolius*. All three tree species are very similar in appearance, chemical constituents and traditional herbal medicine uses. The word *jaborandi* comes from the Tupi Indian language meaning "one that causes slobbering". It does cause excessive salivation.

The active principle of *jaborandi* is pilocarpine.

21. **C.**

22. **B.** ***Additional info:*** Atropine sulfate 2 mg is given hypodermically as a physiological antidote. Stomach should be washed with potassium permanganate. Dehydration may be present due to excessive sweating etc. This may be treated by giving 5% glucose saline drip.

MULTIPLE ANSWER TYPE (PGI, CHANDIGARH PATTERN)

23. **A,B,C,D,E.** Most students know about just choices A and B, and would perhaps tick just these two. However all choices are correct. Vitamin B_{12a} is another name for Hydroxocobalamin. It loses a hydroxyl group and then binds a cyanyl group from the cyanide, forming cyanocobalamin (Vitamin B_{12}). It is thus a unique antidote, which converts a poison into a vitamin! However too much of it is produced, so it is excreted in the urine. Some of it releases the cyanide moiety back in the blood, but at a rate slow enough to be taken care of by normal detoxifying mechanisms of the body.

Remember that hydroxocobalamin is also one of the body's natural mechanism to detoxify cyanide.

Alpha-ketoglutaric acid is a very safe antidote for cyanide, because it binds to cyanide directly without the generation of methemoglobin.

Stroma free methemoglobin provides exogenous methemoglobin for combination with cyanide, without the need to produce it endogenously.

24. **A,B,C,E.** It is common knowledge that cytochrome oxidase is inhibited by CN. However cyanide inhibits many metalloenzymes (including several iron- and copper containing enzymes) because of its ability to form complexes with the metal portion of metalloenzymes. Except acetylcholinesterase, all the above named enzymes are inhibited by cyanide. However it is true that the interaction of cyanide and cytochrome oxidase is best understood currently, and also the major intracellular toxic mechanism in cyanide poisoning.

25. **C,E.** Amyl nitrite is used by inhalation and sodium nitrite is used intravenously. The aim is to produce about 20-30% methemoglobin.

26. **A,D,E.** ***Additional info: Jaborandi*** is *Pilocarpus microphyllus*, whose active principle is the alkaloid pilocarpine. Pilocarpine is a parasympathomimetic drug whose action is very similar to muscarine. Its main symptoms are flushing of the face, perspiration, salivation, lachrymation, excessive secretion of the mucus, contraction of the pupils, slowing of the heart and slow and irregular pulse.

46 Toxic Gases

1. **Burning of fire in a closed room may cause death because it produces:**
   A. Carbon dioxide
   B. Carbon monoxide
   C. Hydrogen sulphide
   D. Smoke

2. **At the following blood CO concentration, the clinical picture will stimulate alcoholic intoxication:**
   A. 10 %
   B. 30 %
   C. 50 %
   D. 70 %

3. **Dry ice is:**
   A. Solid carbon dioxide
   B. Solid carbon monoxide
   C. Ice with dissolved carbon dioxide
   D. Both (A) and (B)

4. **Canaries were once taken by coal miners with them to the mines because they are very sensitive to:**
   A. Carbon monoxide
   B. Methane
   C. Chlorine
   D. Both (A) and (B)

5. **Which toxic gas erupted from Lake Nyos in Nigeria on Aug 21, 1986, killing more than 1700 people and over 3000 cattle?**
   A. Hydrogen sulfide
   B. Carbon monoxide
   C. Chlorine
   D. Carbon dioxide

6. **Cherry red color of blood and tissues is characteristic of poisoning with:**
   A. Carbon monoxide
   B. Carbon dioxide
   C. Hydrogen sulfide
   D. All of the above

7. **Carbon monoxide is:**
   A. A dark red gas heavier than air
   B. A yellow irritant gas with a choking odor
   C. A colorless gas, heavier than air with a faint smell of decaying fish
   D. A colorless, odorless gas that is lighter than air

8. **The affinity of carbon monoxide for hemoglobin is:**
   A. 50 times greater than that of oxygen
   B. 250 times greater than that of oxygen
   C. 1000 times greater than that of oxygen
   D. 50 times lesser than that of oxygen

MULTIPLE ANSWER TYPE (PGI, CHANDIGARH PATTERN)

9. **Which of the following gases act as simple asphyxiants?**
   A. Argon
   B. Ammonia

C. Carbon monoxide
D. Ethane
E. Nitrogen

10. Sewer gas contains:
A. Phosgene
B. H_2S
C. CO_2
D. Methane
E. Phosphine

11. How does carbon monoxide bring about deleterious action on human beings?
A. It causes RBCs to lyse causing hemoglobinuria and kidney failure
B. It combines with cytochrome oxidase within the mitochondria, rendering them inactive
C. It combines with hemoglobin, effectively shutting off its function of oxygen transport
D. It destroys the surfactant of the lungs
E. It irritates the respiratory tract making it impossible to breathe

12. Carbon monoxide poisoning can occur in the following situations:
A. Inhalation of automobile exhaust
B. Mining accidents
C. Environmental degradation of carbon dioxide
D. Inhalation of smoke from a fire, especially when it is lit in confined spaces
E. Bursting of an air-conditioner

ANSWERS

1. B.
2. **B.** When carboxyhaemoglobin levels in blood are around 20%-30%, it is considered mild to moderate carbon monoxide poisoning. The symptoms are quite nonspecific and include headache, dizziness, weakness, nausea, dyspnoea, visual disturbances, irritability and lack of concentration. Physical findings are also non-specific and include tachycardia, tachypnoea, mild systolic hypotension, low grade fever, vomiting, and confusion. Most of these signs and symptoms are seen in acute alcoholic intoxication too. Indeed carbon monoxide poisoning at this concentration may be misdiagnosed as acute ethanol or methanol intoxication.

   Carbon monoxide poisoning at this concentration can also be misdiagnosed as (i) food poisoning (ii) hysteria (iii) acute delirium tremens (iv) migraine headache and (v) cerebral vascular disease.

   Between 40%-60%, there is weakness and inco-ordination of the limbs with mental confusion. The inco-ordination produced by CO is said to resemble that produced by alcoholic intoxication.

   Thus in fact between 30% and 60%, the victim may all along appear like an intoxicated person.
3. **A.** ***Related facts:*** Remember two more facts about dry ice, which may form the basis of other MCQs. Dry ice is whitish in color and it acts as a corrosive.
4. **D.** Canaries are small yellow songbirds, which are very sensitive to both carbon monoxide and methane. Since these gases can leak in mines and cause death in miners, they would take canaries with them as early warning signals. If canaries stopped singing or fell down in their cage, it would indicate that carbon monoxide or methane was leaking from somewhere and the miners would immediately come to the surface. The use of canaries in British mines was phased out as recently as 1986.

   Mice can also be used similarly as they too are very sensitive to these gases, but canaries are better indicators than mice.
5. **D.** Lake Nyos is one of only three lakes in the world known to be saturated with carbon dioxide - the others are Lake Manoun, also in Cameroon about 100km away, and Lake Kivu in Rwanda. Carbon dioxide naturally seeps from geothermal sources below these bodies of water and dissolves under pressure in the cold layers at the bottom of the lakes. In lake Nyos, an estimated 90 million kilograms of CO_2 seeps up through the lake bed annually, and gets dissolved in bottom layers of water. Lake Nyos is thermally stratified, with layers of warm, less dense water near the surface floating on the colder, denser water layers near the lake's bottom. Because of the pressure of tonnes of layers of water above it, water in the lower layers gets supersaturated with carbon dioxide.

   On August 21, 1986, a landslide, or perhaps a small volcanic eruption occurred on the bed of the lake, causing the lake to overturn. In effect the lower supersaturated layers of water came to the top; top layers going to the bottom in one big cataclysmic upheavel. Since the bottom layers were supersaturated with carbon dioxide, the sudden release of pressure, caused the gas to come out of solution. An estimated 1.6 million tonnes of CO_2 were released immediately. Since CO_2

is heavier than air, it kept close to the ground, rushing down two nearby valleys. It displaced all the atmospheric air and suffocated an estimated 1746 people and over 3000 cattle within 20 km of the lake. This has been one of the worst mass disaster caused by a toxic gas in recent times.

Earlier, on August 15, 1984, a similar sudden outgassing of CO_2 had occurred at Lake Manoun, killing 37 local residents.

6. **A.** It is due to the formation of carboxyhaemoglobin.

7. **D.**

8. **B.**

MULTIPLE ANSWER TYPE (PGI, CHANDIGARH PATTERN)

9. **A,D,E.** Toxic gases are divided into (i) simple asphyxiants (ii) systemic asphyxiants and (iii) respiratory irritants. **Simple asphyxiants** simply displace oxygen and kill by making it non-available to the victim. Examples are nitrogen, carbon dioxide, aliphatic hydrocarbon gases such as butane, methane and ethane and noble gases such as xenon, argon, neon etc. **Systemic asphyxiants** do displace oxygen, but that is not the primary mechanism by which they kill. The primary mechanism of producing death is by producing significant systemic toxicity. One of the best example is Carbon monoxide. Hydrocyanic gas is another example. Finally there are **respiratory irritants** which damage the respiratory tract and lungs by destroying the lining cells. Examples are chlorine, ammonia, formaldehyde, ozone, sulfur dioxide and heavy metal gases such as copper fumes, mercury vapor etc.

In the above question ammonia is a respiratory irritant and carbon monoxide is a systemic asphyxiant.

10. **B,C,D.** Sewer gas is a complex mixture of toxic and non-toxic gases that can be present at varying levels depending upon the source. It is formed during the decay of household and industrial waste. Highly toxic components of sewer gas include **hydrogen sulfide** and **ammonia.**

Sewer gas also contains **methane, carbon dioxide, sulfur dioxide**, and **nitrous oxides**. In addition, chlorine bleaches, industrial solvents, and gasoline are frequently present in municipal and privately owned-sewage treatment systems.

Sewer gas can enter a home through a floor drain, from a leaking or blocked plumbing roof vent, or (if the gases are in soil adjacent to the house) through cracks in foundations. Sanitary and farm workers can be exposed to sewer gas during the cleaning and maintenance of municipal sewers, manure storage tanks, and home septic tanks.

The principal risks and effects associated with exposure are (i) hydrogen sulfide poisoning (ii) asphyxiation (methane acts like carbon monoxide, blocking oxygen in the blood, and can similarly cause suffocation and death at high levels) and (iii) explosion and fire (methane and hydrogen sulfide are flammable and highly explosive).

11. **C.**

12. **A,B,D.**

47 War Gases and Chemical Warfare

1. **Mustard gas and lewisite are examples of:**
   A. Vesicant or blistering gases
   B. Asphyxiants
   C. Tear gases
   D. Sternutators

2. **Chemical name for mustard gas is:**
   A. Diphenylchlorarsine
   B. Chlorodiphydrophenarsazine
   C. Methyl isocyanate
   D. Dichlordiethyl sulphide

3. **Lewisite has an odor similar to that of:**
   A. Garlic
   B. Geranium
   C. Rotten eggs
   D. Bitter almonds

4. **Which of the following is also known as "Dew of Death"?**
   A. Hydrogen cyanide gas
   B. Methyl isocyanate
   C. Lewisite
   D. Sulfur mustard

5. **The best treatment for Lewisite would be:**
   A. EDTA
   B. Sodium formaldehyde sulfoxylate
   C. Physostigmine
   D. Dimercaprol

6. **Which of the following groups would phosgene and diphosgene best belong to?**
   A. Vesicants
   B. Lung damaging agents
   C. Nerve agents
   D. Vomiting agents

7. **The chemical formula of phosgene is:**
   A. $COCl_2$
   B. CNCl
   C. $CSCl_2$
   D. COHCl

8. **Main action of phosgene is on:**
   A. Liver
   B. Lung alveoli
   C. Heart
   D. Brain

9. **The odor of phosgene is that of:**
   A. Bitter almonds
   B. Pungent
   C. Newly mown hay or green corn
   D. Rotten eggs

10. **Sternutator is an agent that:**
    A. Causes heart failure
    B. Causes severe pulmonary edema
    C. Induces instantaneous paralysis
    D. Induces sneezing and often lacrimation and vomiting

11. **Death in phosgene poisoning is due to:**
    - **A.** Methemoglobinemia
    - **B.** Severe pulmonary edema
    - **C.** Paralysis
    - **D.** Acute glomerulonephritis

MULTIPLE ANSWER TYPE (PGI, CHANDIGARH PATTERN)

12. **Mustard gas is also called as:**
    - **A.** Yprite
    - **B.** Sulfur mustard
    - **C.** Brown bangles
    - **D.** Nitrogen mustard
    - **E.** Kampfstoff Lost

13. **Phosgene is also known as:**
    - **A.** Carbonic dichloride
    - **B.** Carbon hydrochloride
    - **C.** Carbon oxychloride
    - **D.** Green cross
    - **E.** Yellow cross

ANSWERS

1. A.
2. D. The chemical formula of mustard gas is Cl-CH_2-CH_2-S-CH_2-CH_2-Cl. Depending on how one reads it, it may be called Dichlor-diethyl sulphide, 1,1-thiobis(2-chloroethane) or Bis(2-chloroethyl) sulfide.
3. B. Geranium is a flower of the family *Geraniaceae*. It is a white, pink, or purple flower with elongated styles and glands that alternate with the petals. Lewisite is a rather fragrant compound having the fragrance of geranium blossoms.

   The chemical structure of Lewisite is shown below:

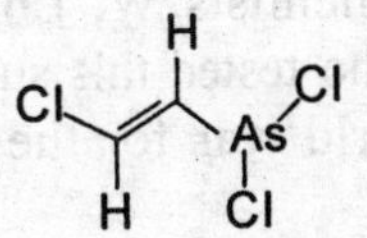

Fig. 47.1: Chemical structure of Lewisite

The chemical name for Lewisite is dichloro (2-chlorovinyl) arsine. Its molecular formula is $C_2H_2AsCl_3$. Industrially-produced Lewisite has a strong penetrating geranium odor, although the pure compound is odorless.

Lewisite was developed in 1918 by a team of Americans headed by Captain Winford Lee Lewis working at Catholic University in Washington DC, in retaliation for German gas attacks during World War I, but was never actually used. It was in the process of manufacture when the armistice was signed. After World War I, the US became interested in Lewisite because it was not flamable. Thus, the US created a large stockpile of the substance. Production also took place in Great Britain, France, Italy, the Soviet Union, and Japan in the immediate post war years.

Fears that Lewisite might be used during the World War II prompted scientists to develop an antidote to it. That antidote is now known as British Anti-Lewisite (BAL), which is widely used for arsenic and several other heavy metal poisonings.

After BAL was discovered, it rendered Lewisite obsolete. The US had no option but to discard its stocks. It neutralized its stockpile (of Lewisite) with bleach and dumped it into the Gulf of Mexico.

4. C.
5. D. Dimercaprol is another name for BAL or British Anti-Lewisite. It is the best treatment for Lewisite, as the name itself would suggest.
6. B.
7. A.
8. B. ***Additional info:*** Damage caused by phosgene is due to the presence of a highly reactive carbonyl group (CO) attached to 2 chloride atoms. The gas dissolves slowly in water. This slow dissolution allows phosgene to enter the pulmonary system without significant damage to the upper airways. However, in the lower airways and alveoli, it combines with water (in the alveoli) to form carbon dioxide and hydrochloric acid.

$$COCl_2 + H_2O \rightarrow CO_2 + 2HCl$$

The HCl sets up intense tissue necrosis and inflammation. After the first few hours of exposure, there is leakage of serum into the alveolar septa. The tissue fills with fluid, causing hypoxia and apnea. Massive amounts of fluid (up to 1 L/h) leak out of the circulation, leading to a noncardiogenic pulmonary edema, with associated hypoxemia and volume depletion.

9. C.

10. **D.** Sternutator is a substance that primarily causes sneezing. The word comes from Latin *sternutare*, to sneeze. Diphenylaminechlorarsine, diphenylchlorarsine, and diphenylcyanarsine are some examples of sternutators. Although sternutators are primarily sneezing agents, they also induce lacrimation, nausea and vomiting. Indeed sometimes sternutators are called 'vomiting agents'.

Additional info: Sternutators are agents used in warfare or riot control.

There are a number of chemical agents used in warfare or riot control. On the basis of their physiologic action, these chemical agents have been classified in five groups as follows:

1. Vesicants (blister gases), which include mustard gas, lewisite, ethyldichlorarsine, and phenyldichlorarsine.
2. Lung irritants (choking gases), which include phosgene, chloropierin, and chorine.
3. Sternutators (sneezing gases), which include diphenylaminechlorarsine, diphenylchlorarsine, and diphenylcyanarsine.
4. Systemic poisons (blood and nerve poisons), which include hydrocyanic acid, cyanogen chloride, and arsine.
5. Lacrimators (tear gases), which include chloracetophenone, chloracetophenone solutions, and brombenzylcyanide.

11. B.

MULTIPLE ANSWER TYPE (PGI, CHANDIGARH PATTERN)

12. **A,B,E.** ***Additional info*:** Mustard gas is a war gas. It was its earlier name. Currently it is more often known as sulfur mustard. The chemical formula of mustard gas is:

$$Cl\text{-}CH_2\text{-}CH_2\text{-}S\text{-}CH_2\text{-}CH_2\text{-}Cl.$$

Its other names include yellow cross, H, HD, yprite, sulfur mustard and Kampfstoff Lost, but the name mustard gas came to be more widely used, because the impure "agent quality" is said to have an odour similar to that of mustard, garlic or horseradish. When pure, it is in fact both odourless and colourless.

"H" refers to undistilled or raw sulfur mustard, which contains a large fraction of impurities. "HD" refers to a distilled or purified form of sulfur mustard.

The name Yprite comes from the fact that it was first used near Ypres in Flanders on 12th July 1917, during the first World War (WW1). It has been used in war as late as the Iran-Iraq War in 1980–1988. "Kampfstoff" means "battle substance" in German. "Lost" comes from the family names of the (German) chemists W. Lommel and W. Steinkopf who tested this substance during the first world war for the usefulness as weapon.

Nitrogen mustard (Also known sometimes as "HN") is *not* a synonym of mustard gas. It is a derivative of sulfur mustard. The only difference in the chemical formula is that the S atom (of sulfur mustard) is replaced by an N atom. Far from being used as a war gas, nitrogen mustard is actually used therapeutically as a cure for Hodgkin's Disease. Nitrogen mustard and Lewisite are related to mustard gas, and hence are known as mustard agents.

The effects of mustard gas exposure include the reddening and blistering of skin, and, if inhaled, will also cause blistering to the lining of the lungs, causing chronic impairment, or at worst, death. Exposure to high concentrations will attack the corneas of the eyes, eventually rendering the victim blind.

Mustard gas is a particularly deadly and debilitating poison, but its real danger when it was first used in WW1, compared to other chemical warfare agents at the time, was the fact that it could penetrate all protective materials and masks that were available at the time. In fact during World War I, it was Phosgene or Carbonyl Chloride ($COCl_2$) which was initially used in combination with chlorine gas for combat purposes by the German army. However the German army had to switch over to mustard gas in 1917 because of the development of effective gas masks. Phosgene could not penetrate these gas masks (making phosgene almost useless as a war gas), while mustard gas could.

One of the reasons that exposure to mustard gas must be prevented, rather than cured, is that detoxification is quite difficult due to its insolubility.

13. A,C,D. Synonyms for phosgene include carbonic dichloride, carbon oxychloride, carbonyl dichloride, chloroformyl chloride, d-stoff, and green cross. Yellow cross is the name given to mustard gas.

Additional info: Crosses were actually code names given to chemical agents used in World War I by the Germans. The Germans marked these agents by colored crosses on artillery rounds to identify them easily. This gave rise to their current popular names. Four colored crosses were used by the Germans: white, blue, green and yellow. Interestingly the color of the cross could indicate which organ would be affected most by that agent.

1. **White Cross** (*Weisskreuz* in German). These were irritants affecting the eyes and other moist tissues. Examples — Bromoacetone, Chloroacetone.
2. **Blue Cross** (*Blaukreuz* in German). These affected the upper respiratory tract. Examples — Diphenyl chloroarsine, Ethyl dichloroarsine.
3. **Green Cross** (*Grünkreuz* in German). These affected the lungs. Examples— Chloropicrin, Phosgene.
4. **Yellow Cross** (*Gelbkreuz* in German). These attacked any exposed surfaces. Examples — Mustard gas.

48 Miscellaneous Poisons

1. **Absorption of ingested kerosene can be slowed by giving:**
   A. Sodium edetate
   B. Activated charcoal
   C. Magnesium sulphate
   D. Plain water
   E. Liquid paraffin
2. **Which of the following can cause harm by acting as mechanical irritants?**
   A. Diamond powder
   B. Powdered glass
   C. Pins and needles
   D. All of the above
3. **Which one of the following poisonings is the most common among the toddlers in India?**
   A. Sodium hydroxide poisoning
   B. Kerosene poisoning
   C. Insecticide poisoning
   D. Mercury poisoning
   E. Nicotine poisoning
4. **Causes of methemoglobinaemia are all *except*:**
   A. Nitrites
   B. Phenacetin
   C. Sulfonamides
   D. Phenytoin
5. **Which of the following chemicals is the main ingredient of "smelling salts"?**
   A. Ammonia
   B. Carbolic acid
   C. Chlorine
   D. Zyklon B
6. **Which of the following is a non irritant gas with systemic toxicity?**
   A. Nitrogen
   B. Carbon monoxide
   C. Ammonia
   D. Chlorine
7. **Which of the following acids is also known as prussic acid?**
   A. Acetic acid
   B. Oxalic acid
   C. Hydrocyanic acid
   D. Nitric acid
8. **Ergot of rye or sclerotium is associated with which of the following poisonous species?**
   A. Ricinus communis
   B. Croton tiglium
   C. *Claviceps purpurea*
   D. Plumbage rosea

9. Linseeds used for cattle/animal feeding can cause accidental poisoning with which of the following poisons?

A. Aconitine
B. Hydrocyanic acid
C. Pilocarpine
D. Atropine

10. Holy Fire or St. Anthony's fire is a syndrome seen in chronic poisoning with:

A. Semecarpus anacardium
B. Abrus precatorius
C. Plumbago Zeylanica
D. *Claviceps purpurea*

11. Sodium nitroprusside is useful in poisoning with:

A. Claviceps purpurea
B. Copper
C. Arsenic
D. Organophosphorus

12. Which important drug of abuse can be synthesized from the poisonous species *Claviceps purpurea*?

A. Heroin
B. THC
C. Cocaine
D. LSD

13. Cage test is used in:

A. Alcohol poisoning
B. Opiate poisoning
C. Datura poisoning
D. Cannabis poisoning

MULTIPLE ANSWER TYPE (PGI, CHANDIGARH PATTERN)

14. The following facts are correct about mechanical irritants:

A. They are quickly absorbed from the stomach mucosa
B. They only have local action
C. They cause irritation of GIT
D. They are most commonly used as homicidal poisons
E. They cause instantaneous death

15. Contents of Brompton's cocktail are:

A. Cocaine
B. Morphine
C. Chlorpromazine
D. *Datura*
E. Alcohol

16. Widmark formula is used for which of the following poisons?

A. Barbiturates
B. Alcohol
C. Dhatura
D. Organophosphorus
E. Aluminum phosphide

17. In which of the following poisonings, erethism is seen?

A. Aconite
B. Sulphuric acid
C. Ratti
D. Claviceps purpurea
E. Mercury

ANSWERS

1. E.

2. D.

3. B.

4. D. ***Related fact:*** The full list of drugs/ chemicals which cause methemoglobinaemia is:

   (A) MEDICATIONS

   i. Amyl nitrite
   ii. Benzocaine
   iii. Dapsone
   iv. Lidocaine
   v. Nitroglycerine
   vi. Nitroprusside
   vii. Phenacetin [Acetaminophen (Paracetamol, Tylenol) is the active metabolite of Phenacetin]
   viii. Phenazopyridine
   ix. Prilocaine (local anaesthetic)
   x. Quinones (e.g. Chloroquine, primaquine)
   xi. Sulfonamides (e.g. sulfanilamide, sulfathiazide, sulfapyridine, sulfamethoxazole)

   (B) CHEMICAL AGENTS

   i. Aniline dye derivates (e.g. shoe dyes, marking inks)
   ii. Butyl nitrite
   iii. Chlorobenzene
   iv. Fires (heat induced denaturation)
   v. Isobutyl nitrite
   vi. Food adulterated with nitrites
   vii. Food high in nitrates
   viii. Naphthalene
   ix. Nitrophenol
   x. Nitrous gases (seen in arc welders)
   xi. Silver nitrate
   xii. Trinitrotoluene
   xiii. Well water (nitrates. Well water can get contaminated by nitrogenous fertilizers, animal organic waste, or seepage from septic tanks).

   Hint: Methemoglobin is an oxidation product of Hemoglobin. So watch out for **oxidising agents**.

5. A.

6. B.

7. C. ***Additional info:*** Prussic acid is an old name for Hydrocyanic acid (HCN). It is so called since it was first obtained in 1783 by the Swedish chemist Karl Wilhelm Scheele (1742-1786), by heating Prussian blue (Potassium ferric hexacyanoferrate) with sulphuric acid.

> Prussian blue, the English translation of French *bleu de Preusse,* is so called in allusion to its blue color and its accidental discovery by Diesbach in 1704 in Berlin, capital of Prussia. [Incidentally Diesbach was a colourmaker, and he was trying to make a red, not a blue. He got a blue, because one of the chemicals he was using was contaminated. This accident gave the world its first modern synthetic color!].
>
> Prussia, former principal state of Germany got its name from Prussians, who dwelt on south-east coast of *Baltic sea.* Their name derives from Lithuanian *prud* meaning pond or lake, alluding to the Baltic sea.

Hydrogen cyanide (H-C ≡ N) is a colorless, very poisonous, and highly volatile liquid that boils slightly above room temperature at 26°C, thereby generating hydrogen cyanide gas.

In its gaseous state, H-C ≡ N is referred to as hydrogen cyanide; in its liquid form it is called prussic acid or hydrocyanic acid. A solution of hydrogen cyanide in water is also referred to as hydrocyanic acid or prussic acid.

8. C. ***Additional info:*** *Claviceps purpurea* is a fungus which is very commonly seen in the grain-fields, especially during the moist, warm weather. Though the fungus affects all cereals, rye is most commonly affected. Its spores are carried by the wind or by insects to the young ovaries of the rye. Within the ovary the spores germinate into hyphal filaments which secrete a ferment and so penetrate the basal portion of the ovary. The tissue of the grain is decomposed by the ferment, leading to the formation of a yellow, viscid substance called honeydew. This attracts insects which in turn spread the fungus to other spikes of rye. The hyphal filaments penetrate deeper into the ovary and the latter disappears, eventually to be replaced by a hardened, curved purple body called the *sclerotium* or *ergot of rye*. The name ergot comes from the old French *argot* meaning 'a cock's spur'. These curved grains resemble the cock's spur and hence the name. An old name for ergot was 'spurred rye'.

9. B. ***Related facts:*** Many plants contain cyanogenetic (or cyanophoric) glycosides, which can yield HCN in the GIT of humans and animals under proper conditions. These plants contain both the cyanogenetic glycoside as well as an enzyme (emulsin), which can convert the glycoside to HCN. However it needs water for conversion, which is present in the stomach. Presence of acids can enhance the reaction (for detailed reaction please see chapter 50). There are other conditions too, when HCN can be produced from these plants. For instance, when plant cells are damaged by wilting, frosting or stunting, the glycoside degrades to form free HCN. HCN poisoning can be a lethal problem for cattle grazing sorghums or other cyanogenetic plants. Some conditions can favor excessive accumulation of these cyanogenetic glycosides. These are conditions of stress such as drought, excessive soil nitrogen, young plants, periods of rapid growth followed by cool, cloudy weather and lush regrowth after cutting for hay, grazing or frost.

Table 48.1 gives details of main cyanogenetic glycosides, their main sources and other necessary details. Note that *Kadwi juar* also produces a cyanogenetic glycoside. This may be mentioned in the question sometimes (instead of linseed as in the current question).

Also note that the botanical name of bitter almond is *Prunus amygdalus amara*. *Prunus amygdalus* produces two varieties, *Prunus amygdalus dulcis*—often with white flowers (normal sweet fragrant almond) and *Prunus amygdalus amara*— often with pink flowers (bitter almond). Cyanogenetic glycoside is present only in the latter variety ***(See Table 48.1 on Next page).***

10. D ***Additional info:*** 'St. Anthony's fire' or ergotism is caused by eating of diseased food grains (usually rye) infected with the fungus *Claviceps purpurea*. In the Middle Ages many poor peasants were forced to eat these grains because of poverty. The victims suffered from acute pain in the limbs and sometimes convulsions. This began by their limbs feeling as if on fire, before turning black like charcoal and falling off. Many a helpless peasant became a victim and suffered a loss of all the four limbs.

It is now known that this disease was caused by the presence of toxic chemicals ergotamine and ergotoxin in the ergot. They are potent constrictors of smooth muscle, causing blood vessels to contract, resulting in gangrene. In ancient times, of course, it was thought that the blackening was due to an invisible fire. A pilgrimage to the shrine of

Table 48.1: Main cyanogenetic glycosides, their main sources, and other relevant data

S.No.	Glycoside	Main source (Botanical name)	Common name	Family	Chemical name
1.	Amygdalin	*Prunus amygdalus amara*	*Bitter Almond*	Rosaceae (rose family)	D(-)-Mandelonitrile-gentiobioside
2.	Dhurrin	*Sorghum vulgare*	*Kadwi Juar, Sudan grass*	Gramineae	β-Glucoside of p-hydroxymandelonitrile
3.	Hydrangin	*Hydrangea macrophylla*	*Bigleaf Hydrangea, Wild hydrangea, Seven Barks*	Saxifragaceae	7-Hydroxycoumarin (7-Hydroxy-2H-1-benzopyran-2-one)
4.	Linamarin	*Linum usitatissimum*	*Linseed (alsi, also known as Flax)*	Linaceae	Acetone-cyanohydrin-glucoside
5.	Manihotoxin	*Manihot utilissima*	*Bitter cassava*	Euphorbiaceae	When isolated, given the name Manihotoxin, but now found identical with linamarin (q.v.)
6.	Phaseolunatin	*Phaseolus lunatus*	*Lima Bean, Sieva Been, Butter Bean*	Leguminosae	When isolated, given the name Phaseolunatin, but now found identical with linamarin (q.v.)
7.	Prulaurasin	*Prunus laurocerasus*	*Cherry laurel*	Rosaceae	DL-Mandelonitrile-D-glucoside
8.	Prunasin	*Prunus serotina*	*Black cherry*	Rosaceae	D(-)-Mandelonitrile-D-glucoside
9.	Sambunigrin	*Sambucus canadensis*	*Elderberry*	Caprifoliaceae	L(+)-Mandelonitrile-D-glucoside
10.	Taxiphyllin	*Henriettella fascicularis*	*None*	Melastomataceae	(2*R*)-α-β-D-Glucopyranosyloxy)-4-hydroxybenzeneacetonitrile ($C_{14}H_{17}NO_7.2H_2O$)
11.	Vicianin	*Vicia angustifolia*	*Common Vetch*	Leguminosae	Mandelonitrile-vicianoside

St. Anthony was believed to bring relief and hence the name 'St. Anthony's fire'.

11. **A.** ***Related fact:*** *Claviceps purpurea* has potent vasoconstrictors such as ergotamine, ergonovine and ergometrine, which can cause hypertension or ischaemia to important organs (e.g. brain and heart). Sodium nitroprusside is a potent vasodilator, quite useful in poisoning caused by *Claviceps purpurea*.

12. **D.** ***Additional info:*** LSD was in fact synthesized accidentally by Dr Albert Hofmann, trying to improve upon various ergot alkaloids, so they could have more desirable pharmacological properties.

13. **A.** A physician who suspects alcohol abuse or dependency have a number of short screening tests available, which a person can take even on his or her own. Because people with alcoholism often deny their problem or otherwise attempt to hide it, the tests are designed to elicit answers related to problems associated with drinking rather than the amount of liquor consumed or other specific drinking habits.

Four questions are asked in CAGE test:

- Have you ever felt you should **C**ut down on your drinking?
- Have people **A**nnoyed you by criticizing your drinking?
- Have you ever felt bad or **G**uilty about your drinking?
- Have you ever had a drink first thing in the morning to steady your nerves or to get rid of a hangover (**E**ye opener)?

Note the bold letters after which the test CAGE is named.

Item responses on the CAGE are scored 0 (negative) or 1 (affirmative), with an affirmative score an indication of alcohol problems. A total score of 2 or greater is considered clinically significant.

Developed by Dr. John Ewing, founding Director of the Bowles Center for Alcohol Studies, University of North Carolina at Chapel Hill, CAGE is an internationally used assessment instrument for identifying alcoholics. It is particularly popular with primary care givers. CAGE has been translated into several languages.

Another test for alcoholism is the T-ACE Test:

T-ACE Test. The T-ACE test is a four-question test that appears to be quite accurate in identifying alcoholism in both men and women. It asks the following questions:

- Does it TAKE (T) more than three drinks to make you feel high?
- Have you ever been ANNOYED (A) by people's criticism of your drinking?
- Are you trying to CUT DOWN (C) on drinking?
- Have you ever used alcohol as an EYE OPENER (E) in the morning?

A positive response to two of these four questions is considered to indicate possible alcohol abuse or dependence.

Other tests are (i) Self-Administered Alcoholism Screening Test (SAAST) (ii) Alcohol Use Disorders Identification Test (AUDIT Test), Michigan Alcoholism Screening Test (MAST) and The Alcohol Dependence Scale (ADS). The details of these tests are beyond the scope of this book.

MULTIPLE ANSWER TYPE (PGI, CHANDIGARH PATTERN)

14. B,C. Mechanical irritants are NOT absorbed from the body.

15. A,B,C,E. Brompton's cocktail is a liquid "cocktail" of morphine (or heroin), cocaine, alcohol (and sometimes other central nervous system depressants), chlorpromazine and flavoring, which probably takes its name from Brompton hospital. It is sometimes provided to patients suffering from pain associated with terminal illness such as cancers.

16. B. For more info on this question, please see Chapter 41 (Inebriant Poisons).

17. E. ***Related facts:*** The word comes from Greek *erethismos*, meaning "irritation". Erethism is seen in chronic mercury poisoning (e.g. in workers in mirror industries). It involves severe mental symptoms occurring in such chronically poisoned patients. There is excessive irritability and sensitiveness, the patient is easily upset, dislikes being watched at work, loses his temper and self control; depression, loss of memory and insomnia many follow. Hallucinations, delusions and mania may occur rarely.

The term was used by John Pearson in 1805 to encompass all manifestations of mercury poisoning. However with the passage of time the term came to be used only for mental symptoms.

49 Drug Dependence and Drug Habituation

1. **Which of the following best defines a drug?**
   A. It is a chemical which can cure a disease
   B. It is a tablet, capsule or syrup that can be bought from the market at a doctor's prescription
   C. It is the name given to any chemical that is ingested by humans
   D. It is any substance other than those required for the maintenance of normal health, that when taken into the living organism may modify one or more of its functions

2. **Which of the following terms best describes a state of periodic or chronic intoxication produced by the repeated consumption of a drug, which is harmful to the individual and to the society?**
   A. Drug habituation
   B. Drug addiction
   C. Drug overdose
   D. Drug abuse

3. **Drug dependence is a term which:**
   A. Includes drug addiction but excludes drug habituation
   B. Includes drug abuse but excludes substance abuse
   C. Includes both drug addiction and drug habituation
   D. Includes drug addiction but excludes drug abuse

4. **The most important qualifying characteristic of drug addiction is:**
   A. There are both physical and psychological dependence
   B. There is physical dependence only
   C. There is psychological dependence only
   D. There is a mere desire to take the drug, but no compulsion

5. **All are adulterants of heroin *except*:**
   A. Chalk powder
   B. Quinine
   C. Charcoal
   D. Fructose

6. **Drug abuser's elbow is the name given to:**
   A. Abrasion of elbows caused by repeated falls
   B. Myositis ossificans developing in drug abusers
   C. Lacerations around elbows due to frequent scuffles in drug abusers
   D. Drug induced arthritis

7. **The term "liquid gold" refers to:**
   A. Urine of a jaundiced patient
   B. Inhalational hydrocarbons which can only be bought by addicts at very high cost in the black market

C. Urine of a person who has ingested yellow sulfide of arsenic
D. Urine of amphetamine abuser

8. "Speed" is the common slang name for which of the following?
A. Amphetamine
B. Morphine
C. Cocaine
D. Ketamine

9. There is a narcotic abuse case with jet black tongue. The cause is:
A. Cocaine poisoning
B. Morphine poisoning
C. Cannabis toxicity
D. LSD poisoning

10. Heroin is the same thing as:
A. Butarphanol
B. Diacetylmorphine
C. Dextromethorphan
D. Codeine

11. Magnan's sign or symptom refers to:
A. Nasal septum perforation in chronic cocaine abuse
B. Pupillary constriction in acute heroin overdose
C. Tactile hallucinations in chronic cocaine abuse
D. Whole body orgasm, often encountered in "crack" abuse

12. "Crack" cocaine refers to:
A. Cocaine hydrochloride
B. Cocaine sulfate
C. Pure cocaine alkaloid
D. Procaine

13. Which of the following is considered an antidote for cocaine poisoning?
A. Benzoylecgonine
B. Diazepam
C. Ethyl alcohol
D. Nitric oxide

14. Cocaine produces its euphoriant effect by:
A. Increasing reuptake of dopamine, serotonin and norepinephrine
B. Blocking reuptake of dopamine, serotonin and norepinephrine
C. Causing increased firing of GABAergic neurons
D. Blocking GABAergic neurons

15. Formication is most typically seen in:
A. Chronic cocaine abuse
B. Mercuric chloride poisoning
C. Amphetamine overdose
D. Mushroom poisoning

16. Perforation of the nasal septum may most commonly be seen in:
A. Amphetamine abuse
B. Cocaine abuse
C. LSD misuse
D. Hallucinogenic mushroom poisoning

17. Which of the following may lead to body packer syndrome?
A. The practice of applying packs of drugs around upper arms so the drugs of abuse could transfuse slowly to give a constant high without fear of detection by the police
B. Many drug addicts packing themselves in a closed room and then smoking drugs of abuse, so they could benefit from drug laden fumes exhaled by their fellow addicts
C. Packing drugs of abuse in household pets and transporting them across nations for the purpose of smuggling
D. Smuggling illicit drugs by ingesting condoms or plastic bags packed with the drug

18. The term "mainlining" refers to:
A. Drug addict getting high and falling into a gutter accidentally asphyxiating himself

B. Pushing the drug directly into a vein
C. Withdrawal symptoms caused when the addict is off the drug
D. Stealing in order to buy illicit drugs

MULTIPLE ANSWER TYPE (PGI, CHANDIGARH PATTERN)

19. The following are common adulterants for drugs of addiction:
A. Gold chloride
B. Lactose
C. Sucrose
D. Potassium cyanide
E. Cantharides

20. Which of the following facts are correct about cotton fever?
A. It is caused by ingesting cotton which is common in drug addicts
B. It is a febrile condition due to inadvertent injection of cotton fibres in their veins by drug addicts
C. It is the name given to a fictitious fever which drug abusers use to get leave
D. It is caused by a bacteria *Enterobacter agglomerans* which thrives in cotton fibres
E. It is the name given to the habit of exchanging drugs among drug pushers, because these drugs are hidden in cotton

ANSWERS

1. D.
2. B.
3. C.
4. A.
5. C. Heroin is a white powder, and the best adulterant for it would be a white colored compound. Charcoal is a black colored substance and obviously can not be used to adulterate heroin.
6. B. Drug abuser's elbow or myositis ossificans is caused by repeated, inept needle punctures; the muscle around the elbow is replaced with scar tissue or with a calcific mass (extraosseous metaplasia).
7. D. ***Explanations and further information:*** Traditionally eastern Siberians would ingest hallucinogenic mushrooms (fly agaric) and would then collect their urine. The urine sometimes still warm, was drunk by those desiring a repeat drug effect. This is an early example of recycling of drugs.

   Some modern users of amphetamines do the same. The logic is that 40% of amphetamine is excreted unchanged in the urine, coupled with the fact that some users have an enormous tolerance of up to 1000 – 2000 mg / day. Thus a person taking 2000 mg a day would be excreting almost 800 mg of amphetamine unchanged in his urine. Theoretically speaking if someone drank this urine, he could get another "kick". To make use of this fact, this urine is collected and sold in vials of yellow fluid called LIQUID GOLD. The reasons for calling it "liquid gold" are (i) it is liquid in state (ii) it is golden yellow in color (in fact all concentrated urine is) (iii) it is sold at very high cost, thus alluding to the price of gold.

   This question is often wrongly asked as follows:

   Urine appears 'Liquid Gold' in which poisoning?

   (a) Heavy metals (b) Barbiturates (c) Organophosphorus (d) Amphetamine.

   The intended answer of course is (d). But this is not a correctly asked question.
8. A.
9. A. ***Related facts:*** The tongue and teeth of the habitual cocaine eater in India are jet black, probably due to the chemical change brought about by lime and saliva acting upon cocaine. This is however a highly controversial feature.
10. B.
11. C. ***Related facts:*** In chronic cocaine abuse, the patient gets a crawling, illusory sensation of a foreign body under the skin. Often he feels that some bugs are crawling under his skin. These are referred to as "cocaine bugs". The patient scratches his skin as a result, causing irregular scratches, excoriation and ulcers. This sign was first described by the French psychiatrist Valentin Jacques Joseph Magnan (1835-1916).
12. C. ***Related facts:*** A coca leaf typically contains less than 2% cocaine. If chewed in such form, it rarely presents the user with any social or medical problems.

    Cocaine sulfate is produced by macerating coca leaves along with water that has been acidulated with sulfuric acid. This is often accomplished by putting the ingredients into a vat and stamping on it, in a manner not dissimilar to the traditional method for crushing grapes. After the cocaine is extracted, the water is evaporated to yield a pastey mass of impure cocaine sulfate (Fig. 49.1).

Cocaine sulfate is an intermediate step to producing cocaine hydrochloride. In South America it (Cocaine sulfate) is commonly smoked along with tobacco, and is known as *pasta, basuco, basa, pitillo*, or simply *paste*. This coca paste is estimated to contain between 20%-85% cocaine sulfate.

Cocaine is however most often used in the form of the salt, cocaine hydrochloride, which is produced by reacting cocaine paste with hydrochloric acid. Cocaine hydrochloride is estimated to contain 90% cocaine. Cocaine hydrochloride is mostly snorted (absorption occurs through nasal mucus membrane) or injected.

Snorting cocaine hydrochloride is considered rather old-fashioned now among users, because it does not give a very strong "high". Normally, only the intravenous route of administration could be expected to deliver the more potent and rapid hit they have been seeking. Yet there are very strong cultural prejudices against injecting recreational drugs. So a smokeable form of cocaine was developed. Smokeable form of cocaine gives a "better" high for two reasons (i) cocaine tends to constrict the capillaries of nasal septum but not those of lungs, so absorption is better and quicker through lungs (ii) from the lungs the drug goes to the left heart and from there directly to the brain; the drug thus reaches the brain immediately and without being diluted by systemic blood.

Cocaine hydrochloride itself can not be smoked since it decomposes at the temperature required to vaporise it. Pure cocaine in alkaloidal form ("free base") however has a much lower vaporising point. Thus cocaine hydrochloride must be converted to pure cocaine. Initially, "free-base" cocaine was typically produced using volatile solvents, usually ether. Unfortunately, this technique is physically dangerous. The solvent tends to ignite. Hence a more convenient method of producing smokeable free-base became popular. Its product is "crack". To obtain crack-cocaine, ordinary cocaine hydrochloride is concentrated by heating the drug in a solution of baking soda until the water evaporates. This type of base-cocaine makes a cracking sound when heated; hence the name "crack". Since base-cocaine vaporises at a low temperature, it can be easily inhaled via a heated pipe.

13. **B.** ***Related facts:*** Diazepam is effective in controlling agitation, CNS stimulation and convulsions often seen in cocaine poisoning.

14. **B.** Increased concentrations of certain amines, especially serotonin (5HT), at neuronal junctions in the brain has been found to be associated with mood elevation. There is an automatic mechanism in the brain

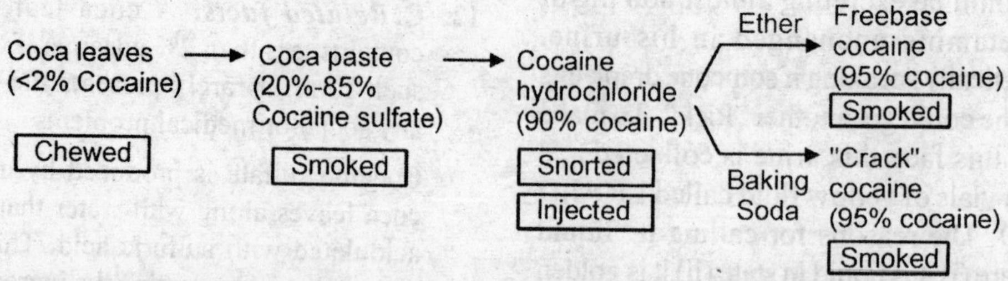

Fig. 49.1: Various forms of cocaine, their manufacture and concentrations and how they are used by addicts

whereby as soon as these amines are released at nerve terminals they are absorbed back (reuptaken, so they could be used again). Agents which block this reuptake are associated with elevation of mood, and are used clinically as antidepressants. These are known as Selective Serotonin Reuptake Inhibitors or SSRIs (e.g. fluoxetine, sertraline, citalopram, paroxetine). Cocaine blocks the reuptake of not only serotonin but also dopamine and norepinephrine.

15. A. ***Related facts:*** Formication (from Latin *formica*, "ant". Interestingly formic acid is so called, because it was first obtained by distilling red ants!) is the hallucination that ants or other insects are creeping on or under the skin. Formication is a feature of some psychotic states as well as drug abuse – most notably cocaine.

> The term must not be confused with "fornication" (note that just one letter is different in this word – "n" in place of "m"), which is also of interest to forensic personnel. Fornication is sexual intercourse that is "illicit" or outside of marriage. The term "fornication" has a close medical relative by the name of "fornix", the word for "arch" in Latin (There are fornices of the conjunctiva as well as vagina, which are anatomically arched structures. In addition, a fibrous tract underneath the corpus callosum is also called fornix for the same reason). In ancient times Roman prostitutes used to hang out under the arches of certain public buildings in order to solicit customers. The act of carrying on an illicit relationship consequently came to be called "going under the arches" or fornication.

Variant: This question has been asked in this variation too→Magnan's symptom is (a) Illusion (b) Delusion (c) Auditory hallucination (d) Formication. The answer is (d) Formication.

16. B. ***Related facts:*** This is because cocaine is frequently taken via nasal route. Cocaine constricts the capillaries of the nasal septum, which in turn may cause perforation in the long run. Another frequently asked related question is about preservation of nasal swabs in cocaine abuse (see chapter 50 for this question).

17. D. Body packer syndrome is the name given to a dangerous and life threatening illness developing in persons who have ingested dangerous amounts of illicit drugs to illegally transport them across nations. This remarkably innovative way of smuggling drugs across nations involves several steps:

i. First the drugs are packed in condoms (usually, but other suitable rubber or polythene containers may be used as well) and tightly sealed.

ii. The person volunteering to smuggle drugs swallows these condoms. Each condom typically contains about 8 to 10 g of drug and it is usual to ingest about 50-100 such packets (although cases of persons carrying more than 200 packets are known). Thus a total of about 1 kg of drug is transported in one instance. Usually the person also takes a constipating agent such as diphenoxylate or loperamide, so he does not feel the need to move his bowels while in transit.

iii. This person flies to the country of destination. He can obviously pass through the customs easily as the drug is within his GIT. Such persons are usually known as body packers. They are also known as "mules", "swallowers", "internal carriers", or "couriers".

iv. On reaching the country of destination, the body packer takes laxatives, cathartics, or enemas to defecate. Defecation is done in a special pan. Body packers know the number of packets they have ingested, and they count them during defecation in order to determine when passage is complete. The packer recovers all condoms, washes them and delivers them to the drug mafia. These body packers reportedly receive several thousand dollars per trip.

v. Occasionally the condoms burst within the GIT while the body packer is in transit (generally the packets tend to leak before they rupture). This suddenly releases great amounts of drug within his system threatening his life. This is known as body packer syndrome. The practice of transporting drugs in this novel manner is known as body packing or body stuffing.

vi. The symptoms would generally give away the drug the body packer was carrying. Heroin overdose causes sedation, miosis, and diminished bowel sounds followed by the onset of lethal respiratory depression. Cocaine overdose causes anxiety, dilated pupils, diaphoresis, tachycardia, and hypertension, followed by hyperthermia, seizures, and cardiovascular collapse. Other drugs also give rise to symptoms typical of them.

Some other facts about body packing or body stuffing, which may help in solving related MCQs are:

- The phenomenon of body packing was first described in 1973 in Toronto, Canada, although anecdotal reports suggest that at the time, the practice had been in vogue for at least a decade.
- In the 1973 case, the mule had swallowed a condom filled with hashish, and he was caught because a small-bowel obstruction had developed. The condom was surgically removed, and the body packer recovered uneventfully.
- Drugs commonly transported by mules include cocaine, heroin, amphetamines, 3,4-methylenedioxymethamphetamine ("ecstasy"), marijuana and hashish. Cases are known where more than one type of drugs are transported.
- Pediatric body packers (children as young as 12 years of age) and pregnant body packers are known. Some packers are known to stuff the drug inside their rectum. Females sometimes stuff the drug in their vaginal tract too.
- Body packers are generally caught for one of three reasons (i) leaking/bursting of condoms and consequent drug-induced toxic effects (ii) intestinal obstruction (iii) medical assessment of the body packer after he was arrested for some other reason.
- The abdominal examination may reveal distention or palpable packets. Gentle rectal and vaginal examinations may also disclose packets. The rest of the physical examination is generally not helpful.
- Helpful special investigations include plain abdominal radiography, computed tomography, contrast-enhanced abdominal radiography and ultrasonography. Urine toxicology testing as an initial screening tool is generally not useful. An MCQ that is frequently asked related to this information is→Which of the following special investigations are likely to be helpful in the identification of a body packer (a) ultrasonography (b) CT scan (c) plain radiography (d) all of the above. The answer is (d) all of the above.
- Packing drugs of abuse in a dead body or household pets and transporting them across nations for the purpose of smuggling is not known till date.

18. B. Vein may be construed as a "main line" through which the drug is injected into the system; hence the term. The student would do well to remember various routes of administration of illicit drugs and their corresponding names. These are:

- Injected intravenously ("mainlining").
- Injected subcutaneously ("skin popping").
- Smoked ("chasing the dragon").
- Sniffed ("snorting").

A person who injects drugs subcutaneously over the years gets irregular shaped ulcers (because of repeated infections), which look much like maps in a geographical atlas. For this reason, they are often known as geographical ulcers. An MCQ may be asked on this piece of information like this→Geographical ulcers are seen in (a) Mainlining (b) Skin popping (c) Chasing the dragon (d) Snorting. The answer is (b) Skin popping.

MULTIPLE ANSWER TYPE (PGI, CHANDIGARH PATTERN)

19. B,C. ***Additional info:*** Gold chloride is too costly a compound as an adulterant. Potassium cyanide is a deadly poison and obviously can not be used to adulterate anything. Cantharides are bright green in color and thus can not be used. A common adulterant must be white in color because most drugs of addiction such as heroin, cocaine etc are white in color. The common adulterants (besides lactose and sucrose) are quinine and talcum powder. Rarely baking soda, mannitol and magnesium silicate are also used.

20. B,D. ***Additional info:*** Cotton plants are heavily colonized by a strain of bacteria known as *Enterobacter agglomerans.* Most injection drug users utilize small pieces of cotton to filter particulate matter from their drug solution before they inject. This introduces small amounts of *Enterobacter agglomerans* into the solution. When it is administered intravenously, this small quantity of bacteria can be enough to cause cotton fever.

This was first noted in the early 1940s with farm workers who breathed in large quantities of unprocessed cotton.

It is commonly believed that it is something about the material (cotton or other) that causes the effects of the fever. This is not so; it is the bacteria found in the cotton. It is certainly true, however, that injecting a cotton fiber which will be broken down in the blood stream is a good way to deliver large amounts of the bacteria into the blood stream.

Cotton fever has specific symptoms that differentiate it from other ailments: fever, chills, and shortness of breath. In Europe, cotton fever is commonly called "the shakes"—a reference to another common symptom of cotton fever. Those with this ailment often experience violent shaking or shivering.

These symptoms normally occur immediately following an injection, but there are reports of lags up to an hour in length. Under most circumstances, cotton fever is relatively benign.

50 Review Test Papers

TEST PAPER I

1. Dicobalt edetate is the drug of choice in the treatment of poisoning by:
A. Aluminum phosphide
B. Opium
C. Cyanide
D. Poisonous Mushroom

2. Blindness and metabolic acidosis are common findings in poisoning by:
A. Carbolic acid
B. Carbon monoxide
C. Phosphorus
D. Methyl alcohol

3. If there is a smell of bitter almonds from the stomach contents, the poisoning is most likely due to:
A. Methyl alcohol
B. Organophosphates
C. Arsenic
D. HCN

4. Wenzell's test is used in:
A. Aconite
B. Strychnine
C. Dhatura
D. Cannabis

5. Streaming of the nuclei may be seen in:
A. Advanced putrefaction
B. Electrocution
C. Hanging
D. Starvation

6. Amygdalin can produce toxic levels of:
A. Arsenic
B. Nicotine
C. Atropine
D. Cyanide

7. Luminous vomit and stools are diagnostic of:
A. Phosphorus poisoning
B. Head injury
C. Impending death
D. Carbolic acid poisoning

8. Clinical picture in which of the following poisoning appears similar to that of acute yellow atrophy of the liver?
A. *Datura*
B. Arsenic
C. Lead
D. Phosphorus

9. Which of the following poisonous plants is sometimes referred to as Monk's hood?
A. *Abrus precatorius*
B. *Atropa belladona*
C. *Aconitum napellus*
D. *Semecarpus anacardium*

10. Woodbury's test is done for:
A. Alcohol in the urine

B. Cocaine in nasal secretions
C. Heroin in bile
D. Strychnine in blood

TEST PAPER II

11. 4-Dimethylaminophenol (4-DMAP) is a useful antidote against which of the following poisonings?
A. Arsenic
B. Cyanide
C. Carbon monoxide
D. Methyl alcohol

12. Optic atrophy is the characteristic feature of poisoning by:
A. Lead
B. Aconite
C. Phosphorus
D. Methyl alcohol

13. In which of the following poisonings is jaundice a major symptom?
A. Sulphuric acid
B. Phosphorus
C. Aluminum phosphide
D. *Datura fastuosa*

14. Ewing's postulates must be fulfilled before trauma may be said to have caused:
A. Malignant disease
B. Myocardial infarction
C. Cerebral concussion
D. A neuropathy similar to that seen in alcoholism

15. Faint letter mark can be made visible by:
A. Infrared photography
B. Spectrophotometer
C. Ordinary light
D. X-rays

16. In a dead body, if blood is not available for grouping, which of the following tissues can be preserved for grouping?
A. Bone
B. Bone marrow
C. Muscle
D. Any of the above

17. *Modus operandi* is:
A. A new method of identification
B. Death on operation table
C. A criminal's characteristic patterns and style of work
D. A new method of online registration of doctors with the MCI

18. "Nobbing fractures" are most characteristic of:
A. Extensive bone deep burns
B. Caffey's syndrome
C. Repeated hits by *lathi*
D. Injury by a glancing bullet

19. Kunkel's test is used for:
A. Carbon monoxide
B. Cocaine
C. Morphine
D. Organophosphorus

20. People suffering from achlorhydria may not suffer from toxic effects of oral ingestion of:
A. Phosphorus
B. Copper sulphate
C. Arsenic trioxide
D. Potassium cyanide

TEST PAPER III

21. A dead body is found to have marks like branching of a tree on front of chest. The most likely cause of death could be due to:
A. Firearm
B. Lightening injury
C. Injury due to bomb blast
D. Road traffic accident

22. Widmark's formula is used to calculate the quantity of which of the following poisons in the body, after attainment of equilibirium between the blood and tissue levels?
A. Methyl alcohol

B. Barbiturates
C. Ethyl alcohol
D. Morphine

23. Running amok is typically seen in poisoning with:
A. Cannabis
B. Cocaine
C. Dhatura
D. Ethyl alcohol

24. Weppen's test is used for:
A. Cannabis
B. Cocaine
C. Morphine
D. Alcohol

25. Hoppe-Seyler's test is for:
A. Mercury
B. Lead
C. Alcohol
D. Carbon Monoxide

26. A farmer who worked in the field the whole day, suddenly took ill and was brought to the hospital with vomiting, diarrhoea, salivation, perspiration, constricted pupils and pulmonary edema. The most likely diagnosis is:
A. Acute left ventricular failure
B. Organophosphorus poisoning
C. Snake bite
D. Aluminium phosphide poisoning

27. Which of the following poisons causes delirium?
A. Strychnine
B. Datura
C. Opium
D. Castor

28. Preservation of nasal swabs may be useful in:
A. Drowning
B. Anaphylaxis
C. Cocaine poisoning
D. Carbon monoxide poisoning

29. Fomepizole is useful in poisoning with:
A. Ethyl alcohol
B. Barbiturates
C. Aluminium phosphide
D. Methyl alcohol

30. Asthma like symptoms are seen in .... poisoning.
A. Arsenic
B. Organophosphorus
C. Lead
D. Gold

TEST PAPER IV

31. A four-and-half-year-old healthy child ingests a bottle containing about 80 ml of clear liquid. He had found the bottle under the kitchen sink at home. The child complained of headache and dizziness and later developed seizures. He was immediately admitted to the hospital, where he was found to have profound acidosis. Ophthalmic examination revealed dilated pupils with sluggish light reaction. Three weeks later, it is noted that the child's visual acuity is markedly decreased. Which of the following chemical substances was most likely present in the liquid ingested by this child?
A. Ethanol
B. Methanol
C. Organophosphate
D. Mercuric chloride

32. Hemoglobinuria is seen in all of the following *except*:
A. Copper sulphat poisoning
B. Viperine bite
C. Clostridium welchii sepsis
D. Thalassemia

33. Hemorrhagic necrosis of putamen is seen in a person who has died of suspicious poisoning. Which of the following poisonings might have occurred?
A. Methanol
B. Carbon monoxide
C. Organophosphates
D. Arsenic trioxide

34. Blood cholinesterase levels should be estimated for three weeks in non fatal cases of poisoning with:
A. Parathion
B. Endrin
C. Thallium sulphate
D. Aresious oxide

35. "Bone pearls" or "wax drippings" may be seen in:
A. Arsenic poisoning
B. Electrocution
C. Hanging
D. Advanced putrefaction

36. Lilly antidote kit is useful against which of the following poisonings?
A. Arsenic
B. Organophosphorus
C. Cyanide
D. Corrosive poisonings

37. Dryness of mouth, dilated pupils and delirium are symptoms of:
A. Chronic lead poisoning
B. Opium addiction
C. Chronic arsenic poisoning
D. Datura poisoning

38. Which of the following poisons resembles the root of horseradish?
A. Marking nut
B. Aconite
C. Ratti
D. Root of castor plant

39. Iatrogenic administration of sodium nitroprusside can give rise to which of the following poisonings?
A. Sodium
B. Cyanide
C. Nitrites
D. Iron

MULTIPLE ANSWER TYPE (PGI, CHANDIGARH PATTERN)

40. Diwali poisoning is due to:
A. Phosphorus
B. Arsenic
C. Mercury
D. Lead
E. Copper

ANSWERS

TEST PAPER I

1. **C.** ***Related fact:*** Dicobalt edetate (Kelocyanor) is a chelator of cyanide. Remember, for Confirmed cyanide poisonings Cobalt is very good. This is because of cobalt's severe adverse effects. The adverse effects include (i) Cardiac dysrhythmias (ii) Hypotension.
2. **D.** Common poisons which cause blindness are:
   i. Methyl alcohol.
   ii. Datura (temporary). Remember the phrase "blind as a bat"! The blindness is due to dilation of pupil and paralysis of ciliary muscles.
   iii. Osmium tetroxide (osmic acid). The vapor of osmium tetroxide deposits a film of metallic osmium on conjunctiva and cornea. Thus the blindness is more physical than chemical.
   iv. Chronic exposure to formalin fumes. Produces bilateral optic neuritis followed by bilateral optic atrophy.
   v. Tamoxifen. This is an antiestrogen usually taken in breast cancer. High doses are associated with retinal degeneration.
   vi. Atoxyl (Sodium para-aminophenylarsonate)–Also known as Soamin or Arsamin. Odorless, slightly saline taste. Causes blindness due to optic atrophy.
   vii. Tobacco–causes tobacco amblyopia. Progressive loss of visual function almost exclusively in heavy smokers.
   viii. Cyanide – Optic nerves are very sensitive to cyanide. In Leber's hereditary optic atrophy, there is congenital deficiency of rhodanese. Exclusively affects males. Results in acute visual failure due to accumulation of cyanide.
   ix. Deferoxamine – may cause nightblindness and other visual disorders.
3. **D.** ***Related fact:*** Hydrocyanic acid (HCN) smells like bitter almonds. Interestingly this odor can only be detected by 60-80% of people. The ability to detect this odor is believed to be a sex-linked recessive trait. The male to female incidence of inability to detect this odor is about 3:1.
4. **B.** ***Related fact:*** Wenzell's test is done for strychnine. The suspected material is treated with a solution of 1 part of potassium permanganate in 2000 parts of sulfuric acid. Strychnine present even in very small proportion, will cause color reactions. Named after William Theodore Wenzell (1829–1913), an American physician.

   Another test for strychnine is the *Sonnenschein's test*. In this test, the suspected substance is dissolved in a drop of sulfuric acid, some cerosoceric oxide is added, and stirred with a glass rod; a deep blue color is formed, changing to violet, and finally to cherry red in the presence of strychnine.

   Wenzell's test is not to be confused with the Wetzel's test which is done for carbon monoxide in blood. To the blood to be examined 4 volumes of water are added and treated with 3 volumes of a 1 per cent tannin solution. If CO is present, the blood becomes carmine red; normal blood slowly assumes a grayish hue. Wetzel's test is named after the German doctor Georg Wetzel (1871–1951).
5. **B.** In electrocution, the cells of the epidermis are often flattened and elongated. These are more eosinophilic and stain darker than

normal cells with haematoxylin and eosin. Gas spaces between the cells – formed by overheating of tissue fluids – may split the cells apart. Large vacuoles may be produced within the cells too for the same reason. The nuclei of these cells – especially those of the lower layers – show a peculiar distortion. They are horizontally stretched and seem to be orientated like the iron filings in a magnetic field; indeed at one time this effect was claimed to be due to electromagnetic effects produced by the current! This peculiar appearance is known as "streaming of the nuclei". Now it is known that this appearance may be seen in purely thermal burns too as well as in some hypothermic lesions.

6. **D** ***Related fact:*** Many cyanogenic plants contain the toxin amygdalin ($C_{20}H_{27}NO_{11}$). Notable among them are bitter almonds, plums, peaches, apricots and seeds of pear and apple. Although found in all parts of the plant, this toxin is found in maximum concentration in young leaves.
Amygdalin, though not harmful on its own, can however be converted to hydrocyanic acid by an enzyme *emulsin*, which is found in the seeds of these plants. Emulsin is also found in certain intestinal bacteria. *Beta-glucosidase*, an enzyme found in human intestines, can also catalyse the same reaction. Thus this reaction can be catalysed even in the absence of seeds.
The reaction is as follows: (See bottom of the page).

7. **A.**

8. **D.**

9. **C.** *Aconitum napellus* or Aconite is a plant which displays an erect terminal spike of blue flowers. These are all helmet shaped, looking rather like the hood of a monk; hence the name. It is also known as Blue rocket – the name deriving from the blue color of its flowers.

10. **A.** ***Related fact:*** To 2 mL of urine 1 mL of sulfuric acid is added, and a crystal of potassium dichromate; a green color will form if alcohol is present in urine.

TEST PAPER II

11. **B.** ***Related fact:*** The use of 4-DMAP is quite popular in Europe. It is not used in US. The usual dose is 3mg/kg IV. It is an oxidizing agent, producing methemoglobin much like sodium nitrite does. However while peak methemoglobin levels in case of sodium nitrite reach in about 30 minutes, with 4-DMAP peak levels are reached in just 5 minutes. As with sodium nitrite, its major adverse effect is excessive methemoglobin production.
In methyl alcohol, the antidote is 4-methyl pyrazole (4MP). The two names are quite similar sounding, and the student must be aware of this.

12. **D.** The optic atrophy is due to formaldehyde, a metabolic product of methyl alcohol.

13. **B.** ***Related fact:*** Phosphorus is a liver poison. Jaundice appears after about 5-6 days of ingestion.

14. **A.** There are five postulates known as *Ewing's postulates*, which must be fulfilled before a malignant disease may be attributed to a previous trauma (i) The part developing the malignant disease must have been normal prior to trauma (ii)The trauma must be sufficient to cause tissue disruption (iii) The tumor must originate on the part of the body that sustained the injury (iv) The tumor must

$$\underset{\text{(Amygdalin)}}{C_{20}H_{27}NO_{11}} + \underset{\text{(water)}}{2H_20} \xrightarrow{\textit{emulsin}} \underset{\text{(glucose)}}{2C_6H_{12}0_6} + \underset{\text{(benzaldehyde)}}{C_6H_5CHO} + \underset{\text{(hydrocyanic acid)}}{HCN}$$

be of the same histologic type, as the cells that were disrupted (v) The tumor must develop within a reasonable amount of time after sustaining the trauma. This period is usually taken as 3 weeks to 3 years after the injury.

15. A.

16. D. *Related fact:* Other tissues that can be preserved are (i) molar or premolar teeth (ii) hair with intact hair roots.

17. C. *Related facts: Modus operandi* (often used in the abbreviated form MO) is a Latin phrase, which approximately translates as "mode of operation". The plural is *modi operandi*. It is a criminal's characteristic patterns and style of work. For instance, a criminal may always want to lure his victims to a secluded place, and then strangulate him with a particular kind of rope. If the police finds many murders occurring roughly in the same area, with the same method, they can reasonably suspect that all murders were being committed by the same man. Thus it is used in police work all over the world to nab criminals.

A criminal's MO can also be used in profiling, where it can be used to find clues to the perpetrator's psychology.

Modus operandi should not be confused with a criminal's "signature behavior". Signature behaviors are behaviors committed by offenders that serve psychological and emotional needs. For instance, a criminal may always want to write the letter "M" (perhaps describing his initials) on the forehead of his victims after murdering them. Or he may always write a letter to the police after murder imploring them to catch him. Note that while Modus operandi is a characteristic method of killing, signature behavior does not signify a particular killing method.

While a criminals MO may change over time, his or her signature will usually stay the same.

18. B Caffey's syndrome is synonymous with "Battered baby syndrome". When the assailant holds the child with both hands and shakes him violently, or when he kneels upon the chest of the child, the posterior ends of the ribs – near their union with vertebrae – get fractured. About 1-2 weeks later when callus is formed, these partially healed fractures appear as a "string of beads" in X-rays. "Nobbing fractures" is thus a radiological finding and is seen in the paravertebral gutter.

19. A. Kunkel's test consists of adding a few drops of 3% tannic acid to patient's blood diluted 1:10 with distilled water. The appearance of a crimson red coagulum indicates the presence of COHb. The test is sometimes known as tannic acid test too.

Kunkel has done pioneer work in carbon monoxide poisoning. He was the first investigator to write – as early as in 1888 – about dizziness in chronic CO poisoning.

20. D. *Related facts:* This is because hydrochloric acid in the stomach is supposed to convert potassium cyanide to hydrocyanic acid which is poisonous. In the absence of hydrochloric acid, potassium cyanide may not exert its poisonous effect. In fact it is asserted by some historians that Rasputin (1872-1916) did not die despite being given cyanide pastries by his enemies, because he was suffering from achlorhydria.

TEST PAPER III

21. B. For detailed explanation and similar questions, please see Chapter 15 (Electrocution, atmospheric lightening, radiation injury).

22. C. For more info on this formula, please refer to Chapter 41 (Inebriant poisons).

23. A.

24. C. *Related facts:* This is a very old test (Weppen described it in 1874), and no one uses it now. It is included here simply

because it has been asked so many times in MCQs, and students are quite stumped with this question. Weppen's test is basically a color test not only for morphine but for other opium alkaloids as well.

The most widely used colour reactions for morphine (and other opium alkaloids) are those in which a solution of some substance x in concentrated sulphuric acid is used as a reagent. This reagent is added to a minute portion of the solid opium alkaloid (say morphine) and the resulting colour changes noted. Many substances have been suggested for this purpose by different authors and the tests are named after those authors. The main tests and the substances are given in the following table (Table 50.1).

25. **D.** ***Related facts:*** The test was developed by the German physiologist and chemist Ernst Felix Immanuel Hoppe-Seyler (1825–1895). It is a simple color test used to detect if the person died of carbon monoxide poisoning. It is done as follows: Add to blood twice its volume of a solution of sodium hydroxide of 1.3 specific gravity. Normal blood will form a dingy brown mass with a green shade if spread thin on a white surface; but if carbon monoxide is present, the mass is red.

26. **B.**

27. **B.**

28. **C.** ***Related facts:*** This is because cocaine is frequently "snorted", i.e. taken by the nasal route.

29. **D.** ***Related facts:*** Fomepizole is the trade name of 4-methyl pyrazole. For its mechanism of action see Chapter 41 (Inebriant poisons).

30. **B.**

TEST PAPER IV

31. **B.** ***Related facts:*** Damage to retina is produced by metabolites of methanol, namely formic acid. The damage is not immediate, but occurs afters some gap.

32. **D.** In all the above cases, except thalassemia, there is intravascular hemolysis, giving rise to hemoglobinuria. In Thalassemia there is extravascular hemolysis.

33. **A.** ***Related facts:*** Necrosis of putamen – either hemorrhagic or nonhemorrhagic – is seen in methanol poisoning. Necrosis of

Table 50.1: Various tests for morphine, the reagents used and the colors produced [Note: The arrow (→) indicates that the color changes to the subsequent color soon. Thus "Fine purple red→ Violet→ blue" means that first a fine purple red color is produced, which rapidly changes to violet and then finally to blue.]

Name of the test	*Concentrated Sulphuric acid added to the following substance to make the reagent*	*Color given by morphine with this reagent*
Marquis' test	Formaldehyde	Fine purple red →Violet→blue
Fróehde's test	Ammonium molybdate	Violet→blue→light green
Mecke's test, Lafon's test	Selenious acid	Blue green →grey green
Wasicky's test	p-dimethyl-aminobenzaldehyde	Orange
Reichard's test	Sodium tungstate	Violet
Flueckiger's test	Titanium dioxide	Deep purple
Schneider's test, Weppen's test (often known as Schneider-Weppen test)	Sucrose	Pink

globus pallidus has been described in carbon monoxide poisoning.

34. A.

35. B. This highly doubtful finding in electrocution is thought to be caused by calcium phosphate in the bone melting due to high temperature produced by the current, and then fusing as round balls. This is typically seen radiologically as round density foci known as "osseus pearls", "bone pearls" or "wax drippings". They are supposed to be the size of a pea.

36. C. ***Related fact:*** Also known as Lilly Cyanide Kit (because it was made by Eli Lilly), it is the only FDA (Food and Drug Administration) approved antidote in the US today. It has three components (i) Amyl nitrite pearls (ii) Solution of 3% sodium nitrite and (iii) Solution of 25% sodium thiosulfate. The kit has an expiration date, with amyl nitrite having the shortest shelf life.

This cyanide kit is no more made by Eli Lilly. It is now available from Taylor pharmaceuticals, a Division of Akorn, Inc.

37. D. Symptoms of **D**atura poisoning (a poison starting with "D") may best be remembered by the following D's:

Delirium
Dilated pupils (with blurred vision)
Diplopia
Disorientation
Drunken gait
Dry mouth
Dry skin
Dysarthria
Dysphagia
Drowsiness (occurs in late stages).

38. B. The root of aconite is conical, stout and dark, with longitudinal wrinkles and resembles that of horseradish. It may be differentiated from it by scraping it and exposing it to air. Root of aconite is whitish at first, but becomes pink on exposure to air; no such change is noted in horseradish. All differences between the two roots are given below (Table 50.2).

39. B. ***Related fact:*** Sodium nitroprusside is a potent vasodilator used as an antihypertensive. One molecule of sodium nitroprusside contains five cyanide moieties [$Na_2Fe(CN)_5NO$], which can be released in the body. Normally (i.e. in the therapeutic dose of 2-10 microgram/kg/min) the mitochondrial enzyme rhodanese is able to detoxify cyanide (this is done by transfering a sulfur atom from normal thiosulfate reserves of the body to the cyanide ions, converting them into harmless thiocyanate). However if thiosulfate reserves are depleted, as in infants, malnourished or postoperative patients, cyanide may begin to accumulate even at therapeutic doses. Manifestations which may occur in hours or days consist of alteration in mental status and acidosis. Concurrent administration of thiosulfate or hydroxocobalamin with nitroprusside prevents toxicity.

Table 50.2: Differences between root of aconite and the root of horseradish

Characteristics	*Root of Aconite*	*Root of Horseradish*
Shape	Conical	Less conical
Taste	Slightly sweetish. Causes tingling and numbness of mouth, tongue and lips	No tingling occurs. The taste is rather pungent
Cut surface	White at first; becomes pink on exposure to air	No such change

MULTIPLE ANSWER TYPE (PGI, CHANDIGARH PATTERN)

40. A,C,E. At the outset, it must be said that the term "Diwali poisoning" is not an internationally recognized term, and no international toxicologist is known to use it. This is understandable since Diwali is not celebrated internationally. However even in an Indian context, this is not a generally recognized term and should best be avoided. The only reason this question has been taken up here is because it has appeared in the examinations many times.

The meaning of the term Diwali poisoning is at best ambiguous, but can be construed as poisoning occurring due to crackers lit on the festival of Diwali. Crackers contain a number of chemicals and if a curious child ingests these crackers, he may get poisoning from any of these chemicals. These chemicals have an amazingly vast range (Aluminum, Ammonium nitrate, Ammonium perchlorate, Antimony trisulfide, Barium salts, Black powder, Calcium oxalate, Copper salts, Phosphorus (both red and white), Potassium chlorate, Potassium dichromate, Potassium hydrogen phthalate, Strontium salts, Sulfur, Titanium and zinc) and poisoning can occur because of any of these salts. Since the term Diwali poisoning can refer to poisoning by any of these chemicals, it should best be avoided.

Copper acetoarsenite as well as several other salts of copper emit very rich blue flame and are often used in fireworks. Similarly both red and white phosphorus are used in fireworks.

Mercury is most often used in fireworks as dried pellets of mercuric sulphocyanate [$Hg(CNS)_2$]. This is a combustible substance which in burning gives off a poisonous vapor (mercury) and leaves a peculiar brownish black voluminous residue (composed of foamed carbon mixed with HgS) which is expelled in a serpentine form. Since significant Hg vapor is released, these should preferably be used only in well ventilated areas. These crackers are used in Diwali as *Pharaoh's serpents* and are also employed as scientific toys. These crackers are available either as little cones or as tablets. They can be ignited with a match or put on a very hot surface to get the desired serpents.

Arsenic and lead are usually not known to be of any use in Diwali crackers.

Index

Important note: This index has been prepared for easy location of questions by students. For obvious reasons, keywords appearing in the answer section do not appear in this index as a rule. However where it is thought that the keyword is so important that it must be included, even if it appears in the answer section, it has been so indicated against the entry. Students may want to be cautious while exploring such key terms, because they may reveal the answer to a question straightaway.

B

C

G

H

K

L

N

O

Q

R

T